RHEUMATIC DISEASES
AND THE
ENVIRONMENT

RHEUMATIC DISEASES

AND THE

ENVIRONMENT

Editors

Lee D. Kaufman, M.D.
Associate Professor of Medicine
Chief, Division of Rheumatology
State University of New York at Stony Brook
Stony Brook, New York

John Varga, M.D.
Chief, Section of Rheumatology
Department of Medicine
University of Illinois at
Chicago College of Medicine
Chicago, Illinois

A member of the Hodder Headline Group

LONDON · SYDNEY · AUCKLAND

Co-published in the USA by Oxford University Press, Inc., New York

First published in Great Britain in 1999 by
Arnold, a member of the Hodder Headline Group,
338 Euston Road, London NW1 3BH

http://www.arnoldpublishers.com

Co-published in the United States of America by
Oxford University Press Inc.,
198 Madison Avenue, New York, NY10016
Oxford is a registered trademark of Oxford University Press

Whilst the advice and information in this book are believed to be true and
accurate at the date of going to press, neither the authors nor the publisher
can accept any legal responsibility or liability for any errors or omissions
that may be made. In particular (but without limiting the generality of the
preceding disclaimer) every effort has been made to check drug dosages;
however, it is still possible that errors have been missed. Furthermore,
dosage schedules are constantly being revised and new side-effects
recognized. For these reasons the reader is strongly urged to consult the
drug companies' printed instructions before administering any of the drugs
recommended in this book.

British Library Cataloguing in Publication Data
A catalogue record for this book is available from the British Library

Library of Congress Cataloging-in-Publication Data
Rheumatic diseases and the environment / editors, Lee D. Kaufman, John Varga.
     p.   cm.
     Includes bibliographical references and index.
     ISBN 0-412-07911-9
     1. Rheumatism—Environmental aspects.   2. Connective tissues—
Diseases—Environmental aspects.   3. Arthritis—Environmental
aspects.   I. Kaufman, Lee.   II. Varga, John.
     [DNLM: 1. Rheumatic Diseases—etiology.   2. Rheumatic Diseases—
physiopathology.   3. Environmental Exposure.   WE 544R4706 1998]
RC927.R4525   1998
616.7′23—dc21
DNLM/DLC
for Library of Congress   98-19472
                                                                            CIP

ISBN 0 412 07911 9

1 2 3 4 5 6 7 8 9 10

Printed and bound in Great Britain by The Bath Press, Bath, Avon

What do you think about this book? Or any other Arnold title?
Please send your comments to feedback.arnold@hodder.co.uk

To Marjorie, Joshua, and Adam, who complete the circle,
and to Bob Dylan, whose clarity of vision
will always be a beacon in the high muddy water

Lee D. Kaufman, M.D.

To my wife Julie
and my sons Peter and Andrew,
who always remind me of what it's all about

John Varga, M.D.

Contents

Part V: Rheumatic Syndromes and the Workplace

Part VI: Surveillance, Regulatory, and Legal Approaches to Environmental Exposure-Associated Rheumatic Disease

Contributing Authors

Louis Bessette, M.D., F.R.C.P., M.S.
Assistant Professor of Medicine
Division of Rheumatology
Centre Hospitalier
Universitate de Québec
Pavillon CHUL
Laval University
2705 boul. Laurier, Ste-Foy, Québec
Canada G1V 4G2

David G. Borenstein, M.D.
Clinical Professor of Medicine
Division of Rheumatology
Department of Medicine
The George Washington University Medical
    Center
2021 K Street, NW, Suite 300
Washington, D.C. 20006

Leonard H. Calabrese, D.O.
Vice Chairman
Department of Rheumatic and Immunologic
    Diseases
The Cleveland Clinic Foundation
9500 Euclid Avenue
Cleveland, Ohio 44195

Huan J. Chang, M.D.
Assistant Professor of Medicine
Section of Rheumatology
University of Illinois at Chicago College of
    Medicine, Chicago
MC-733
1160 Molecular Biology Research Building
900 S. Ashland Avenue
Chicago, Illinois 60607

Daniel J. Clauw, M.D.
Associate Professor of Medicine and Orthopaedics
Chief, Division of Rheumatology, Immunology,
    and Allergy
Georgetown University Medical Center
3800 Reservoir Rd. NW
Washington, D.C. 20007

Mark R. Cullen, M.D.
Professor of Medicine and Public Health
Director, Yale Occupational and Environmental
    Medicine Program
Yale University School of Medicine
135 College Street, Rm 366
New Haven, Connecticut 06510

Jack J. Cush, M.D.
Medical Director—Arthritis Center
Presbyterian Hospital of Dallas
Clinical Associate Professor of Internal Medicine
The University of Texas Southwestern Medical
    Center
Dallas, Texas
8200 Walnut Hill Lane
Dallas, Texas 75213

David T. Felson, M.D., M.P.H.
Professor of Medicine
Boston University Arthritis Center
Boston University Medical Center
80 E. Concord Street
Boston, Massachusetts 02118

Allan Gibofsky, M.D., J.D., F.C.L.M.
Professor of Medicine
Division of Rheumatology
Hospital for Special Surgery
Cornell University Medical College
1300 York Avenue
New York, New York 10021

Gerald J. Gleich, M.D.
Professor of Immunology and Medicine
Department of Immunology
The Mayo Clinic and Foundation
200 First Street, SW
Rochester, Minnesota 55905

Juan J. Gómez-Reino, M.D., Ph.D.
Chief Service of Rheumatology
Complejo Hospitalario
Universitario Santiago de Compostela
Spain

Marc C. Hochberg, M.D.
Professor of Medicine
Head, Division of Rheumatology
Department of Medicine
University of Maryland School of Medicine
10 South Pine Street, Room 834
Baltimore, Maryland 21201

Mariana J. Kaplan, M.D.
Fellow
Division of Rheumatology
Department of Medicine
University of Michigan
R4540 Kresge 1, Box 0531
200 Zina Pitcher Place
Ann Arbor, Michigan 48109

Jeffrey N. Katz, M.D., M.S.
Associate Professor of Medicine
Robert B. Brigham Multipurpose Arthritis
   Disease Center
Brigham and Womens Hospital
Harvard Medical School
75 Francis Street
Boston, Massachusetts 02115

Lee D. Kaufman, M.D.
Chief, Division of Rheumatology
Associate Professor of Medicine
The State University of New York at Stony Brook
School of Medicine
Health Sciences Center
Stony Brook, New York 11794

Lauren B. Krupp, M.D.
Associate Professor
Department of Neurology and Psychology
State University of New York at Stony Brook
School of Medicine
Health Sciences Center
Stony Brook, New York 11794

Lori A. Love, M.D., Ph.D.
Director, Clinical Research and Review Staff
Office of Special Nutritionals
Center for Food Safety and Applied Nutrition
Food and Drug Administration
200 C Street, NW, HFS-452
Washington, D.C. 20204

Carlo L. Mainardi, M.D.
Professor of Medicine
University of Maryland School of Medicine
655 West Baltimore Street
Baltimore, Maryland 21201

Brian F. Mandell, M.D., Ph.D.
Program Director
Department of Rheumatic and Immunologic
   Diseases
Senior Associate Program Director
Internal Medicine Residency Program
Cleveland Clinic Foundation
A50
9500 Euclid Avenue
Cleveland, Ohio 44195

Maravillas Izquierdo Martinez, M.D.
Staff, Toxic Oil Unit
Ciudad Sanitaria Doce de Octubre
Carretera de Andalucia Km 5.4
28041 Madrid
Spain

Alfonse T. Masi, M.D., Dr.P.H.
Professor of Medicine
Department of Medicine
University of Illinois College of Medicine, Peoria
One Illini Drive
P.O. Box 1649
Peoria, Illinois 61656

Frederick W. Miller, M.D., Ph.D.
Senior Investigator and Medical Officer
Laboratory of Molecular and Developmental
   Immunology
Division of Monoclonal Antibodies
Center for Biologics Evaluation & Research
Food & Drug Administration
NIH Building 29B, Room 2G11, HFM-561
8800 Rockville Pike
Bethesda, MD 20892

Theodore Pincus, M.D.
Professor of Medicine and Microbiology
Division of Rheumatology and Immunology
Vanderbilt University Medical Center
230 Oxford House
1313 21st Avenue South
Nashville, Tennessee 37232

Dean A. Pollina, Ph.D.
Research Assistant Professor
Department of Neurology
State University of New York at Stony Brook
School of Medicine
Health Sciences Center
Stony Brook, New York 11794

Bruce C. Richardson, M.D., Ph.D.
Associate Professor of Medicine

Chief, Arthritis Division
Veterans Affairs Hospital
University of Michigan
R4540 Kresge 1, Box 0531
200 Zina Pitcher Place
Ann Arbor, Michigan 48109

Patricia J. Rohan, M.D.
Medical Officer
Hematology Products Branch, Division of Blood
  Applications
Office of Blood Research and Review,
  Food and Drug Administration
FDA/HFM-380
1401 Rockville Pike
Rockville, MD 20852

Lewis J. Rubin, M.D.
Professor of Medicine and Physiology
Head, Division of Pulmonary and Critical
  Care Medicine
University of Maryland School of Medicine
655 West Baltimore Street
Baltimore, Maryland 21201

Robert L. Rubin, Ph.D.
Associate Professor
Department of Molecular and Experimental
  Medicine
The Scripps Research Institute
10550 North Torrey Pines Road
La Jolla, California 92037

Marina Rull, M.D.
Research Fellow in Rheumatology
Department of Arthritis Research
Veterans Affairs Medical Center
University and Woodland Avenues
Philadelphia, Pennsylvania 19104;
Division of Rheumatology
Hospital of the University of Pennsylvania
34th and Spruce Street
Philadelphia, Pennsylvania 19104

H. Ralph Schumacher, Jr., M.D.
Professor of Medicine
University of Pennsylvania School of Medicine
34th and Spruce Street
Philadelphia, Pennsylvania 19104;
Chief, Division of Rheumatology

Veterans Affairs Medical Center
University and Woodland Avenues
Philadelphia, Pennsylvania 19104

Alan J. Silman, M.D.
Professor
AOR Epidemiology Research
University of Manchester
Oxford Road
M13 9PT, Manchester
England

Jack W. Snyder, M.D., J.D., Ph.D.
Associate Professor
Departments of Emergency Medicine and
  Laboratory Medicine
Jefferson Medical College of Thomas
  Jefferson University
1025 Walnut Street
Philadelphia, Pennsylvania 19107

Snezana Trajkovic, M.D.
Fellow in Rheumatology
Department of Medicine
University of Maryland School of Medicine
655 West Baltimore Street
Baltimore, Maryland 21201

John Varga, M.D.
Professor of Medicine, Biochemistry and
  Molecular Biology
Chief, Section of Rheumatology
Department of Medicine
University of Illinois at Chicago
  College of Medicine
MC-733
1160 Molecular Biology Research Building
900 Ashland Avenue
Chicago, Illinois 60607

Frederick Wolfe, M.D.
Clinical Professor of Internal Medicine and
  Family and Community Medicine
University of Kansas School of Medicine, Witchita
1010 North Kansas
Witchita, Kansas 67214;
Director, Witchita Arthritis Research and
  Clinical Centers
1035 N. Emporia, Suite 230
Witchita, Kansas 67214

Preface

The relationship between environmental exposure (broadly defined in this volume as exposure to foods, drugs, chemicals, biologicals, radiation, noise, and emotional and physical stresses) and the development of human disease has been of great interest for many years. The rising incidence of autoimmune and rheumatic diseases suggests the possible influence of an increasing lifetime burden of environmental exposures, due both to increased life expectancy and to greater environmental contamination.

In general, environmentally associated rheumatic diseases are characterized by a variable degree of similarity to their "idiopathic" counterparts, a period of exposure to the putative offending agent, latency between exposure and development of symptoms and signs, and, in certain cases, by the "dechallenge" phenomenon of improvement or resolution upon removal of the etiologic agent. Furthermore, the variable "attack rate" of an environmental agent (i.e., the heterogeneous host response to an environmental exposure) reflects the role of immunogenetic and pharmacogenetic susceptibility. Indeed, our increasing awareness of genetic susceptibility in the development of human disease suggests that, in a broader sense, most rheumatic disorders may represent "environmentally associated diseases."

This volume brings together up-to-date discussions of the potential pathogenetic mechanisms underlying environmental exposure-associated rheumatic diseases, epidemiologic and surveillance approaches for the recognition and characterization of environmental exposure-associated rheumatic diseases, legal versus scientific notions of causality, approaches to the regulatory oversight of environmental agents potentially implicated in the development of rheumatic diseases, along with illustrations of specific environmental exposure-associated rheumatic diseases.

In light of the relentless accumulation of novel physical and biological agents introduced into our environment, it is likely that discussions of environmental exposure-associated rheumatic diseases will continue to take place in the mass media and the courts, as well as in the clinic and in academia. This book is written for physicians and other health care providers, biomedical scientists, epidemiologists, toxicologists, regulators, lawmakers, and members of the legal profession dealing with environmental associated rheumatic diseases. It is our hope that this broad community will be motivated to engage in this important and timely dialogue.

Lee D. Kaufman, M.D.
John Varga, M.D.

Acknowledgments

The editors of this book wish to express their gratitude to Joyce-Rachel John, Cathy Felgar, Gill Kent, Jim Geronimo, and to Lauren Enck. Their enthusiastic support and tireless efforts have guided this project to its successful conclusion. We are deeply grateful to our expert contributors for taking a significant amount of time from their busy schedules to create this unique and important contribution to the literature. On a personal note, we warmly thank our mentors who, throughout our careers, have provided immeasurable inspiration and encouragement: Mark Needle, Kendrick Lance, Allen Kaplan, Ervin Varga, Eric J. Hall, Tom Cooper, Elliot Rosenstein, and Sergio Jimenez.

RHEUMATIC DISEASES
AND THE
ENVIRONMENT

I

Overview of Epidemiology and Differential Diagnosis

Epidemiology of Environmental and Occupational Connective Tissue Diseases

Alan J. Silman and Marc C. Hochberg

This chapter reviews epidemiological approaches to investigating the relationship between environmental exposures and the development of rheumatic diseases. The first part of the chapter is devoted to a review of the different methodologies available and their relative strengths and weaknesses for investigating this topic. The second part of the chapter critically reviews the data linking two exposures, L-tryptophan and silicone breast implants, in relation to their role in the development of autoimmune disease.

WHAT ARE ENVIRONMENTAL EXPOSURES?

At a simple level, "environmental exposures" covers all those susceptibility factors that are not inherited. It is perhaps useful, however, to separate out those factors that are "constitutional," such as body height, menopause, age and other comorbidities. "True" environmental exposures, as such, can be usefully subdivided into those that might be considered macroenvironmental and those that are microenvironmental. Under the heading of the former are included those exposures over which individuals have no control and which reflect the environment in which they live. Examples include atmospheric pollution and water contamination. The importance of this distinction from an epidemiological perspective is two-fold. First, the individual would not be aware of the exposure and therefore would be unable to provide accurate and verifiable data. Second, within a population all individuals are likely to receive the same level of exposure, and therefore the appropriate epidemiological method (*vide infra*) would be an ecological study comparing populations rather than comparing individuals within populations.

By contrast, microenvironmental exposures consequently describe those exposures which are under the control of the individual and which discriminate between individuals. Typical exposures include those that occur in the workplace, diet, leisure time and other activities, in addition to "unplanned exposures" such as infection with microorganisms. When individuals vary within a population with respect to their exposure level, it is then possible to conceive an epidemiological study design that investigates exposure at an individual level.

EPIDEMIOLOGICAL STUDY DESIGNS

There are several study designs that can be used to investigate environmental health effects. These are listed in Table 1.1.

Case Series

The existence of many possible environmental associations is first suggested by either a single case report or a case series. This may be valuable but, of course, could represent the random co-occurrence of a disease and an exposure which are not causally related. It is important, therefore, to consider what factors might indicate a greater likelihood of cause and effect relationship (listed in Table 1.2): first, if the clinical outcome is extremely rare and would not be expected to occur sporadically; second, if the exposure itself was considerably greater than would be considered appropriate (for example, an individual in the workplace who had been involved in an accident involving massive exposure); third, if multiple cases had been reported of the same exposure with the same relatively rare clinical consequence; fourth, if there was a biological plausibility linking the exposure to the development of the disease. There are several examples where a case series has been the only available data linking rheumatic disease with environmental exposure yet the relationship is considered sufficiently strong to be accepted as an association.[1-6]

Table 1-1 Epidemiological approaches to studying environmental effects

---

Case series
Ecological Study
Case control: within cohort
                       independent controls
Cohort study: prospective
                    retrospective

Table 1-2 Factors suggesting case reports might represent true cause and effect

---

- Rarity of clinical outcome
- Rarity of magnitude (duration/concentration) of exposure
- Multiple similar cases reported
- Cases with similar exposure exhibit clinical similarity
- Temporal sequence appropriate
- Consistent with epidemiological data
- Biological plausibility

Ecological Study

As is discussed above, it is very difficult to investigate macroenvironmental influences on the development of autoimmune rheumatic diseases. The classic epidemiological approach is to look for geographical clustering with a nonrandom distribution of cases in space, the hypothesis being that there is a point or multiple point source(s) of environmental exposure that is associated with the development of disease in that high-risk area. Such an example is shown for systemic sclerosis (SSc) (Figure 1.1), where the hypothesis was raised that the occurrence of SSc was increased in areas in close proximity to large airports.[7] The ecological study is, of course, subject to the problems that there may be other differences between populations as well as the hypothesized exposure. These confounding factors may not be known or measured during the course of the investigation, and a spurious cause and effect is concluded.

Analytical Approaches: Necessity and Sufficiency

The standard epidemiological approach to investigating environmental exposure is to undertake an analytical study either comparing the exposure status in cases with the disease with that of an appropriate control group—that is, the case-control study—or comparing the occurrence of disease in an exposed group with that in a group not exposed to the risk factor—the cohort study. Traditionally, case-control studies are useful for studying common exposures in relatively rare diseases, whereas cohort studies are useful for studying the occurrence of a fairly common disease following exposures that are relatively rare, for example in occupa-

tionally derived groups. The difficulty in establishing a relationship to many of the putative environmental agents and rheumatic diseases is that both the diseases and the putative exposure(s) are rare.

It is useful here to consider the concepts of *necessity* and *sufficiency* in relation to exposures. If an exposure is *necessary,* this would mean that the disease would not occur in its absence. If the exposure is *sufficient,* then no other risk factor, including genetic, need be present. There are four possible disease exposure relationships, as illustrated in Figure 1.2. Typically, not all individuals in a given population would neatly fall into either of categories *a* or *d*—that is, the exposure always results in disease, and the disease never occurs in the absence of exposure. Specifically, with many of the environmental hazards postulated for connective-tissue disease, the converse is the case: predominantly most individuals fall into categories *b* and *c*. These will be illustrated using the example of organic solvents and SSc. Thus the vast majority of individuals who are exposed to organic solvents do not develop SSc; therefore the exposure to solvents alone is insufficient to explain disease onset (category *b*). Furthermore, most individuals who develop SSc have not been exposed to solvents (category *c*). Another example is the possible link between cocaine abuse and the development of SSc.[8,9] The vast majority of individuals with scleroderma are not cocaine abusers, and the vast majority of cocaine abusers do not develop SSc. Under these circumstances, it has to be accepted that it is very difficult epidemiologically, using either a case-control or cohort approach, to investigate such associations.

Case-Control Approach

There are two approaches to undertaking case-control studies. The optimal method is to identify an entire population of individuals, such as one defined by geography or from an occupational role, and then select the cases by some form of screening to ensure that all cases within the population have been ascertained and the controls are either the entire nondiseased population or, much more efficiently, a random sample of such individuals. Such an approach is, however, in practice difficult to apply in rare connective-tissue diseases because the cases themselves are normally recruited over a period of time from specialist clinics without there being a coherent population source from which to select the controls. Controls are therefore selected from friends, neighbors, or random population lists, and clearly these are subject to all sorts of biases in relation to how they were selected. Detailed discussion of control selection in such studies is given elsewhere.[10] If an occupational exposure is suspected, the case-control approach cannot be undertaken within an occupational grouping *per se,* because all the subjects, both the cases and the controls, will have been exposed and therefore will have been "overmatched" for exposure. However, if the

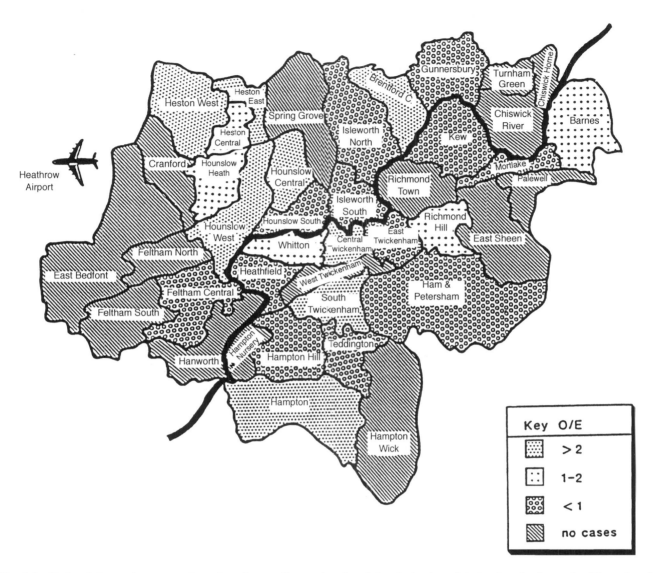

Fig. 1-1 Ratio of observed to expected number of cases of systemic sclerosis by electoral ward, in two London boroughs. (Reproduced with permission, Silman et al. 1990.)

putative occupational exposure itself is extremely rare, then it does not make sense to use random population controls to look for exposures in this particular occupation. An alternative strategy, therefore, would be to use the case-control approach, but where the exposure is not considered primarily as working in the occupation, some indication of "dosage" of occupational exposure is utilized. This could be done by stratifying exposure by duration or intensity of exposure. It is then possible to undertake an analysis of differing levels of exposure, looking for a trend of increasing risk with increasing dose. This is illustrated in Table 1.3, with three exposure levels: low, moderate and heavy. The risk of disease in each of two highest-exposure groups is calculated relative to the risk in the lowest-exposure group. In a case-control study this is done by calculating odds ratios, as

shown in Table 1.3, with the risk in "low" group being set as 1. The chi-squared test for trend is a useful statistical test to determine a linear trend of increasing risk. Statistically, it is most efficient to stratify into equal-sized groups (by quintiles, and so on). Biologically, it might be more coherent to stratify by specific levels of exposure (occupational grade) and to combine groups if the numbers are too small.

Cohort Study

The cohort study can avoid many of the biases associated with the case-control study, particularly the timing of exposure in relation to disease onset. This also avoids the possibility of recall bias, especially where cases are being asked

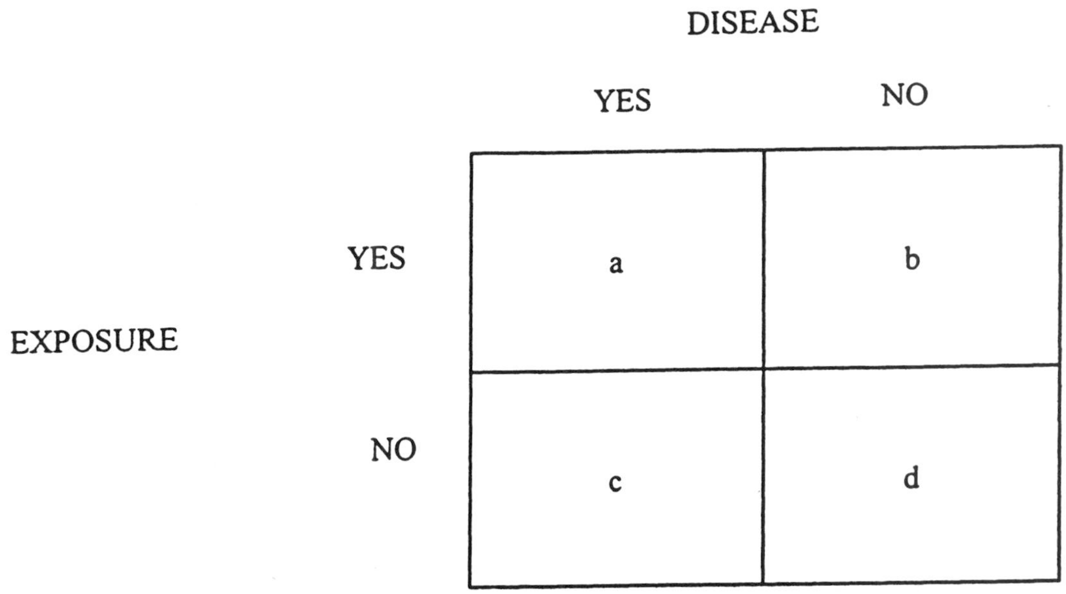

DISEASE

YES   NO

EXPOSURE

YES

| a | b |

NO

| c | d |

Fig. 1-2 Conceptual classification of putative environmental exposure associated disorders (reviewed in text).

Table 1-3 Calculation of odds ratio with multiple levels of exposure: example with three levels of exposure

Exposure Level	Cases	Controls	Odds Ratio
Low	a_L	b_L	$\dfrac{a_L b_L}{a_L b_L} = 1$
Moderate	a_M	b_M	$\dfrac{a_M b_L}{a_L b_M}$
Heavy	a_H	b_H	$\dfrac{a_H b_L}{a_L b_H}$

Reproduced by permission, Silman 1996.[10]

to recall their own exposure, and there may be differing recall between cases and noncases in this respect.

The alternative approaches are to select a cohort of individuals, examine their exposure status, and then prospectively follow up to determine the subsequent risk of disease. This can be achieved either by receiving continuing notification of new cases from physician record systems or, in the case of undiagnosed disorders, by screening the study population at the end of the study. By contrast, another approach is to identify retrospectively a cohort of individuals, which provides information on their baseline exposure risk, and to determine their current disease status (the "retrospective" study). The advantage of this latter approach is its timeliness since the cases of disease have already occurred. The disadvantage, however, is that such cohorts may not be readily available and indeed the quality of the data on baseline exposure risk may be limited. Quite often it is possible to use existing cohorts collected for other reasons to examine particular risk factors. One recent example is the evaluation of

the relation of silicone breast implants and connective-tissue disease, which was analyzed within the Nurses Health Study.[11] The major problem inherent in cohort study designs in this area is their low statistical power with rare diseases. An example of this is in a disease like SSc with a population incidence of approximately ten to twenty per million person-years at risk: most studies will indicate wide confidence intervals around any putative increased risk, and it is difficult under such circumstances to exclude either a positive or even a negative effect. This is one of the major problems in the studies undertaken thus far on the relationship between silicone breast implants and SSc (*vide infra*).

In summary, therefore, in this brief methodological overview it is clear that there are considerable difficulties in establishing a presence of association between rare exposures and rare diseases. A number of different approaches may need to be used and the results from different studies perhaps should be pooled, using meta-analyses in order to obtain a much more robust estimate of an effect than could be obtained from a single study. These principles are illustrated in the following brief discussion of epidemiologic issues relating to the purported association of silicone breast implants and connective-tissue disease.

SILICONE BREAST IMPLANTS AND RHEUMATIC DISEASE

Prevalence of Silicone Breast Implants

Polydimethylsiloxane gel, in which individual chains of the polymer are cross-linked with varying degrees of free fluid polymer, has been used as a filling of breast implants since 1962.[12] Silicone elastomer, which contains chemically treated amorphous fumed silica, is also added to the envelope of some implants to increase their tensile strength, lessening the potential for implant rupture.[13] The reader is referred to Chapter 7 for a discussion of the clinical and immunopathological aspects of silicone and rheumatic disease.

Three studies have examined the prevalence of silicone breast implants among women in the United States.[14–16] As part of the 1988 National Health Interview Survey, the Food and Drug Administration Centre for Devices and Radiological Health included a Medical Device Implant Survey.[14] This survey collected information on many different types of medical devices, including breast implants. In the respondent sample, 143 women reported having at least one breast implant; this corresponded to a prevalence of 3.3 implant recipients per 1000 women aged 18 years and above, and a weighted estimate of 304,000 women in the United States. This is likely to be an underestimate, because subjects may be reluctant to answer sensitive questions in face-to-face interviews.

In a postal survey funded by Dow Corning Corporation, questionnaires were mailed to a stratified sample of 40,000 representative American households by geographic region, household income, population density, age of occupants and household size.[15] The response rate was 70.7%. Two hundred and forty households, approximately 1% of responding households, reported that a female occupant aged 15 years or above had a breast implant. The estimated prevalence of breast implants was 8.19 per 1000 women aged 15 years and above; age-specific prevalence had a unimodal distribution, with the peak in the 45 to 54 year age group at a ratio of 16.26 per 1000. Prevalence increased with increasing income, reaching 16.9 per 1000 among women with a household income of $75,000 or above, and was higher among white women living in the South and West than those in the East or Midwest. Using data from the National Centre for Health Statistics, the authors estimated that there were 815,700 women aged 15 years and above in the United States with breast implants.

The utilization of silicone breast implants was studied in a population-based cohort of women in Olmsted County, Minnesota.[16] During a 28-year period, 749 women aged 15 years and above who were Olmsted County residents and received a first breast implant were identified. The averaged annual rate of implantation between 1964 and 1991 was 72 per 100,000. There was a temporal trend with increasing annual rates from 1964 to 1979, with stability in the estimate thereafter. The estimated prevalence of breast implants among Olmsted County women aged 15 years and above on January 1, 1992 was approximately 1%.

Case Reports and Case Series

The initial report of presumed autoimmune connective-tissue disease related to silicone was of patients who received injections of liquid preparations containing silicone, paraffin or other compounds for cosmetic breast augmentation.[17] Series of cases of women who had injections of silicone, paraffin or other compounds for breast augmentation and developed connective-tissue diseases and connective-tissue-like syndromes were collected from the Japanese literature and recently summarized.[18,19] A computerized search of the English-language literature through June 1993 identified 293 patients with rheumatic symptoms developing after receiving silicone-gel-filled breast implants.[19] Fifty-seven patients fulfilled criteria for a definite connective-tissue disease, and 15 individuals had a possible connective-tissue disease. Since the publication of this review, data have been reported on over 400 additional patients who developed rheumatic symptoms following augmentation mammoplasty with silicone-gel-filled breast implants.[20–25] The vast majority of these patients did not have typical connective-tissue disease but, rather, symptoms of incapacitating fatigue, myalgia, arthralgia and sicca complex.

It has been emphasized that inferences regarding causation of connective-tissue disease by silicone-gel-filled breast implants cannot be made in the absence of properly conducted epidemiologic studies.[26–31] Furthermore, these reports and/or series all share one or more of the following deficiencies that preclude appropriately drawn inferences: 1) poor or absent case definition; 2) failure to apply conventional diagnostic criteria; 3) unknown health status of patient prior to implant; and 4) lack of consistent latent period.[32]

Epidemiologic Studies

Thirteen epidemiologic studies have been published examining the possible association between augmentation mammoplasty with silicone-gel-filled breast implants and the development of connective-tissue disease.[33–45] Two of these studies did not have an internal control group; one used published data to estimate the number of expected cases,[33] while the other used record linkage analysis to estimate the number of expected cases.[41] Neither found an excess of connective-tissue disease. The latter study, however, noted an apparent increased incidence of systemic sclerosis in breast implant recipients. This finding was based on only two cases, one of which was subsequently noted to have had breast reduction rather than breast augmentation.[32]

Three studies relied on self-reporting from mailed questionnaires to determine disease status in women with breast implants and in controls.[35,37,44] Two of these studies, with women who had undergone cosmetic procedures not involving silicone implantation at controls, failed to demonstrate an association between breast implantation and connective-tissue diseases or symptoms.[36,37] The third study found a significant association between breast implantation and self-reported connective-tissue disease.[44] This latter study involved analysis of questionnaires returned by over 400,000 female health professionals out of an initial mailing to 1.75

million women conducted between September 1992 and May 1995 to recruit participants for the Women's Health Study. Two hundred and thirty one of 10,830 women with breast implants reported the development of a connective-tissue disease after the year of implantation, compared to 11,574 of 384,713 women who did not have breast implants. The relative risk (RR) for connective-tissue disease, derived from a Cox proportional hazards model, was 1.24 (95% confidence intervals [CI]: 1.08, 1.41). The authors suggested that these results "... exclude large risks of connective-tissue disease following breast implants." These results, however, need to be interpreted with caution because of numerous potential biases. Important among these is the possibility of differential overreporting of connective-tissue diseases among women with breast implants, and the recognized low validity of self-reported connective-tissue disease.[46,47]

Case-Control Studies

In a case-control study of 349 women with newly diagnosed rheumatoid arthritis and 1456 similarly aged control women in the United States, only one of 300 cases with available data reported breast implantation, compared to 12 controls.[34] The odds ratio (OR) for the association of breast implantation with rheumatoid arthritis in this study was 0.41 (95% CI: 0.05, 3.13).

Another case-control study of 251 women with systemic sclerosis and 289 similarly aged control women living in Australia found four cases and five controls who reported augmentation mammoplasty.[39] The OR, adjusted for differences in socioeconomic status, was 0.89 (95% CI: 0.23, 3.41).

In a case-control study of 274 women with systemic sclerosis and 1184 controls living in Michigan, two cases and 14 controls reported augmentation mammoplasty.[40] The OR, adjusted for age, race and income, was 0.35 (95% CI: 0.05, 2.74).

In a case-control study of 195 patients with systemic lupus erythematosus and 143 controls, only one case and no controls had a breast implant.[42]

One case-control study from a single private rheumatology practice evaluated the association of breast implantation with rheumatoid arthritis and connective-tissue diseases.[43] Of 4229 female patients identified in the practice registry, 150 had breast implants and 721 had a diagnosis of either rheumatoid arthritis or a definite connective-tissue disease. The 150 women with breast implants were younger at the initial visit, had a higher mean income, and were more likely to have been seen between 1986 and 1992 rather than between 1982 and 1985. After adjusting for these possible confounders, the OR for the association between breast implants and rheumatoid arthritis or connective-tissue disease was 0.41 (95% CI: 0.22, 0.77). This finding of a reduced odds ratio may be due to the use of patients from the rheumatology practice with other

diagnoses, including musculoskeletal pain syndromes and fibromyalgia, as controls.

Finally, in a case-control study of 837 women with systemic sclerosis followed at three large university-based referral practices, these women were compared with 2507 controls matched for age and race.[45] Eleven cases and 31 controls had augmentation mammoplasty. The adjusted OR for the association between augmentation mammoplasty and systemic sclerosis was 1.07 (95% CI: 0.53, 2.13).

Cohort Studies

The incidence of connective-tissue disease, diagnosed by a rheumatologist was determined in 250 women who had undergone breast implantation and 353 women who had undergone reconstruction without implants after surgery for breast cancer.[35] One patient in each group developed a connective-tissue disease during follow-up. The estimated RR of 1.08 did not differ from unity.

A retrospective cohort study evaluated 749 women with breast implants and 1498 age-, sex- and race-matched unexposed control women who were residents of Olmsted County, Minnesota.[38] Over a mean follow-up of eight years, five exposed and ten unexposed women developed a connective-tissue disease. The adjusted RR, derived from a multivariate Cox proportional hazards model, was 1.10 (95% CI: 0.37, 3.23). None of the exposed women developed rheumatoid arthritis, systemic lupus erythematosus (SLE), systemic sclerosis or inflammatory muscle disease. The only symptom which occurred with a significantly increased incidence in the women with implants compared to unexposed women was morning stiffness: adjusted RR = 1.80 (95% CI: 1.10, 2.93).

Finally, an analysis of longitudinal data from 87,501 women with information on exposure to breast implants who were participants in the Nurse's Health Study was performed.[11] During over one million person-years of follow-up, a diagnosis of connective-tissue disease was reported by over 5000 women, but was confirmed in only 516 women after review of relevant medical records. Three of the 1183 women with a breast implant developed a confirmed connective-tissue disease and all had rheumatoid arthritis. The adjusted RR for development of confirmed connective-tissue disease was 0.6 (95% CI: 0.2, 2.0). The adjusted RR for development of self-reported connective-tissue disease was 0.7 (95% CI: 0.5, 1.0); this can be compared with that derived from the Women's Health Study (*vide supra*).

Meta-analysis

Most of the studies summarized above had inadequate statistical power to demonstrate a significant association between breast implants and connective-tissue disease, because of either the relatively low frequency of breast implantation or the low incidence rates of connective-tissue disease. A meta-analysis of the published epidemiologic studies of confirmed connective-tissue disease was recently performed.[48] The pooled adjusted OR for the association of augmentation mammoplasty with confirmed connective-tissue disease was 1.03 (95% CI: 0.60-1.62). This result suggests that although one cannot reject the null hypothesis (that is, that there is no causal association between breast implants and confirmed connective-tissue disease), if a causal association does exist, then the excess risk is low.

SUMMARY

Epidemiological approaches play an important role in investigating possible links between environmental exposures and the development of rheumatic diseases. A number of different study designs may be used, depending on the nature of the association, the relative frequency of occurrence of the exposure, and the disease under investigation. Whereas results from epidemiological investigation can provide estimates of the magnitude of increased risk, they cannot with any degree of certainty prove a cause-and-effect relationship to an individual.

REFERENCES

[1]Erasmus LD. Scleroderma in gold miners on the Witwatersrand with particular reference to pulmonary manifestations. *S A J Lab Clin Med.* 1957;3:209–231.

[2]Franzinelli A, Marcolongo R. Epidemiologia dell'artrite, reumatoide e del fattore reumatoide. *Reumatismo.* 1971;23:222–235.

[3]Veltman C, Lange CE, Juhe S, *et al.* Clinical manifestations and course of vinyl chloride disease. *Ann NY Aca Sci.* 1975;246:6–17.

[4]Walder BK. Do solvents cause scleroderma? *Int Soc Trop Dermatol.* 1983;22:157–158.

[5]Haustein UF, Ziegler V. Environmentally induced systemic sclerosis-like disorders. *Int J Dermatol.* 1985;24:147–151.

[6]Olivieri I, Gherardi S, Bini C, *et al.* Trauma and seronegative spondyloarthropathy: Rapid joint destruction in peripheral arthritis triggered by physical injury. *Ann Rheum Dis.* 1988;47:73–76.

[7]Silman AJ, Howard Y, Hicklin AJ, Black CM. Geographical clustering of scleroderma in south and west London. *Br J Rheumatol.* 1990;29:92–96.

[8]Trozak DJ, Gould WM. Cocaine abuse and connective tissue disease. *J Am Acad Dermatol.* 1984;10:525.

[9]Kilaru P, Kim W, Sequeira W. Cocaine and scleroderma: Is there an association? *J Rheumatol.* 1991;18:1753–1755.

[10]Silman AJ. *Epidemiological Studies: A Practical Guide.* Cambridge; Cambridge University Press, 1996.

[11]Sanchez-Guerrero J, Colditz GA, Karlson EW, *et al.* Silicone breast implants and the risk of connective-tissue diseases and symptoms. *N Engl J Med.* 1995;332:1666–1670.

[12]Cook RR, Harrison MC, LeVier RR. The breast implant controversy. *Arthritis Rheum.* 1994;37:153–157.

[13]Lane TH, Burns SA. Silica, silicon and silicones . . . unravelling the mystery. In: Potter M, Rose NR, eds. *Immunology of Silicones. Current Topics in Microbiology and Immunology,* No 210. Berlin: Springer-Verlag, 1995;3–12.

[14]Bright RA, Jeng LL, Moore RM Jr. National survey of self-reported breast implants: 1988 estimates. *J Long-Term Effects Med Implants.* 1993;3:81–89.

[15]Cook RR, Delongchamp RR, Woodbury MA, Perkins LL, Harrison MC. The prevalence of women with breast implants in the United States—1989. *J Clin Epidemiol.* 1995;48:519–526.

[16]Gabriel SE, O'Fallon WM, Beard CM, Kurland LT, Woods JE, Melton LJ III. Trends in the utilization of silicone breast implants, 1964-1991, and methodology for a population based study of outcomes. *J Clin Epidemiol.* 1995;48:527–536.

[17]Myoshi K, Miyaoka T, Kobayashi Y, *et al.* Hypergammaglobulinemia by prolonged adjuvanticity in man: Disorders developed after augmentation mammoplasty. *Ijishimpo.* 1964;2122:9–14.

[18]Kumagai Y, Shiokawa Y, Medsger TA Jr, Rodnan GP. Clinical spectrum of connective tissue disease after cosmetic surgery: Observations of eighteen patients and a review of the Japanese literature. *Arthritis Rheum.* 1984;27:1–12.

[19]Sanchez-Guerrero J, Schur PH, Sergent JS, Liang MH. Silicone breast implants and rheumatic disease: Clinical immunologic and epidemiologic studies. *Arthritis Rheum.* 1994;37:158–168.

[20]Borenstein D. Siliconosis: A spectrum of illness. *Semin Arthritis Rheum.* 1994;24(suppl 1):1–8.

[21]Vasey FB, Havice DL, Bocanegra TS, *et al.* Clinical findings in symptomatic women with silicone breast implants. *Semin Arthritis Rheum.* 1994;24(suppl 1):22–28.

[22]Solomon G. A clinical and laboratory profile of symptomatic women with silicone breast implants. *Semin Arthritis Rheum.* 1994; 24(suppl 1):29–37.

[23]Freundlich B, Altoman C, Sandorf N, Greenberg M, Tomaszewski J. A profile of symptomatic patients with silicone breast implants: A Sjögren's-like syndrome. *Semin Arthritis Rheum.* 1994;24(suppl 1):44–53.

[24]Fenske TK, Davis P, Aaron SL. Human adjuvant disease revisited: A review of eleven post-augmentation mammoplasty patients. *Clin Exp Rheumatol.* 1994;12:477–481.

[25]Shoaib BO, Patten BM, Calkins DS. Adjuvant breast disease: An evaluation of 100 symptomatic women with breast implants or silicone fluid injections. *Keio J Med.* 1994;43:79–87.

[26]Germain BF. Silicone breast implants and rheumatic disease. *Bull Rheum Dis.* 1991;41:1–4.

[27]Hochberg MC. Cosmetic surgical procedures and connective tissue disease: The Cleopatra syndrome revisited. *Ann Intern Med.* 1993;118:981–983.

[28]Edelman DA, Grant S, van Os WAA. Autoimmune disease following the use of silicone gel-filled breast implants: A review of the clinical literature. *Semin Arthritis Rheum.* 1994;24:183–189.

[29]Spiera RF, Gibofsky A, Spiera H. Silicone gel-filled breast implants and connective tissue disease: an overview. *J Rheumatol.* 1994;21:239–245.

[30]Hochberg MC. Silicone breast implants and rheumatic disease. *Br J Rheumatol.* 1994;33:601–604.

[31]Lamm SH. Silicone breast implants and long-term health effects: When are data adequate? *J Clin Epidemiol.* 1995;48:507–511.

[32]Kurland LT, Homburger HA. Epidemiology of autoimmune and immunological diseases in association with silicone implants: Is there an excess of clinical disease or antibody response in population-based or other "controlled" studies? In: Potter M, Rose NR, eds. *Immunology of Silicones. Current Topics in Microbiology and Immunology,* No 210. Berlin: Springer-Verlag, 1995;428–430.

[33]Weisman MH, Vecchione TR, Albert D, Moore LT, Mueller MR. Connective tissue disease following breast augmentation: A preliminary test of the human adjuvant disease hypothesis. *Plast Reconstr Surg.* 1988;82:626–630.

[34]Dugowson CE, Daling J, Koepsell TD, Voigt L, Nelson JL. Silicone breast implants and risk for rheumatoid arthritis. *Arthritis Rheum.* 1992;35(suppl):S66.

[35]Schusterman MA, Kroll SS, Reece GP, *et al.* Incidence of autoimmune disease in patients after breast reconstruction with silicone gel implants versus autogenous tissue: A preliminary report. *Ann Plast Surg.* 1993;31:1–6.

[36]Wells KE, Cruse CW, Baker JL Jr, *et al.* The health status of women following cosmetic surgery. *Plast Reconstr Surg.* 1994;93:907–912.

[37]Giltay EJ, Bernelot Moens HJ, Riley AH, Tan RG. Silicone breast prostheses and rheumatic symptoms: A retrospective follow-up study. *Ann Rheum Dis.* 1994;53:194–196.

[38]Gabriel SE, O'Fallon WM, Kurland LT, Beard CM, Woods JE, Melton LJ III. Risk of connective tissue diseases and other disorders after breast implantation. *N Engl J Med.* 1994;330:1697–1702.

[39]Englert HJ, Brooks P. Scleroderma and augmentation mammoplasty—a causal relationship? *Aust NZ Med J.* 1994;24:74–80.

[40]Burns CG. The epidemiology of systemic sclerosis: A population-based case-control study. PhD thesis. University of Michigan, Ann Arbor, 1994.

[41]McLaughlin JK, Fraumeni JF Jr, Olsen J, Mellemkjaer L. Breast implants, cancer and systemic sclerosis. *JNCI.* 1994;86:1424.

[42]Strom BL, Reidenberg MM, Freundlich B, Schinnar R. Breast silicone implants and risk of systemic lupus erythematosus. *J Clin Epidemiol.* 1994;47:1211–1214.

[43]Goldman JA, Greenblatt J, Boines R, White L, Aylward B, Lamm SH. Breast implants, rheumatoid arthritis and connective tissue diseases in a clinical practice. *J Clin Epidemiol.* 1995;48:571–582.

[44]Hennekens CH, Lee IM, Cook NR, *et al.* Self-reported breast implants and connective tissue diseases in female health professionals: A retrospective cohort study. *JAMA.* 1996;275:616–621.

[45]Hochberg MC, Perlmutter DL, Medsger TA Jr, *et al.* Lack of association of augmentation mammoplasty with systemic sclerosis (scleroderma). *Arthritis Rheum.* 1996;39:1125–1131.

[46]Star VL, Scott J, Sherwin R, Hochberg MC. Validity of self-reported physician-diagnosed rheumatoid arthritis for use in epidemiologic studies. *Arthritis Rheum.* 1993;36(suppl):S100.

[47]Hochberg MC, Perlmutter DL, Medsger TA Jr, *et al.* The prevalence of self-reported physician-diagnosed systemic lupus erythematosus in the United States. *Lupus.* 1995;4:454–456.

[48]Hochberg MC, Perlmutter DL. The association of augmentation mammoplasty with connective tissue disease, including systemic sclerosis (scleroderma): A meta-analysis. In: Potter M, Rose NR, eds. *Immunology of Silicones. Current Topics in Microbiology and Immunology,* No 210. Berlin: Springer-Verlag, 1995;411–417.

2

Laboratory Testing and the Diagnosis of Selected Rheumatic Diseases

Brian F. Mandell and Leonard Calabrese

INTRODUCTION

The clinical utility of any laboratory test is no greater than the skill and knowledge of the clinician who interprets it. Rarely, if ever, is a single immunologic test diagnostic of a specific rheumatic or autoimmune disease. A test result must be viewed in the context of the patient's clinical situation, and interpreted with knowledge of the test's characteristics, limitations and a sense of how the test relates to the pathophysiology of the disease(s) in question.

Clinicians easily understand the cause and effect relationship between the presence of an infectious agent and specific clinical syndromes. Examination of an adequate sputum sample showing abundant neutrophils with intracellular *Streptococcus pneumonia* obtained from a febrile, coughing patient with an infiltrate on chest radiograph provides sufficient evidence confidently to diagnose pneumococcal pneumonia and initiate therapy. Leukocytosis, an elevated erythrocyte sedimentation rate (ESR) and elevated serum transaminase levels are common findings in patients with pneumococcal pneumonia. But they are *associated* findings not specific enough to confirm the diagnosis. The clinician does not rely on them to make the diagnosis (although these and other indirect studies may be somewhat useful in determining prognosis or identifying comorbid conditions). A rise in the titer of antipneumococcal antibodies would be expected to accompany the pneumonia. Antibody levels are not routinely checked, however, because the etiologic agent can be directly detected by gram stain and/or culture. Furthermore, indirect serologic testing may be difficult to interpret due to the presence of antibodies in currently uninfected patients from prior infection, or nonspecific (polyclonal) hypergammaglobulinemia occurring in the setting of inflammation.

In contrast to infection, the etiology and pathogenesis of most rheumatic or autoimmune diseases are not well defined. Hence, our "diagnostic" armamentarium is limited, and is often less specific. Much of the testing employed in the diagnosis of autoimmune disorders is analogous to the use of a chest radiograph, white blood cell count, ESR and antipneumococcal antibodies to diagnose pneumococcal pneumonia.

The most appropriate use of the immunology laboratory in diagnosing rheumatic diseases is to *support* a clinical diagnosis. Some tests are very sensitive and are best used to exclude particular diagnoses. For example, a positive fluorescent antinuclear antibody (ANA) test is present in 95% of patients with systemic lupus erythematosus (SLE). Therefore, a negative ANA decreases the likelihood of SLE. Furthermore, since an ANA is frequently present with other disorders, it is not specific, and cannot be used to distinguish between SLE and related diseases. *A single serologic test should rarely, if ever, be accepted in isolation as definitive proof of any specific rheumatic/autoimmune disease.*

TEST CHARACTERISTICS

The clinical utility of a given laboratory test is determined by the accuracy with which it identifies or excludes a specific disorder. No test is perfect; virtually all have some false negatives (less than 100% sensitive for a specific disease) and false positives (less than 100% specific). Sensitivity and specificity are significantly influenced by the nature of the control and patient groups used in deriving these values. More importantly, test results must be interpreted within a specific clinical situation. For example, if an ANA test ordered on a patient suspected of having SLE (on the basis of arthralgia, clinical findings such as Raynaud phenomenon, anemia, fatigue and an erythematous skin eruption) is found to be "negative," it would make the diagnosis of SLE quite unlikely. If it is "positive," this would intuitively support the diagnosis of SLE since the test ideally should be abnormal in a small minority of control individuals. However, the patient presented might have one of several other disorders such as dermatomyositis, systemic sclerosis or lymphoma which may also be associated with a positive ANA. Since a positive ANA test is infrequently found in normal controls, but may be found in several other disease states, it is relatively *non-specific* and cannot be used as a discriminating test.

The principal factor which must be considered in the evaluation of a given test is the pretest likelihood of the clinical diagnosis. If a clinical diagnosis is strongly considered despite a negative "diagnostic" test result, the possibility of a *false-negative* test should be entertained. The initiation of subsequent studies or a therapeutic trial will depend upon the disease severity, the potential side effects of therapy and the potential risks from untreated disease.

The alternative problem of *false-positive* testing is well exemplified by the individual with a positive serologic test for Lyme disease, nonspecific symptomatology and no exposure to an endemic area. In this case the pretest likelihood of the disease is low, and the positive serologic test alone should not influence the clinician to embark upon a course of prolonged therapy with potential medical (or financial) risk.

A clinical test should also be reproducible and precise. There are technical and biological aspects that may alter the results of a specific diagnostic study and must be considered in the interpretation of test results. These factors, which are disease-independent, include transportation time, collection technique, prior intramuscular injections (causing elevation of serum creatine kinase and serum aldolase), iatrogenic hemolysis during phlebotomy (increasing serum levels of lactic dehydrogenase, aldolase) and age (aldolase, angiotensin converting enzyme, ESR).

SPECIFIC LABORATORY TESTS

Antinuclear Antibodies

The screening test for the presence of ANAs is a fluorescent antibody technique in which a tissue culture cell line is overlaid with patient diluted serum, washed, and then reincubated with a fluorescein-tagged antihuman immunoglobulin. The fluorescent antibody binds the test serum immunoglobulin which has adhered to the cultured cells' nuclear antigens. The pattern and strength of nuclear fluorescence is analyzed by fluorescent microscopy. Some laboratories are beginning to use automated techniques which will require extensive restandardization of normal values. As the methodologies become more sensitive, it is likely that a large proportion of the "control" population will have low levels of these autoantibodies. The pattern of immunofluorescence correlates with the nature of the nuclear antigen (that is, rim pattern = DNA, homogeneous = histone, speckled = ribonuclear proteins). Some patterns correlate somewhat with specific conditions (rim = SLE, nucleolar = scleroderma, anticentromere = limited systemic sclerosis), but immunofluorescent patterns are *not* disease-diagnostic by themselves. Furthermore, a positive ANA may be found in

Table 2-1   Conditions associated with the presence of antinuclear antibodies

SLE
Scleroderma/CREST
Sjögren's syndrome
Autoimmune myositis
Rheumatoid arthritis
Healthy relatives of patients with SLE
Antiphospholipid antibody syndrome
ITP
TTP
Lymphomas
Autoimmune thyroid disease
Sarcoidosis
Interstitial lung disease
Primary pulmonary hypertension
Autoimmune hepatitis
Primary biliary cirrhosis
Drug-induced syndromes
Infectious mononucleosis
HIV infection (low titer)
Subacute bacterial endocarditis
Pauciarticular JRA
Healthy individuals

healthy individuals, particularly those with a family history of SLE or other autoimmune disorders.[1] Conditions associated with a positive ANA are outlined in Table 2-1. In addition, some drug- and chemical exposures are associated with the induction of ANA (reviewed in Chapter 9).

If the ANA is positive in a patient suspected of having an autoimmune disease, additional serological testing may be of value. The detection of antinative DNA antibodies provides additional support for the diagnosis of SLE. Anti-DNA antibody testing is not as sensitive as the ANA in patients with SLE, but it is more specific since these antibodies are less commonly found in patients with other connective-tissue disorders. Anti-DNA antibody titers, unlike the ANA, may vary with lupus activity in some patients, particularly those with renal involvement.[2]

Anti-Ro and anti-La (SSA and SSB) are found in patients with autoimmune disorders characterized by B cell hyperactivity (SLE, RA). Specific syndromes associated with the presence of these antibodies include sicca complex (xerostomia and xerophthalmia), subacute cutaneous lupus, neonatal lupus and congenital complete heart block. Disease-specific autoantibodies have also been identified for systemic sclerosis (anti-SCL-70 or anti-topoisomerase 1) and polydermatomyositis (anti-acyltransferase myositis-specific autoantibodies). Treatment recommendations should not be based upon the presence or absence of a specific pattern of ANA. Treatment decisions depend upon the clinical manifestations. However, characterization of the ANA pattern may assist the clinician in determining how aggressively to monitor for development of future problems and, perhaps, how aggressively to consider immunosuppressive therapy.[3] *The presence of circulating antinuclear antibodies is not sufficient evidence for the presence of an autoimmune or rheumatic disease.*

Selected autoantibodies and their disease associations are listed in Table 2-2.

Rheumatoid Factor

Rheumatoid factors (RF) are antibodies that bind to the Fc (constant) portion of IgG, but usually only if the IgG is

Table 2-2 Autoantibodies associated with specific rheumatic diseases

Disease	Autoantibody	
Systemic lupus erythematosus	ANA	Anti-Ro
	Anti-dsDNA	Anti-La
	Anti-Sm	Anti-Ribosomal
	Anti-histones	P protein
	Anti-RNP	
Drug-induced lupus (or asymptomatic drug-induced ANA)	ANA	
	Antihistones	
Mixed connective-tissue disease	Anti-RNP (without Anti-DNA or Sm)	
	ANA	
Polymyositis	ANA	
	Anti-aminoacyl synthetase (JO1, PL-12)*	
	Anti-SRP	
Dermatomyositis	ANA	
	Anti-Mi-2	
Systemic sclerosis	ANA	
	Anti-Scl-70 (topoisomerase 1)	
CREST Syndrome**	Anticentromere	
Sjögren's syndrome	ANA	
	Anti-Ro (SS-A)	
	Anti-La (SS-B)	
	Rheumatoid factor	
Wegener's granulomatosus	C-ANCA (anti-PR3)	
Microscopic polyarteritis	P-ANCA (anti-myeloperoxidase)	
Autoimmune thyroid disease	Anti-microsomal	
	Anti-thyroglobulin	
Hypercoagulability	Anti-GP1 associated antiphospholipid antibody	
Neonatal lupus	Anti-Ro	
Rheumatoid arthritis	Rheumatoid factor	
	ANA	
Sarcoidosis	Rheumatoid factor	
	ANA	

*Antisynthetase subset of polymyositis: fever, Raynaud phenomenon, interstitial lung disease, "mechanic's" hands and myositis.
**Calcinosis, Raynaud phenomenon, esophageal dysmotility, sclerodactyly, and telangiectasia.
SRP = signal recognition protein.

aggregated or bound to antigen via its Fab (variable, antigen-binding) region. Although classic RF refers to IgM anti-IgG, IgA and IgG RFs also occur. RF is detected in approximately 80% of patients with rheumatoid arthritis (RA). However, the presence of RF in peripheral blood does not establish a diagnosis nor reliably predict the development of RA or any other type of inflammatory arthritis. Since RFs by definition react with certain antigen-antibody complexes, they may appear in individuals with chronic immune complex formation, for example, chronic infections (osteomyelitis, subacute bacterial endocarditis, or hepatitis C). In these conditions, RF levels may be strikingly high and then resolve with successful eradication of the infection. Rheumatoid factors are also frequently present in other rheumatic disorders, including sarcoidosis, SLE, Wegener's granulomatosus and Sjögren's syndrome. Low-titer RF may also develop in association with aging. *The major utility of the rheumatoid factor assay is to support the clinical diagnosis of RA. It should not be utilized as a screening test.*

The Erythrocyte Sedimentation Rate (ESR) and C-Reactive Protein

In response to many infections and as a consequence of tissue damage, malignancy and immune activation, inflammatory cells release cytokines capable of stimulating a specific pattern of protein synthesis by the liver. This *acute phase response* is comprised in part by the increased synthesis of specific proteins (acute phase reactants) and the slightly suppressed synthesis of albumin. The acute phase proteins include the fairly short-lived C-reactive protein (CRP), fibrinogen, transferrin, serum amyloid A, ferritin, haptoglobin and many others. This response can be measured directly in many circumstances by quantitation of serum CRP levels.[4]

The acute phase response can be indirectly assessed by measuring the ESR, an assay based on the principle that in the presence of increased amounts of asymmetric macromolecules (for example, fibrinogen and gammaglobulins), erythrocytes will settle in a standardized, narrow, vertically placed tube at a faster rate. This test is inexpensive, universally available and reproducible. However, it is significantly affected by the time that the blood is stored prior to transport, the type of anticoagulant and *in vivo* variables including estrogen concentration, severe anemia, presence of paraproteins and erythrocyte morphology. The ESR is not always elevated in patients with systemic inflammatory disease, and an elevated ESR does not equate with the presence of infection, malignancy or inflammatory disease. While it has been used as a "sickness index," the ESR cannot substitute for careful clinical judgment.[5]

In some settings, the acute phase response can be used to follow disease activity: Hodgkin's disease, bacterial infection, and some (but not all) patients with temporal arteritis, polymyalgia rheumatica, rheumatoid arthritis and Wegener's granulomatosus. A sudden rise in the ESR does not help the clinician to distinguish between increased disease activity and secondary infection in these disorders. Certain diseases are well recognized to demonstrate at times a striking discordance between disease activity and the ESR: SLE, systemic sclerosis, Takayasu's arteritis, Henoch-Schonlein purpura, disseminated intravascular coagulation (as the fibrinogen is depleted the ESR falls) and trichinosis.

Complete Blood Counts

There are few results obtained from the complete blood count that firmly aid in the diagnosis of specific autoimmune or rheumatic diseases. The relatively mild anemia of chronic inflammation (hypoproduction with slightly increased erythrocyte RDW, slight resistance to erythropoietin, marrow redistribution of adequate iron stores away from erythroid precursors) is a frequent component of rheumatic disorders, as is thrombocytosis. Leukopenia and thrombocytopenia do not routinely accompany the inflammatory response and they are not present in the primary vasculitic syndromes. Their presence in the setting of an apparent systemic disorder should raise suspicion of a primary or secondary marrow process such as malignancy, thrombotic thrombocytopenic purpura, cobalamin deficiency, SLE, paroxysmal nocturnal hemoglobinuria, hypersplenism and Felty syndrome. Hemolysis should be directly investigated by examination of the peripheral smear and reticulocyte count.

The multiple causes of eosinophilia (more than or equal to 500 total eosinophil per mm^3) include atopy, Churg Strauss syndrome, some drug allergies, eosinophilia myalgia syndrome, eosinophilic fasciitis, and occasionally rheumatoid arthritis, scleroderma, lymphoma, cholesterol embolization syndrome, tissue invasion with parasites and, rarely, carcinoma. Extremely high blood and tissue levels of eosinophils can result in the hypereosinophilic syndrome with associated organ (predominantly cardiac and neurologic) dysfunction.

Muscle enzymes

A number of primary autoimmune diseases as well as exogenous substances, including prescribed medications, can produce muscle damage with or without necrosis. Clinical symptoms of inflammatory and toxic myopathies include proximal greater than distal muscle weakness, occasionally with significant myalgias. Objective detection of subtle weakness early in the course of the disease process can be difficult, especially in young children and athletic or very muscular adults. Laboratory testing can be useful in the recognition of muscle damage if several caveats are recognized. The degree of muscle enzyme activity in the blood has no direct correlation with the degree of weakness. Even in the setting of clear-cut, active, biopsy-documented polymyositis, normal muscle enzyme levels may occur. The commonly

measured transaminases (ALT and AST) are present in skeletal (as well as smooth and cardiac) myocytes. Thus they may be elevated in the serum of patients with inflammatory muscle disease (myositis) or toxic muscle damage, and may be incorrectly interpreted as liver damage. Aldolase, an enzyme of the glycolytic pathway, is present in most tissues including liver, erythrocytes and muscle. Aldolase elevation is therefore *not* a specific marker of muscle damage. On the other hand, creatine phosphokinase (CPK) is not present to a significant degree in liver or erythrocytes and, if brain and kidney infarction are excluded, elevations of CPK are the most specific marker routinely available for myonecrosis. The MB isoenzyme of CPK, frequently used as a marker for myocardial infarction, is also present in regenerating skeletal muscle and may be found in the serum of patients with some dystrophies and chronic myositis.

Chemical and medication causes of myopathy or myositis with elevated levels of muscle enzyme activities include adulterated L-tryptophan, hemlock, cimetidine, HMG-Co A reductase inhibitors, clofibrate, azidothymidine, colchicine, D-penicillamine, alcohol, chloroquine and hydroxychloroquine. Primary or chemical-induced neuropathies generally do not significantly increase the serum level of muscle enzymes. Corticosteroid-induced myopathy is also not associated with elevated serum muscle enzyme activities. Serum CPK activity may also be increased in patients with hypothyroidism.

DIAGNOSIS OF SELECTED SPECIFIC DISORDERS: EXAMPLES

The diagnosis of specific autoimmune and rheumatic disorders is not established on the basis of a single laboratory study. Diagnoses are made taking into consideration the constellation of clinical symptoms and findings, supporting this information with appropriate laboratory studies. For clinical research purposes, to assure a more homogeneous study patient population, committees of the American College of Rheumatology (formerly known as the American Rheumatism Association) and other organizations have attempted to define diagnostic criteria for several rheumatic disorders. Because of the emphasis on specificity of diagnosis, these criteria may not be ideal for the initial diagnosis in a given patient. At the onset of disease sufficient specific features may not have had time to develop in order to meet full criteria, yet the diagnosis may be apparent to experienced clinicians. Despite these limitations, diagnostic criteria serve a useful purpose when attempting to define disease associations, as with external (environmental) triggers.

Systemic Lupus Erythematosus (SLE)

SLE is an idiopathic autoimmune multisystem disorder which affects primarily women. The estimated prevalence of SLE in the United States is between 15 and 50 per 100,000.

The more common manifestations of SLE include constitutional features such as fever and fatigue, arthralgia or polyarthritis, a variety of skin rashes and oral/nasal ulcerations, photosensitivity, mild to moderately severe Raynaud phenomenon, glomerulonephritis, serositis, leukopenia, anemia and thrombocytopenia. A positive ANA is present in more than 90% of patients, and anti-DNA antibodies are present in 70% of patients. The 1982 revised criteria for the diagnosis of SLE are shown in Table 2-3.[6] In the clinic, the diagnosis of SLE is frequently made in the absence of four or more criteria (the suggested minimum). Most importantly, alternative defined diagnoses must be excluded. Endocarditis, HIV infection and other potential conditions with similar features can often be rapidly excluded. However, other autoimmune diseases such as scleroderma may take months before the distinctive characteristics develop and the diagnosis becomes apparent. Renal biopsy, with immune staining as well as histopathology, may occasionally be necessary to distinguish SLE from alternative diagnoses and to plan therapeutic intervention.

Systemic Sclerosis (SSc)

Systemic sclerosis is a rare disorder. If mild cases are included, there may be 100,000 cases in the United States. Hospital and billing records suggest a significantly lower prevalence. It is a fibrosing disorder associated with often severe Raynaud's phenomenon and small vessel obliterative disease. A varying degree of progressive distal and proximal skin thickening is the hallmark of the disease. Other common manifestations include esophageal and intestinal dysmotility, myositis, cardiac conduction disease and bibasilar pulmonary fibrosis. Several clinical subsets of the disease have been described.

Skin thickening proximal to the metacarpophalangeal joints was the single major criterion for classification of systemic sclerosis.[7] The presence of two or more of the following features contributed further as minor criteria: sclerodactyly, digital pitting scars of fingertips or loss of digital finger pad substance, and bibasilar pulmonary fibrosis. Proximal skin thickening may occur in unrelated disorders and alternative diagnoses must be excluded. At times, especially in patients who present with diffuse distal symmetric edema prior to developing cutaneous induration, the initial diagnosis is unclear and may appear to be polyarthritis. Antinuclear antibodies are present in more than 90% of patients whereas anti-DNA antibodies are generally not detected.

Idiopathic Inflammatory Muscle Disease (Myositis)

Myositis can accompany various rheumatic disorders including SLE, SSc, sarcoidosis, Sjögren's syndrome and rheumatoid arthritis. Polymyositis is a primary inflammatory disease of proximal greater than distal skeletal muscle, which may also be associated with esophageal dysfunction, bibasilar pulmonary fibrosis and occasionally polyarthritis. Dermatomyositis also involves proximal muscle but is asso-

Table 2-3 The 1982 revised American Rheumatism Association criteria for diagnosis of SLE

Criterion	Definition
1. Malar rash	Fixed erythema, flat or raised, over the malar eminences.
2. Discoid rash	Erythematous raised patches with adherent keratotic scaling and follicular plugging.
3. Photosensitivity	Skin rash as a result of unusual reaction to sunlight, by patient history or physician observation.
4. Oral ulcers	Oral or nasopharyngeal ulceration, usually painless, observed by a physician.
5. Arthritis	Nonerosive arthritis involving two or more peripheral joints.
6. Renal disorder	(a) Persistent proteinuria greater than 0.6 per day.
	(b) Cellular casts.
7. Serositis	(a) Pleuritis.
	(b) Pericarditis.
8. Neurologic disorder	(a) Seizures—in the absence of offending drugs or known metabolic derangement.
	(b) Psychosis—in the absence of offending drugs or known metabolic derangement.
9. Hematologic disorder	(a) Hemolytic anemia with reticulocytosis; or
	(b) Leukopenia—less than 4000/mm^3 on more than two occasions; or
	(c) Lymphopenia—less than 1500/mm^3 on more than two occasions; or
	(d) Thrombocytopenia—less than 100,000/mm^3 in the absence of offending drugs.
10. Immunologic disorder	(a) Positive LE cell preparation; or
	(b) Anti-DNA; or
	(c) Anti-Sm: presence of antibody to Sm nuclear antigen; or
	(d) False-positive serologic test for syphilis known to be positive for at least 6 months.
11. Antinuclear antibody	An abnormal titer of antinuclear antibody by immunofluorescence or an equivalent assay at any point in time in the absence of drug therapy.

From Tan, *et al.*[6]

ciated with characteristic skin lesions on the eyelids and over the extensor tendons, photosensitivity, and an increased frequency of malignancy in patients older than 40 years of age. Diagnosis is most definitively made by muscle biopsy in the setting of proximal muscle weakness and elevated serum levels of muscle enzymes. In the absence of muscle biopsy, diagnosis is suggested by the appropriate clinical pattern of muscle involvement, elevated muscle enzymes, and an abnormal electromyogram. The ANA is frequently positive, and specific autoantibodies define clinical disease subsets (Table 2-2).

REFERENCES

[1]Talal N, Pillarisetty RJ, DeHoratius RJ, Messner RP. Immunologic regulations of spontaneous antibodies to DNA and RNA. 1. Significance of IgM and IgG antibodies in SLE patients and asymptomatic relatives. *Clin Exp Immunol.* 1976;25:377–382.

[2]Lloyd W, Schur PH. Immune complexes, complement, and anti-DNA in exacerbations of systemic lupus erythematosus (SLE). *Medicine.* 1981;60:208–217.

[3]Targoff IN, Johnson AE, Miller FW. Antibody to signal recognition particle in polymyositis. *Arth Rheum.* 1990;33:1361–1370.

[4]Kushner I. C Reactive protein in rheumatology. *Arthritis Rheum.* 1991;1065–1068.

[5]Bedell SE, Bush ET. Erythrocyte sedimentation rate: From folklore to facts. *Am J Med.* 1985;78:1001–1010.

[6]Tan EM, Cohen AS, Fries JF, *et al.* The 1982 revised criteria for the classification of systemic lupus erythematosus. *Arthritis Rheum.* 1982;25:1271–1277.

[7]Subcommittee for Scleroderma Criteria of the American Rheumatism Association Diagnostic and Therapeutic Criteria Committee. Preliminary criteria for the classification of systemic sclerosis (scleroderma). *Arthritis Rheum.* 1980;23:581–590.

II

Etiopathogenetic Considerations

3

Mechanisms of Autoimmunity in Environmentally Induced Connective Tissue Diseases

Mariana J. Kaplan and Bruce C. Richardson

INTRODUCTION

Certain molecules found in environmental, pharmacologic or food sources can induce and perpetuate autoimmunity. These compounds are known as xenobiotics. Autoimmunity induced by xenobiotics is a recognized health hazard that affects genetically predisposed individuals. Well-characterized examples include drugs like procainamide and hydralazine, which induce a lupuslike disease, and gold salts, which induce an immune-complex-mediated nephropathy. Many other xenobiotics exist or remain to be identified. The examples of the better-characterized xenobiotics are useful, because they provide insights into mechanisms by which other agents could trigger autoimmune diseases. The purpose of this chapter is to review mechanisms by which known xenobiotics may interact with cells of the immune system and induce autoimmunity.

Xenobiotics are a chemically heterogenous group of low-molecular-weight molecules. The mechanisms by which many of these agents cause autoimmunity vary widely and, in humans, are often unclear. However, studies of xenobiotic-induced autoimmunity in animal models have provided useful information. Often, the manifestations are sufficiently similar in humans and animals to allow some insights into the human disease. Table 3-1 lists some animal models of xenobiotic-induced autoimmunity, together with their predominant clinical manifestations and the corresponding human disease. These animal models, together with others summarized elsewhere in this book, form the foundation of many of our current concepts regarding the role of xenobiotics in autoimmunity.

The number of drugs and chemicals capable of eliciting autoantibody (autoAb) formation and autoimmune disease is still growing, in part due to an increased awareness of this problem. Table 3-2 provides some examples of these chemicals and their associated diseases. In this chapter, we first review basic mechanisms contributing to the development of autoimmunity. We then discuss specific mechanisms associated with xenobiotic-induced autoimmunity. Finally, we emphasize some particularly well-studied models, such as mercury and procainamide, that add insight into the pathogenic mechanisms of these entities. Examples of other xenobiotics known or proposed to induce autoimmunity are addressed in other chapters (Chapter 5 for rapeseed oil, Chapter 6 for tryptophan, Chapter 7 for silica and silicon and Chapter 9 for drug-induced lupus).

TOLERANCE AND AUTOIMMUNITY

Many mechanisms been proposed by which xenobiotics produce autoimmunity.[1] Some, such as the inhibition of complement components by nucleophilic compounds including procainamide, hydralazine and D-penicillamine, have been observed *in vitro*. However, the relevance of mostly *in vitro* observations to the induction of autoimmunity *in vivo* is not always clear. In contrast, mechanisms which disrupt immunological tolerance *in vivo* have been more persuasively implicated in the development of autoimmunity. This review will be directed at mechanisms by which xenobiotics may modify lymphocytes and antigen-presenting cells (APC) to disrupt tolerance and initiate an *in vivo* autoimmune state.[2–4]

During development, cells capable of responding to self-determinants, referred to as autoreactive, are deleted or rendered anergic. This phenomenon is known as immune tolerance. Tolerance, an active process continuously maintained throughout life, is mediated by multiple mechanisms.[5] This results in an immune system which recognizes and responds to foreign molecules, but ignores self-molecules. Autoimmunity develops when autoreactive T and B lymphocytes recognize and respond to self-antigens. This concept is supported by a large body of experimental evidence demonstrating that T and B cells capable of responding to self-mole-

Table 3-1 Animal models of autoimmunity triggered by xenobiotics

Xenobiotic	Animal Species/Strain	Autoimmunity	Human Counterpart
Mercury	Rats		
	(BN, DZB, MAXX)	Antilaminin antibodies	SLE
	(PVG)	Antihistone antibodies	GMN
	Mice (SJL/J)	Antifibrillarin, histone	SSc
Gold	Rats	IC-renal disease	GMN
	Rabbits	IC-renal disease	
	Guinea pigs	IC-renal disease	
Penicillamine	Mice	Ab ACh receptor	MG
	Rats (BN)	Anti-GBM, -TBM, laminin	GMN
	Guinea pigs	Myositis, MG	
L-canavanine	Monkeys	ANA	SLE
	Mice		
Hydralazine	Mice	ANA	SLE
Procainamide	Mice	ANA, IC-GMN	
		alveolitis, SLE	

Ab: antibody; ACh: acetylcholine; ANA: Antinuclear antibody; BN: Brown-Norway; GMN: glomerulonephritis; GBM: glomerular basement membrane; IC: immune complex; IC-GMN: IC-glomerulonephritis; MG: myasthenia gravis; TBM: tubular basement membrane; SSc: systemic sclerosis.

cules can induce various forms of autoimmunity. One particularly persuasive model is murine chronic graft-versus-host (GvH) disease. Chronic GvH disease is induced by the adoptive transfer of CD4+ T cells from a parent strain into the F1 hybrid of histoincompatible parental strains. The transferred cells respond to host Ia molecules *in vivo*. Mice with chronic GvH develop a syndrome clinically resembling human systemic lupus erythematosus (SLE), with immune complex glomerulonephritis, splenomegaly, lymphadenopathy and immunoglobulin deposition at the dermal-epidermal junction.[6] These mice also develop hypergammaglobulinemia and autoantibodies to native and single-stranded DNA, histones, ribonuclear proteins, thymocytes and erythrocytes. This model clearly demonstrates that major histocompatibility complex (MHC) responsive T cells can cause a lupuslike disease. Other well-established models of autoimmunity include the induction of antibody responses to the acetylcholine receptor, producing a disease resembling human myasthenia gravis, and experimental allergic encephalomyelitis (EAE), where T cells responding to determinants on myelin basic protein cause a multiple-sclerosis-like disease.[7] The identification of similar autoreactive T and B lymphocytes in patients with autoimmune diseases further demonstrates that the mechanisms maintaining tolerance can sometimes break down, resulting in diseases like SLE, myasthenia gravis or multiple sclerosis.[7,8]

Both genetic and environmental factors contribute to tolerance breakdown. Genes of the MHC complex clearly predispose to the development of autoimmunity.[9] Other genetic influences exist. Examples include homozygosity for the gene controlling activity of hepatic acetyltransferase, which contributes to some forms of drug-induced lupus (DIL).[10] Less well understood genetic influences include female sex[9], and certain families display a strong tendency to develop autoimmunity, although the genes contributing to familial autoimmunity are not yet known. In addition to genetic influences, environmental factors play a role in triggering the autoimmune process. These factors include infectious agents such as viruses and bacteria, ultraviolet (UV) light, and xenobiotics such as drugs and heavy metals. Current models support the concept that exposure to the inciting agent, in a host of the proper genetic background, may result in the development of autoimmunity.

The development of autoimmunity requires that the interaction between genetically regulated elements and the environmental agent causes the breakdown of "self" tolerance. This results in the activation and expansion of self-reactive T and B lymphocyte clones. The T cells orchestrate the autoimmune response by a variety of pathways including direct cytotoxic actions on target cells, the secretion of cytokines and the activation of autoreactive B lymphocytes.[2] The autoreactive B cells secrete autoantibodies forming immune complexes with the target antigen, which results in the production of other inflammatory mediators triggered by the immune complexes. The key step in this process is the breakdown of tolerance. Alternative and non-mutually exclusive possibilities have been proposed to explain how tolerance is maintained and how it may be impaired. These are discussed in the sections below. The abundance of possible routes through which tolerance may be disrupted and the experi-

Table 3-2 Chemicals associated with autoimmunity

Methyldopa	Autoimmune cytopenias
Allopurinol	SLE-like disease
Amiodarone	Autoimmune thyroid disease
Bleomycin	Scleroderma, Raynaud syndrome
Cadmium	Renal disease
Carbamazepine	SLE-like syndrome
Chloropromazine	Hemolytic anemia, SLE-like syndrome
Cocaine	SLE-like syndrome, vasculitis
Dapsone	SLE-like syndrome
Ethosuximide	SLE-like syndrome, scleroderma, myositis
Gold	Nephropathy, cytopenias, SLE-like syndrome
Hydantoins	SLE-like syndrome
Hydralazine	SLE-like syndrome
Isoniazid	SLE-like syndrome
L-canavanine	Hemolytic anemia, SLE-like syndrome
L-tryptophan	Eosinophilia myalgia syndrome
Lovastatin	SLE-like syndrome
Mercury	Nephropathy
Nitrofurantoin	SLE-like syndrome
Penicillamine	SLE-like syndrome, cytopenias, myasthenia, myositis
Penicillin	SLE-like syndrome, cytopenias
Phenylbutazone	SLE-like syndrome
Procainamide	SLE-like syndrome, cytopenias
Quinidine	Cytopenias, SLE-like syndrome, arthritis
Silicon	Sclerodermalike disease
Sulfasalazine	SLE-like syndrome
Sulfonamides	SLE-like syndrome
Tartrazine	SLE-like syndrome
Tetracyclines	SLE-like syndrome
Trilene	Systemic sclerosis
Vinyl chloride	Systemic sclerosis

mental evidence supporting these routes suggest that there are likely to be multiple mechanisms leading to autoimmunity.[4]

Mechanisms Leading to Impaired Tolerance

Some mechanisms known to be implicated in the development of impaired immune tolerance are summarized in Table 3-3. An important mechanism responsible for maintaining tolerance is the deletion of autoreactive lymphocytes. For T cells this occurs in the thymus, where cells bearing high-affinity receptors for self-determinants are deleted by apoptosis. It is likely that autoreactive T cells are also deleted extrathymically, although the mechanisms involved are not well understood. For B cells, surface immunoglobulin interacting with molecules on adjacent cell surfaces can also trigger apoptosis.[11] Failure to delete autoreactive lymphocytes is

Table 3-3 Mechanisms leading to impaired immunologic tolerance

1. Failure to delete autoreactive lymphocytes
2. Failure to tolerate autoreactive lymphocytes
3. Modified self-antigen
4. Presentation of cryptic epitopes
5. Antigenic mimicry
6. Abnormal cytokine secretion
7. Abnormal MHC molecule expression
8. Abnormal adhesion molecule expression
9. Presentation of normally sequestered antigens
10. Idiotypic networks

one mechanism causing autoimmunity. This is best demonstrated in the *lpr* and *gld* murine lupus models, characterized by mutations in the molecules signaling apoptosis which prevent the deletion of autoreactive T cells.[12] In another model, transgenic mice with B cells expressing the antiapoptotic Bcl2 gene products fail to delete autoreactive B cells, resulting in the production of autoantibodies.[13]

A related form of tolerance is clonal anergy, which occurs in both T and B cells. Anergic cells bear receptors for their respective ligands but are unable to respond to stimuli. In T cells, a lack of necessary costimulatory signals by the APC, such as those mediated through CD28 on the T cell and the B7 molecules on the APC, can lead to anergy.[14] B cells may be similarly tolerated by a relatively weak, costimulator-deficient, antigenic stimulus such as some soluble antigens.[15,16]

It is also possible that some T lymphocytes with potentially self-reactive receptors may ignore self-antigen because of low-affinity APC interactions, low-level MHC expression on the APC or the absence of necessary cytokines. Overexpression of adhesion molecules on T cells can induce autoreactivity *in vitro* and autoimmunity *in vivo,*[17,18] suggesting that overstabilization of T cell-APC interactions can interfere with tolerance. This mechanism may contribute to human SLE.[19] Enhanced expression of MHC molecules on APC, induced by gamma interferon, has also been shown to abrogate immune unresponsiveness.[15] This mechanism has been implicated in some diabetes models.[15] Potentially autoreactive B cells may fail to respond to stimuli because of insufficient presentation of autoantigens but secrete autoantibody under other circumstances. Experiments demonstrating the generation of autoantibodies induced by nonspecific polyclonal B cell activators support this concept.[20]

Another mechanism proposed for the abrogation of tolerance is the modification of self-antigens. Self-antigens modified by chemical reactions such as oxidation may be perceived by the immune system as "foreign," triggering a response.[1] There is also evidence suggesting that some molecules bear immunologically "cryptic" epitopes which are not exposed to the immune system until degraded by the antigen-presenting cell and presented in the context of self-

MHC molecules.[21] This has recently been demonstrated for the CD4 molecule in an HIV model (21) as well as in other systems.

Antigenic mimicry has been proposed as another mechanism capable of breaking tolerance. In this model, a molecule on an invading microorganism initiates an immune response cross-reactive with host molecules. This leads to a response directed at the host molecule. Recent evidence suggests that molecular mimicry may play a role in the development of multiple sclerosis, where T cell clones reactive with myelin basic protein are activated by bacterial and viral peptides.[15]

Contributing to the modified self-antigen, the antigenic mimicry and the cryptic epitope hypotheses is the phenomenon of epitope spreading. In epitope spreading, the immune response directed at an epitope on a self-antigen, initiated by one or more of these mechanisms, spreads to other epitopes within the molecule and even to physically distinct but noncovalently linked molecules. Epitope spreading clearly contributes to the development of autoantibody responses in experimental models of autoimmunity, and in humans.[22]

Idiotype networks are also implicated in impaired tolerance. This hypothesis states that T and B cell receptors recognize receptors on other B and T cells without development of tolerance, forming what is referred to as the idiotype network. Under normal conditions, this network may stimulate or suppress immune responses through idiotype-anti-idiotype interactions. This concept is illustrated by an early experiment which demonstrated that antibodies to tobacco mosaic virus (TMV) could be induced by immunizing mice with rabbit antibodies to idiotypes on anti-TMV antibodies.[23] This mechanism has relevance to autoimmunity because in some systems anti-idiotypic responses appear to cross-react with self-antigens, leading to or augmenting autoimmunity.[1]

Finally, immune responses to self-antigens for which T cell tolerance is normally not established may be implicated in the development of autoimmunity.[3] Proteins have been implicated as key autoantigens in organ-specific autoimmunity, such as thyroid peroxidase in the case of thyroiditis, and glutamic acid decarboxylase in human insulin-dependent diabetes mellitus and the nonobese diabetic mouse model. These proteins are not expressed in the normal thymus, leading to the retention of potentially autoreactive T cells in the periphery. These cells may then become activated during inflammatory responses involving the relevant organs, such as the thyroid or pancreas, leading to an autoimmune response.[15]

MECHANISMS FOR XENOBIOTIC-INDUCED AUTOIMMUNITY

The mechanisms for disrupted immune tolerance discussed above very likely play a role in the development of xenobiotic-induced autoimmunity. Much of the evidence supporting this statement derives from *in vitro* and *in vivo* model systems. However, a few cautionary words are in order regarding the design and interpretation of *in vitro* and *in vivo* xenobiotic models. Confounding variables include the possibility that metabolites may be responsible for inducing autoimmunity and that there exists genetic heterogeneity in the metabolism of some compounds. For example, impaired sulfoxidation of D-penicillamine increases the risk of adverse renal effects, thrombocytopenia and cutaneous lesions. Similarly, individuals who are genetically slow acetylators of procainamide or hydralazine have an increased risk of developing DIL. For other drugs, it is still uncertain whether their immunomodulating potential is due to the unmetabolized agents, their metabolites, or both. Bioavailability, as determined by the vehicle, may influence chemical reactivity of some low-molecular-weight compounds after oral exposure. Finally, compounds dissolved in aqueous media are more readily taken up in the circulation, whereas agents in an oil matrix are more likely to be conveyed by chylomicrons to the lymph. This level of heterogeneity confounds the task of sorting out exactly how xenobiotics trigger autoimmunity. However, progress has been made. Some of the mechanisms proposed, based on this work, are discussed below.[1,24–26]

Binding of a Drug or its Metabolite(s) to Self-Molecules to Form Novel Autoantigens

A chemically reactive substance may combine with a host molecule to modify its structure, creating new epitopes no longer recognized as "self" by the immune system. Host T lymphocytes may then react with the novel determinants and induce autoantibodies through "helper" effects. For example, when small molecules (or "haptens") like dinitrophenol are coupled to thyroglobulin and used to immunize mice, antibodies reactive with determinants on thyroglobulin are produced. This probably involves the principle of epitope spreading. T cells are essential for the production of these autoantibodies. T cells responding to haptenic determinants may also contribute to autoimmunity through mechanisms independent of B cells. In the case of nitrofurantoin, which can cause a lupuslike disease, there is evidence for cell-mediated reactions to the drug, but no evidence of drug binding by immunoglobulin. This is consistent with the idea that the drug functions as a T-cell-specific hapten. In nickel-induced contact dermatitis, cloned CD4+ T cells from the skin lesions are stimulated by autologous class II MHC molecule-bearing cells and nickel. Proliferation can be abrogated by anti-class II monoclonal antibodies, suggesting that the cells are responding to nickel-modified molecules presented by class II molecules.

Another example is phenytoin, which triggers the development of lymphoid hyperplasia, plasmacytosis and the production of autoantibodies. Metabolites of this drug may attach to the surface of lymphoid cells and covalently modify their MHC antigens. T lymphocytes then recognize the modified molecules as "foreign." The kinetics and morphology of the phenytoin-induced reactions bear resemblance to GvH.[27]

Xenobiotic-induced conformational changes can also expose previously hidden antigenic determinants. Under certain experimental conditions, procainamide, hydralazine, L-canavanine, isoniazid and D-penicillamine bind polynucleotides and induce a stable transition of DNA from the B (right-handed) to Z (left-handed) conformation. The Z conformation of DNA is more immunogenic and may contribute to the formation of some anti-DNA antibodies.[28]

Molecular Mimicry

Although usually associated with exposure to microorganisms, this phenomenon hypothetically could occur following exposure to certain inorganic and organic molecules which possess determinants cross-reactive with self-antigens. For xenobiotics, this may represent a variation on the modified self-antigen hypothesis discussed above, where the xenobiotic resembles a modified self-molecule.

Generation of Cryptic Epitopes

This phenomenon has been implicated in autoimmunity induced by gold and other metals. A recent study has shown that alteration of bovine ribonuclease A by the Au (III) form of gold results in T cell sensitization to cryptic peptides of this protein.[29] It appears that gold alteration of proteins disrupts antigen processing mechanisms leading to presentation of cryptic peptides. This mechanism could contribute to autoimmunity by generation of an immune response to the cryptic epitopes and subsequent epitope spreading.

Inhibition of Clonal Deletion

Environmental agents may affect thymic selection or may directly modify mature T cells to produce autoimmunity. For example, some xenobiotics may inhibit elimination of autoreactive T cells from the thymus or periphery, allowing release or generation of self-reactive T cells. Total lymphoid irradiation can trigger organ-specific autoimmunity in rodents by this mechanism.[3] Another example is cyclosporin; irradiated hosts transplanted with syngeneic or even autologous bone marrow cells and treated with cyclosporin develop a lupuslike disease after the cyclosporin has been withdrawn. This phenomenon has been described in humans, rats and mice. The autoimmune disease is transferable by T cells from affected animals. Removal of the thymus from the transplanted recipients prevents autoimmunity, but the thymus is

required for the appearance of cyclosporin-induced autoreactive T cells in the donors. When injected into newborn mice, cyclosporin can also induce autoimmunity, presumably by a similar mechanism: autoreactive T cells have been found in the peripheral blood of these mice.[30]

Overexpression of Lymphocyte Adhesion Molecules

Overexpression of the adhesion molecule lymphocyte function-associated antigen LFA-1 (CD11a/CD18) is another mechanism causing T cell autoreactivity *in vitro* and autoimmunity *in vivo*.[17] Some xenobiotics such as 5-azacytidine and procainamide can increase T cell LFA-1 expression, most likely by inhibiting DNA methylation, a mechanism regulating gene expression.[17] Murine T cells overexpressing LFA-1, caused indirectly by treatment with 5-azacytidine or procainamide or directly by transfection, become autoreactive and cause a lupuslike disease in syngeneic recipients.[18,31] DNA in T cells from patients with idiopathic SLE is hypomethylated, and a subset of T cells overexpresses LFA-1, supporting a role for overexpression of adhesion molecules in human autoimmunity.[19,32] This topic is discussed more fully below.

Polyclonal B Lymphocyte Activation

Polyclonal B cell activation may contribute to systemic autoimmunity. A large number of molecules, particularly of microbial origin, have been found to act as polyclonal B cell activators and induce autoantibodies along with antibodies of other specificities. Polyclonal activation may play a role in the pathogenesis of mercury-induced autoimmunity in animal models (*vide infra*). However, the primary importance of exogenous polyclonal B cell activators in the induction of systemic disease is still questioned, and it may be that polyclonal B cell activators exacerbate autoimmunity but are insufficient by themselves to cause it. This is supported by the fact that expression of autoimmune diseases in animal models requires T cell participation and that autoantibodies induced by polyclonal B cell activators are primarily low-affinity IgM molecules, while tissue damage in systemic autoimmune diseases such as SLE involves high-affinity IgG autoantibodies.[33]

Modification and Abnormal Expression of MHC II Class Molecules and/or Cytokines

Some xenobiotics alter second messenger systems, in some cases acting as cofactors and increasing MHC expression and cytokine production. If aberrant expression of class II MHC molecules occurs, presentation of self-antigens can lead to activation of autoreactive T cells. This mechanism has been proposed for the induction of autoimmune thyroiditis and diabetes.[3] Abnormal expression of class II MHC molecules by specific cells of target organs has also been reported in inflammatory bowel disease and in Sjögren's syndrome. Interferon-alpha has been implicated in the development of a lupuslike human autoimmune disease, possibly by altered expression of class II MHC molecules.[34]

The activation of adenyl cyclase can increase expression of class II MHC molecules. Mercurials, zinc and lead may enhance *in vitro* MHC class II expression by altering different signal transduction mechanisms.[35] The increase of MHC class II expression could then lead to presentation of endogenous antigens, stimulating autoreactive T cells by mechanisms similar to those for autoimmune diabetes.

Defects in Apoptosis

Three independent mutations involving the Fas (CD95) receptor or its ligand have been described which lead to lupuslike diseases in different strains of mice.[36–38] An example is the lpr/lpr mouse, in which a defect in the Fas gene, encoding a molecule triggering apoptosis, prevents the deletion of autoreactive T cells. The response of these autoreactive cells to self determinants *in vivo* appears to contribute to the development of a lupuslike disease. However, in humans only a few cases of defects in the expression or function of Fas receptors have been clearly identified to date.[39] One example recently reported is the Canale-Smith syndrome.[40] A role for abnormal apoptosis caused by xenobiotics is theoretically possible but has not yet been demonstrated.

T Cell Mutations

T cells from patients with rheumatoid arthritis and SLE have an increased frequency of mutations. In the case of SLE, total duration of active disease, past highest disease activity index and number of flares correlate with the number of T cells with mutations.[41] These studies have largely focused on the hypoxanthine phosphoribosyl transferase gene because of the relative ease in detecting mutations of this enzyme. Whether mutations in other genes occur and are pathogenic is not clear. However, these observations raise the possibility that mutations due to radiation or chemicals could modify T and B cell gene expression, potentially contributing to disease processes.[41]

Modification of Lymphocyte Function

Oxidizing agents may inactivate T cells. The activity of lymphocytes is influenced by the status of the thiols on the cell surface. The reduction of thiols or the breaking of protein cross-links through disulfide exchange eliminates disulfide bridges, which in turn is associated with enhanced cellular activity. This can be reversed by oxidizing agents.[1] It has been proposed that some of the compounds known to trigger autoimmunity, such as mercury, vinyl chloride and toxic oils, directly interact with cellular thiols, inactivating T cells. The oxidizing capacity of phagocytic cells is also thought to play a role in the generation of immunogenic drug metabolites. These reactive intermediates can modify T cells via reactions with cellular proteins. An example of this is procainamide, where reactive metabolites have been indirectly implicated in the development of autoimmunity.[42] This is discussed more fully in the chapter on DIL.

EXAMPLES OF XENOBIOTIC-INDUCED AUTOIMMUNITY

Heavy Metals

Autoimmunity induced by heavy metals such as mercury, gold and others has been extensively studied using animal models and may contribute to human disease by multiple mechanisms.[43–46] These heavy metals can bind to carboxyl, nitryl, sulfhydryl and phosphoryl groups, thus rendering self-molecules immunogenic. This mechanism has been proposed to explain the immune-complex glomerulonephritis associated with exposure to mercury in certain animal strains (*vide infra*). Nuclear antigens modified by metals may also become immunogenic, contributing to the development of autoantibodies to these structures in the mercury model system.

Metals can also modify the cells of the immune system. One effect is the differentiation of polyclonal B cells into antibody-secreting cells. This may be mediated either by a direct effect of metals on B cells or by activating T cells to drive the B cell differentiation. One example of this mechanism is the modification of Ia molecules by metals such as nickel and lead, which may then be recognized as modified self-antigens. These metals have been reported to stimulate T cells responsive to the modified Ia molecules. The model of chronic GvH disease indicates that this response can lead to the development of an autoimmune illness with counterparts in a number of human diseases, including SLE, rheumatoid arthritis, Sjögren's syndrome and systemic sclerosis (SSc).[47]

Metals like cadmium, lead, zinc, lithium and mercury can affect signal transduction involving protein kinases, adenylate cyclase and calcium-dependent pathways. Heavy metals are able effectively to substitute for calcium in calmodulin.[48] Activation of calmodulin by these metals may disturb its normal regulation by calcium. Mercury and nickel have been shown to interact directly with the T cell receptor and activate T cells, which could affect immune processes. Mercury has also been found to interfere with the transport of protons through the plasma membrane, blocking proton pumps and enhancing the permeability of the T cell membrane. By this mechanism, mercury might interfere with the activation of pH-dependent kinases and increase protein phosphorylation and DNA transcription. Lead, zinc and cadmium can inhibit membrane ouabaine-sensitive ATPase, favoring the transformation of ATP to cAMP and enhancing protein kinase A-induced protein phosphorylation. Subsequent induction of DNA synthesis might then play a role in lymphocyte activation and proliferation.[49,50]

A role for metal-binding molecules in the nucleus is also possible. Nuclear receptors have been described for mercury and beryllium, but the significance of this interaction is not entirely clear. In addition, receptor-ligand interactions may be altered by a metal, inhibiting normal signaling events. Hypothetically, metals might also mimic the signals generated by these receptor-ligand interactions or might modulate the intracellular generation of second messengers.[43]

It is apparent that metals may have a wide variety of effects on the immune response *in vitro*. Of the metals studied, mercury and gold salts are most clearly shown in animal models to induce autoimmunity *in vivo*. These two will be described in greater detail.

Mercury

Mercurial compounds have been used as therapeutic agents in the past and are still used as pharmacologically active compounds or as a preservative in ointments and skin-lightening creams. Currently, the main sources of exposure to this metal are dental amalgams, electrical products exposed to mercury, pharmaceuticals, paper and pulp mills, and fish consumption. In industrial and laboratory workers, cases of membranous nephropathy and hypersensitivity reactions have been reported, and ointments that contain mercury have been reported to cause immune-mediated glomerulonephritis.[51,52] The possibility of health hazards induced by dental amalgams has been proposed but not proven. Interestingly, dental students have been found to have elevated numbers of T cells, which may indicate occupational exposure to mercury.[53-55] Similar findings have been reported in workers exposed to mercury vapors.

A role for mercury in the pathogenesis of human primary biliary cirrhosis has also been proposed. This disease is characterized immunologically by antimitochondrial antibodies. The main mitochondrial autoantigen, dihydrolipoamide acetyltransferase, is the E2 subunit of pyruvate dehydrogenase, whose antigenic portions contain disulfides and thiols. It has been proposed that, through a series of interactions with disulfide or thiol groups, mercury may affect the bile duct cells, disrupting the mitochondria and neutralizing antioxidant mechanisms. This may alter the structure of mitochondrial enzymes and increase their immunogenicity. However, the role of the antimitochondrial antibodies in the pathogenesis of the bile duct lesions is uncertain.[56,57] Similarities between mercury intoxication and Kawasaki's disease, including fever, erythematous mucosa, lymphadenopathy and increased levels of IgE, have been noted.[58,59] Whereas some researchers have not found increased levels of mercury in the hair of children with mucocutaneous lymph node syndrome, others have detected increased urinary excretion of mercury in patients with this disease.[58-60]

Animal models of mercury-induced autoimmunity are well characterized. Genetically susceptible animals develop autoantibodies and transient renal disease following exposure to mercury.[61] Autoantibodies to a variety of antigens have been reported, including DNA, type II collagen and thyroglobulin.[62,63] However, only a few of these autoantibodies appear to play a pathogenic role. For example, the elution of antinucleolar antibodies from kidneys of mice indicates their possible pathogenic role in the renal lesion. Fibrillarin, a component of the U3, U8 and U13 small nuclear ribonucleoproteins (snRNPs), has been proposed to be the major target for mercury-induced antinuclear antibodies.[64-66] Anti-fibrillarin antibodies are detected in 4% to 7% of North American and 4% of Japanese patients with systemic sclerosis. In black patients, a much higher frequency (21% to 43%) has been described.[67] However, there is no persuasive evidence that mercury-containing compounds play a role in initiating this disease.

Susceptibility to mercury-induced autoimmunity is genetically controlled.[68,69] Mercury-induced anti-glomerular basement membrane (GBM) autoantibodies and immune-complex disease are linked to specific MHC class II genes. Susceptibility to the development of antifibrillarin autoantibodies in mercury-treated mice is determined by the I and S regions of the H-2 complex. Undefined non-H-2 genes might play a role as well. In SJL mice the tendency to develop antinucleolar antibodies during mercury treatment resides in the H-2^a locus, is inherited in a codominant fashion in crosses with murine strains carrying the H-2^b and H-2^d haplotypes (C57BL/6N and DBA/2), and is strongly modulated by non-H-2 genes. Rats that carry the RT1 haplotype (Lewis, Fischer 344) do not develop autoimmunity following mercury exposure in contrast to those with the RTn haplotype, which develop anti-GBM/laminin autoantibodies. Rats with other haplotypes show intermediate susceptibility.

T cells are important in the mercury-induced autoimmunity model.[70,71] Adoptive transfer of CD4+ T cells from mercury-injected to normal BN rats transfers the disease. If recipients are treated with monoclonal antibodies to the CD8+ T cell subset, the disease is exacerbated, suggesting that host CD8+ cells modulate the disease.[72] T-cell-depleted rats (BN rnu/rnu and BN "B" rats) do not develop autoimmunity following mercury injections. When these rats are reconstituted with normal T cells, they develop autoimmune manifestations similar to normal BN rats. Finally, mercury-induced autoimmunity in this strain can be prevented or treated with low doses of cyclosporin A. Since cyclosporin is relatively specific for T cells, this observation again highlights the importance of T cells in this disorder.[73-75]

Using limiting-dilution analysis it can be shown that mercury induces the expansion of at least two different autoreactive T helper cell populations.[76] The first is observed beginning on day 4 and is specific for T helper cells exposed to mercury.[77] The second, found beginning on day 6, responds to Ia-positive cells, presumably on B cells and macrophages. T cells exposed to mercury *in vivo* induce a local GvH disease when injected in the footpad of naive syngeneic BN recipients, with a significant increase in cellularity in the draining popliteal lymph node, supporting the relevance of the autoreactivity observed *in vitro*. The precise mechanism for loss of tolerance and induction of T cell autoreactivity still needs to be determined but may represent modification of Ia molecules. Mercury reacts with sulfhydryl groups on proteins and nonprotein thiols, and other agents such as gold salts and D-pencillamine, which can have similar immunological effects, share this characteristic.[1,78,79] A T cell response to modified Ia antigens could produce an autoimmune disease by a mechanism similar to that causing chronic GvH disease. It has also been proposed that the initial activation of T cells recognizing mercury in combination with nuclear self-proteins (for example, fibrillarin) eventually results in activation of T cells specific for the unaltered self-proteins, possibly by epitope spreading.

Similarities between the mercury model of autoimmunity and chronic GvH disease are striking. An excess of T cell help appears in both conditions; parental T cells stimulate allogeneic Ia-bearing B cells in the GvH disease model, and autoreactive T cells stimulate self-Ia-bearing B cells in the mercury model. Both models are also characterized by preferential activation of the Th2 subset of helper T cells.[80] An imbalance between the Th1 and Th2 compartments has been proposed to mediate the exacerbation of autoimmune symptoms after the exposure to this metal. Up-regulation of IL-4, which promotes differentiation of Th2 cells, and inhibition of interferon-gamma, which inhibits Th2 development, may cause an immunoregulatory imbalance towards the Th2 compartment.[81–84] Evidence also exists that mercury up-regulates the production of nitric oxide in the spleen of susceptible rats. Nitric oxide might, in turn, stimulate the production of Th2 cytokines.[80]

Gold

Gold salts used in the treatment of rheumatoid arthritis can induce an autoimmune renal disease.[85] Proteinuria is observed in 6% to 17% of rheumatoid arthritis patients treated with gold salts; this tends to disappear following withdrawal of the drug.[85,86] Gold-induced kidney disease is more prevalent in rheumatoid arthritis patients who are HLA-DR3-positive, indicating an MHC link to this xenobiotic-induced disease. The same genetic linkage predisposes to the development of membranous nephropathy in patients receiving D-penicillamine (*vide infra*). In most cases, gold-induced human renal disease is characterized by a membranous nephropathy, although minimal-change glomerulonephritis has been observed in 10%. The former manifestation is considered to be mediated by immune complexes, while the latter is a T-cell-mediated response. Gold inclusions in the lysosomes of the proximal convoluted tube and in the glomerular cells have been observed in both conditions. The histological findings in gold-induced glomerular disease are similar to those seen in idiopathic membranous nephropathy, and immune complexes are identified in the glomeruli. Interstitial changes in renal biopsies from patients who had received gold have also been reported.

Several mechanisms have been proposed to explain the development of the renal disease in patients treated with gold. For example, Au (III), a reactive metabolite, can be generated by mononuclear phagocytes exposed to Au (I). It was proposed that oxidation of nuclear proteins ensues, with subsequent sensitization of T cells to the modified antigen.[87–89]

Studies in animal models have suggested other mechanisms of gold-induced autoimmunity.[90] BN rats injected with aurothiopropanolsulfonate sodium salt develop an autoimmune disease characterized by polyclonal B cell activation, lymphoproliferation, IgE hypergammaglobulinemia and the production of autoantibodies. A glomerulonephritis is seen, initially associated with anti-GBM deposition and later with the formation of granular deposits, occasionally resulting in a typical membranous nephropathy. Antitubular basement membrane antibodies deposited in a linear fashion along the tubular basement membrane have been described in association with an immune-complex-mediated glomerulonephritis.[91] Anti-brush-border antibodies are also involved. Lewis rats do not exhibit a glomerulopathy, but instead develop interstitial nephritis and some degree of polyclonal B cell activation response to gold. It has been proposed that, depending on the animal strain examined, gold triggers different B cell clones, thereby inducing different degrees of autoimmunity. A direct toxic effect of gold on the proximal convoluted tubules which might not be immunologically mediated has also been proposed.

DNA Methylation Inhibitors

Substantial evidence suggests that interfering with DNA methylation can contribute to autoimmunity.[31,92] Drugs such as procainamide and hydralazine may cause a lupuslike disease by inhibiting methylation of newly synthesized DNA in T cells. Methylation is a postsynthetic modification of DNA which can suppress gene expression.[93] Inhibiting the methylation of newly synthesized DNA induces or increases expression of genes regulated by this mechanism. Procainamide, hydralazine and UV light, all associated with triggering lupuslike diseases, inhibit T cell DNA methylation.[17] Inhibiting T cell DNA methylation by these agents or the prototypic DNA methylation inhibitor 5-azacytidine results in overexpression of LFA-1 (CD11a/CD18) on the cell surface.[17] Overexpression of LFA-1 makes antigen-specific CD4+ T cells responsive to self-class II MHC determinants without antigen, either by overstabilizing the normally low-affinity interaction between the T cell receptor and MHC molecules, or by transmitting an augmented activation signal. The response of these cells to MHC determinants without specific antigen resembles that in cells mediating chronic GvH disease.[18] Importantly, adoptive transfer of polyclonal murine (DBA/2) T cells made autoreactive by treatment with DNA methylation inhibitors into syngeneic recipients causes a lupuslike disease characterized by anti-DNA and antihistone antibodies, a positive lupus band test and an immune-complex glomerulonephritis. These studies have been reproduced using a cloned Th2 line and syngeneic (AKR) recipients. These mice developed a more severe disease with anti-dsDNA antibodies, scarring glomerulonephritis, pulmonary alveolitis, central nervous system lesions and liver lesions resembling primary biliary cirrhosis. Together these studies suggest that agents which inhibit T cell DNA methylation can induce autoimmunity by modifying adhesion molecule expression.[17,18,31]

This model is supported by other studies demonstrating that T cells from SLE patients have impaired DNA methylation and overexpress LFA-1 on an autoreactive T cell subset with a similar self-MHC specificity.[19,32] The similarity of the clinical manifestations in this DNA methylation inhibitor-induced animal model with human autoimmune disease, together with the similarity in biochemical and immunologic abnormalities in humans with the *in vitro* observations, suggest adhesion molecule over expression as a plausible mechanism for some forms of DIL. Whether other xenobiotics also inhibit DNA methylation is unknown.

Vinyl Chloride and Other Organic Solvents

Several case reports published over the last three decades indicate that exposure to organic compounds, particularly organic solvents, is associated with SSc.[94,95] The most frequently reported link has been with vinyl chloride.[96,97] Human genetic studies have implicated HLA-DR5, of haplotype A1 B8, and HLA-DR3 as risk factors.[98] The major mechanism proposed for inducing autoimmunity is oxidative cell damage with increased immunogenicity of "self" molecules. The oxidized metabolites of this resin are highly reactive and could bind to sulfhydryl and amino groups, modifying antigenicity and/or function. Vinyl chloride has also been shown to bind to nucleotides, which could also play a role in the generation of antinuclear antibodies. Studies in animal models have shown that rats fed vinyl chloride over prolonged periods develop thickening of the skin due to collagen deposition.[99]

L-canavanine

Reversible autoimmune hemolytic anemia and pancytopenia was described in 1981 in a man who ingested alfalfa seeds.[100] The anemia disappeared after discontinuing the product. A possible role for the amino acid L-canavanine, found in alfalfa, was proposed. Subsequently the same group reported that a lupuslike disease was induced in monkeys within several weeks to months of oral treatment with alfalfa seeds, alfalfa sprouts or L-canavanine.[101] Withdrawal of alfalfa seeds from the diet resulted in clinical improvement and return to normal hematologic parameters, although antinuclear and anti-dsDNA antibodies remained detectable for up to two years. Notably, L-canavanine is also found in peas, soybeans and clover.[102,103]

L-canavanine competes with L-arginine for the charging of tRNA-Arg, with subsequent formation of canavanyl proteins. The isoelectric point of canavanine is lower than that of arginine, leading to structural and functional changes in the resulting proteins. The effect that these changes might have in the immune system is not clear but they could enhance immunogenicity of some molecules.[104,105] Canavanine is also known to affect B cell function. This amino acid inhibits DNA synthesis in murine leukocytes at high doses and at lower doses inhibits B cells selectively. Incubation of murine leukocytes with canavanine alters surface charges of B cells from autoimmune-prone strains of mice, while T cells of the same strain and B and T cells from normal mice are not affected. This may be due to the activated status of B cells in these mice. The high metabolic activity may have resulted in increased incorporation of canavanine into surface membrane proteins, modifying the surface charge.[106]

Alternatively, as mentioned above, L-canavanine may stabilize DNA in the Z-configuration, enhancing DNA antigenicity and contributing to the development of anti-DNA antibodies.[1]

D-penicillamine

D-penicillamine is derived from the hydrolysis of penicillin and contains free carboxyl, sulfhydryl and amino groups which may react with macromolecules to alter their antigenicity. D-penicillamine is used in the treatment of rheumatoid arthritis, SSc and Wilson's disease. A variety of autoimmune responses have been associated with penicillamine. Chronic ingestion can result in SLE, myasthenia gravis, myopathies, pemphigus, obliterative bronchiolitis, Goodpasture syndrome, Sjögren syndrome, lymphadenopathy, cytopenias and IgA deficiency.[107]

D-penicillamine is able to bind to the surface of lymphoid cells, creating a neoantigen that stimulates T cells from mice sensitized by injection of either D-penicillamine or D-penicillamine-modified syngeneic spleen cells.[108] The drug sensitizes CD4+ T cells of normal BALB/c mice such that they can be restimulated *in vitro* on coculture with D-penicillamine-modified spleen cells. This may lead to T cell responses similar to the ones found in GvH, with increased class II MHC expression, Th2 cytokine production and subsequent B cell activation.

In vitro studies indicate that D-penicillamine has immunomodulatory effects on lymphocytes and macrophages. D-penicillamine exerts nonspecific mitogenic effects on murine splenic B cells and on murine peripheral B and T cells. It has been proposed that the drug may act as a reducing agent, cleaving disulfide bonds and rendering proteins immunogenic. It might also act as a hapten by binding cysteine-containing proteins, which may then produce autosensitization.[1]

Incubation of peripheral blood mononuclear cells from SLE patients with D-penicillamine results in increased ANA synthesis in some cases. This was observed in patients who were spontaneously low or nonproducers of ANA, while high producers showed decreased synthesis after being exposed to the drug. The enhancement of ANA production required the removal of CD4+ T cells, suggesting a suppressor effect. Pertinent to these observations are reports that D-penicillamine can induce the formation of antibodies to double-stranded DNA in patients with rheumatoid arthritis.

Animal models have proved useful in studying the immunological effects of this xenobiotic. When administered to BN rats, 73% develop weight loss and dermatitis, and die due to disseminated intravascular coagulation (DIC).[114] Pathologic studies reveal widespread granulomatous and necrotic lesions, immune complex deposition and linear deposits of IgG along the glomerular basement membrane. Furthermore, BN rats that receive low doses of D-penicillamine initially do not develop the disease, suggesting the development of tolerance. No adverse effects have been found in other strains, such as Lew and SD rats. The changes described in BN rats are similar to the ones associated with mercury. These changes also bear some resemblance to human disease, although DIC is not a common feature in patients who develop toxicity from this drug. Wistar rats injected with D-penicillamine develop a membranous glomerulopathy, while LEW rats are resistant to the toxicity of this drug.[109]

A transient increase in the number of splenic B cells and CD4+ T cells has been observed in BN rats. Autoreactive class-II-specific T cells, able to proliferate in the presence of syngeneic B cells, have been detected after exposure to D-penicillamine, and spontaneous regulation seems to occur with disappearance of autoreactive T cells in that rat strain. These observations raise the possibility that autologous T cells may be activated by drug-modified membrane determinants on B cells or macrophages in association with autologous MHC class II molecules. These may contribute to the development of autoimmunity by a mechanism similar to chronic GvH disease.

CONCLUSION

It is now well established that low-molecular-weight compounds and chemicals have the potential to induce autoimmunity in man. As is apparent from this review, the mechanisms by which this happens remain incompletely characterized. Nevertheless, important advances have been made.

Recent improvements in molecular and cellular biological techniques show promise for bringing new approaches and new insights into the understanding of the pathogenetic mechanisms of environmentally induced rheumatic diseases.

REFERENCES

[1]Yoshida S, Gershwin ME. Autoimmunity and selected environmental factors of disease induction. *Sem Arth Rheum.* 1993;22:399–419.

[2]Finkelman FD. Relationships among antigen presentation, cytokines, immune deviation and autoimmune disease. *J Exp Med.* 1995;182:279–282.

[3]Jones DEJ, Diamond AG. The basis of autoimmunity: An overview. In: P. Kendall-Taylor, ed. *Bailliere's Clinical Endocrinology and Metabolism.* 1995;9:1–23.

[4]Theofilopoulos AN. The basis of autoimmunity: Part I. Mechanisms of aberrant self-recognition. *Immunol Today.* 1995;16:90–98.

[5]Nossal GJV. Negative selection of lymphocytes. *Cell.* 1994;76:229–239.

[6]Gleichmann E, Pals ST, Rolink AG, Radaszkiewicz T, Gleichmann H. Graft-versus-host reactions: Clues to the etiopathology of a spectrum of immunological diseases. *Immunol Today.* 1984;5(11):324–332.

[7]Steinman L. Escape from "Horror Autotoxicus": Pathogenesis and treatment of autoimmune disease. *Cell.* 1995;80:7–10.

[8]Miller JFAP. Tolerance and autoimmunity in the peripheral T- cell repertoire. In: Coutinho A, Kazatchkine MD, eds. *Autoimmunity: Physiology and Disease.* New York; Wiley-Liss, Inc., 1994;191–202.

[9]Luppi P, Rossiello MR, Faas S, Trucco M. Genetic background and environment contribute synergistically to the onset of autoimmune diseases. *J Mol Med.* 1995;73:381–393.

[10]Yung RL, Richardson BC. Drug induced lupus. *Rheum Dis Clin North Am.* 1994;20:61–86.

[11]Abbas AK. Die and let live. Eliminating dangerous lymphocytes. *Cell.* 1996;84:655–657.

[12]Putterman C, Naparstek Y. Murine models of spontaneous systemic lupus erythematosus. In: Cohen JR, Miller A, eds. *Autoimmune Disease Models. A Guidebook.* San Diego, CA: Academic Press, Inc., 1994;217–244.

[13]Strasser A, Whittingham S, Vaux DL, *et al.* Enforced bcl2 expression in B-lymphoid cells prolongs antibody responses and elicits autoimmune disease. *Proc Natl Acad Sci USA.* 1991;88:8661–8665.

[14]Reiser H, Stadecker MJ. Costimulatory B7-molecules in the pathogenesis of infectious and autoimmune diseases. *N Engl J Med.* 1996;335;18:1369–1377.

[15]Goodnow CC. Balancing immunity and tolerance: Deleting and tuning lymphocyte repertoires. *Proc Natl Acad Sci USA.* 1996;93:2264–2271.

[16]Weaver CT, Unanue ER. The costimulatory function of antigen-presenting cells. *Immunol Today.* 1990;11:49–55.

[17]Richardson B, Powers D, Hooper F, Yung RL, O'Rourke K. Lymphocyte function-associated antigen 1 overexpression and T cell autoreactivity. *Arthritis Rheum.* 1994;37:1363–1372.

[18]Yung R, Powers D, Johnson K, *et al.* Mechanisms of drug-induced lupus: II. T cells over-expressing lymphocyte function-associated antigen 1 become autoreactive and cause a lupuslike disease in syngeneic mice. *J Clin Invest.* 1996;97:2866–2871.

[19]Richardson B, Strahler J, Pivirotto T, *et al.* Phenotypic and functional similarities between 5-azacytidine-treated T cells and a T cell subset in patients with active systemic lupus erythematosus. *Arthritis Rheum.* 1992;35:647–662.

[20]Izui S, Lambert P-H, Fournie GJ, Turler H, Miescher PA. Features of systemic lupus erythematosus in mice injected with bacterial lipopolysaccharide. Identification of circulating DNA and renal localization of DNA-anti-DNA complexes. *J Exp Med.* 1977;145:1115–1130.

[21]Lanzavecchia A. How can cryptic epitopes trigger autoimmunity? *J Exp Med.* 1995;181:1945–1948.

[22]James JA, Gross T, Scofield RH, Harley JB. Immunoglobulin epitope spreading and autoimmune disease after peptide immunization: Sm B/B′-derived PPPGMRPP and PPPGIRGP induce spliceosome autoimmunity. *J Exp Med.* 1995;453–461.

[23]Francotte M, Urbain J. Induction of anti-tobacco mosaic virus antibodies in mice by rabbit anti-idiotypic antibodies. *J Exp Med.* 1984;1485–1494.

[24]Descotes J. Drug-induced immune diseases. In: Dukes MNG, ed. *Drug-Induced Disorders.* Amsterdam, Netherlands; Elsevier, 1990; Vol. 4.

[25]Kammuller ME, Bloksma N, Seimen W. Autoimmunity and toxicology. Immune disregulation induced by drugs and chemicals. In: Kammuller ME, Bloksma N, Seimen W, eds. *Autoimmunity and Toxicology: Immune Disregulation Induced by Drugs and Chemicals.* Amsterdam, Netherlands; Elsevier, 1989;3–29.

[26]Gleichmann E, Kimber I, Purchase IF. Immunotoxicology: Suppressive and stimulatory effects of drugs and environmental chemicals on the immune system. A discussion. *Arch Toxicol.* 1989;63:257–273.

[27]Gleichmann H. Studies on the mechanism of drug sensitization: T-cell-dependent popliteal lymph node reaction to diphenylhydantoin. *Clin Immunol Immunopathol.* 1981;18:203–211.

[28]Lafer EM, Valle RP, Moller A, *et al.* Z-DNA-specific antibodies in human systemic lupus erythematosus. *J Clin Invest.* 1983;71:314–321.

[29]Griem P, Panthel K, Kalbacher H, Gleichmann E. Alteration of a model antigen by Au (III) leads to T cell sensitization to cryptic peptides. *Eur J Immunol.* 1996;26:279–287.

[30]Sakaguchi S, Sakaguchi N. Organ-specific autoimmune disease induced by elimination of T cell subsets. V. Neonatal administration of cyclosporin A causes autoimmune disease. *J Immunol.* 1989;142:471–480.

[31]Yung RL, Quddus J, Chrisp CE, Johnson KJ, Richardson BC. Mechanisms of drug-induced lupus I. Cloned Th2 cells modified with DNA methylation inhibitors in vitro cause autoimmunity in vivo. *J Immunol.* 1995;154:3025–3035.

[32]Richardson B, Scheinbart L, Strahler J, *et al.* Evidence for impaired T cell DNA methylation in systemic lupus erythematosus and rheumatoid arthritis. *Arthritis Rheum.* 1990;33:1665–1673.

[33]Theofilopoulus AN, Dixon FJ. Murine models of systemic lupus erythematosus. *Adv Immunol.* 1985;37:269–390.

[34]Fattovich G, Betterle C, Brollo L, *et al.* Autoantibodies during alpha-interferon therapy for chronic hepatitis B. *J Med Virol.* 1991;34:132–135.

[35]Kowolenko M, McCabe MJ Jr, Lawrence DA. Metal-induced alterations of immunity. In: DS Newcombe, Rose NR, Bloom JC, eds. *Clinical Immunotoxicology.* New York; Raven Press Ltd, 1992;401–419.

[36]Watanabe-Fukunaga R, Brannan CI, Copeland NG, Jenkins NA, Nagata S. Lymphoproliferation disorder in mice explained by defects in fas antigen that mediates apoptosis. *Nature.* 1992;356:314–317.

[37]Allen RD, Marshall JD, Roths JB, Sidman CL. Differences defined by bone marrow transplantation suggest that lpr and gld mutations of genes encoding an interacting pair of molecules. *J Exp Med.* 1990;172:1367–1375.

[38]Cohen PI, Eisenberg RA. lpr and gld: Single gene models of systemic autoimmunity and lymphoproliferative disease. *Annu Rev Immunol.* 1991;9:243–269.

[39]Myaler E, Bini P, Drappa J, *et al.* The apoptosis-1/Fas protein in human systemic lupus erythematosus. *J Clin Invest.* 1994;93:1029–1034.

[40]Drappa J, Vaishnaw AK, Sullivan KE, Chu JL, Elkon KB. Fas gene mutations in the Canale-Smith syndrome, an inherited lymphoproliferative disorder associated with autoimmunity. *N Engl J Med.* 1996;335:1643–1649.

[41]Dawisha SM, Gmelig-Meyling F, Steinberg AD. Assessment of clinical parameters associated with increased frequency of mutant T cells in patients with systemic lupus erythematosus. *Arthritis Rheum.* 1994;37:270–277.

[42]Rubin RL. Autoimmune reactions induced by procainamide and hydralazine. In: Kammuller ME, Bloksma N, Seinen H, eds. *Autoimmunity and Toxicology.* New York; Elsevier, 1989;119–142.

[43]Pelletier L, Tournade H, Druet P. Immunologically mediated manifestations of metals. In: Dayan AD, *et al.* eds. *Immunotoxicity of Metals and Immunotoxicology.* New York; Plenum Press, 1990;121–137.

[44]Balazs T. Immunogenetically controlled autoimmune reactions induced by mercury, gold and D-penicillamine in laboratory animals: a review from the vantage point of premarketing safety studies. *Toxicol Ind Health.* 1987;3:331–336.

[45]Bigazzi PE. Autoimmunity and heavy metals. *Lupus.* 1994;3:449–453.

[46]McCabe MJ, Lawrence DA. Effects of metals on lymphocyte development and function. In: Schook LB, Laskin DL, eds. *Xenobiotics and Inflammation.* San Diego, CA; Academic Press, Inc, 1994;213–232.

[47]Santos GW, Hess AD, Vogelsang GB. Graft versus host reactions. *Immunol Rev.* 1984;88:169–192.

[48]Cheung WY. Calmodulin: its potential role in cell proliferation and heavy metal toxicity. *Fed Proc.* 1984;43:2995–2999.

[49]Halliwell B, Gutteridge JM. The importance of free radicals and catalytic metal ions in human diseases. *Mol Aspcts Med.* 1985;8:89–193.

[50]Druet P, Pelletier L, Rossert J, Druet E, Hirsch F, Sapin C. Autoimmune reactions induced by metals. In: Kammuller ME, Bloksma N, Seinen W, eds. *Autoimmunity and Toxicology. Immune*

Disregulation Induced by Drugs and Chemicals. Amsterdam, Netherlands; Elsevier, 1989;347–361.

[51]Roger J, Zilikens D, Burg G, Gleichmann E. Systemic autoimmune disease in a patient with long standing exposure to mercury. *Eur J Dermatol.* 1992;2:168–170.

[52]Tubbs RR, Gephardt GN, McMahon JT, *et al.* Membranous glomerulonephritis associated with industrial mercury exposure. *Am J Clin Pathol.* 1982;77:409–413.

[53]Eedy DJ, Burrows D, Clifford T, Fay A. Elevated T cell subpopulations in dental students. *J Prosthet Dent.* 1990;53:593–596.

[54]Enestrom S, Hultman P. Does amalgam affect the immune system? A controversial issue. *Int Arch Allergy Immunol.* 1995;106: 180–203.

[55]Schrallhammer-Benkler K, Ring J, Przbilla B, Meurer M, Landthaler M. Acute mercury intoxication with lichenoid drug eruption followed by mercury contact allergy and development of antinuclear antibodies. *Acta Derm Venereol.* (Stockholm) 1992;72: 294–296.

[56]Gershwin ME, Mackay IR. Primary biliary cirrhosis: Paradigm or paradox for autoimmunity. *Gastroenterology.* 1991;100:822–833.

[57]Gregus Z, Stein AF, Varga F, *et al.* Effect of lipoic acid on biliary excretion of glutathione and metals. *Toxicol Appl Pharmacol.* 1992; 114:88–96.

[58]Aschner M, Aschner JL. Mucocutaneous lymph node syndrome: Is there a relation to mercury exposure? *Am J Dis Child.* 1989;143: 1133–1134.

[59]Adler R, Boxstein D, Schoff P, Kerly D. Metallic mercury vapour poisoning simulating mucocutaneous lymph node syndrome. *J Pediatr.* 1982;14:967–968.

[60]Orlowski JP, Mercen RD. Urine mercury levels in Kawasaki disease. *Pediatrics.* 1980;66:633–636.

[61]Hultman P, Enestrom S. Mercury-induced antinuclear antibodies in mice: Characterization and correlation with renal immune complex deposits. *Clin Exp Immunol.* 1988;71:269–274.

[62]Aten J, Veninga A, Brujin JA, Prins FA, de Heer E, Weening JJ. Antigenic specificities of glomerular-bound autoantibodies in membranous glomerulopathy induced by mercuric chloride. *Clin Immunol Immunopathol.* 1992;63:89–102.

[63]Hultman P, Johansson U, Turley SJ, Lindh U, Enestrom S, Pollard KM. Adverse immunological effects and autoimmunity induced by dental amalgam and alloy in mice. *FASEB J.* 1996;8:1183–1190.

[64]Robinson CJG, Abraham AA, Balazs T. Induction of anti-nuclear antibodies by mercuric chloride in mice. *Clin Exp Immunol.* 1984; 58:300–306.

[65]Lubben B, Rottmann N, Kubicka-Muranyi M, Gleichmann E, Luhrmann R. The specificity of disease-associated anti-fibrillarin autoantibodies compared with that of HgCl2-induced autoantibodies. *Mol Biol Rep.* 1994;20:63–73.

[66]Hultman P, Enestrom S, Pollard KM, Tah EM. Anti-fibrillarin autoantibodies in mercury-treated mice. *Clin Exp Immunol.* 1989; 31:525–532.

[67]Okano Y, Steen VD, Medsger TA Jr. Autoantibody reactive to U3 nucleolar ribonucleoprotein (fibrillarin) in patients with systemic sclerosis. *Arthritis Rheum.* 1992;35:95.

[68]Hultman P, Bell LJ, Enestrom S, Pollard KM. Murine susceptibility to mercury. II. Autoantibody profiles and renal immune deposits in hybrid, backcross, and H-2 congenic mice. *Clin Immunol Immunopathol.* 1993;68:9–20.

[69]Sapin C, Mandet C, Druet E, Gunther E, Druet P. Immune complex type disease induced by HgCl$_2$ in Brown Norway rats: Genetic control of susceptibility. *Clin Exp Immunol.* 1982;48:700–704.

[70]Kubicka-Muranyi M, Behmer O, Uhrberg M, Klonowski H, Bister J, Gleichmann E. Murine systemic autoimmune disease induced by mercuric chloride (HgCl$_2$): Hg-specific helper T-cells react to antigen stored in macrophages. *Int J Immunopharmacol.* 1993;15: 151–161.

[71]Kubicka-Muranyi M, Kremer J, Rottman N, *et al.* Murine systemic autoimmune disease induced by mercuric chloride: T helper cells reacting to self proteins. *Int Arch Allergy Immunol.* 1996;109: 11–20.

[72]Pelletier L, Rossert J, Pasquier R, Vial MC, Druett P. Role of CD8+ T cells in mercury-induced autoimmunity or immunosuppression in the rat. *Scan J Immunol.* 1990;31:65–74.

[73]Pelletier L, Pasquier R, Vial MC, *et al.* Mercury-induced autoimmune glomerulonephritis: Requirement for T cells. *Nephrol Dial Transplant.* 1987;1:211–218.

[74]Pelletier L, Pasquier R, Rossert J, Vial MC, Mandet C, Druet P. Autoreactive T cells in mercury-induced autoimmunity. Ability to induce the autoimmune disease. *J Immunol.* 1988;140:750–754.

[75]Baran D, Vendeville B, Vial MC, Bascou C, Teychenne P, Druet P. Effect of cyclosporine A on mercury-induced autoimmune glomerulonephritis in the Brown Norway rat. *Clin Nephrol.* 1986; 25(suppl):175–180.

[76]Rossert J, Pelletier L, Pasquier R, Druet P. Autoreactive T cells in mercury-induced autoimmunity. Demonstration by limiting dilution analysis. *Eur J Immunol.* 1988;18:1761–1766.

[77]Bowman C, Green C, Borysiewicz L, Lockwood CM. Circulating T-cell populations during mercuric-chloride-induced nephritis in the Brown Norway rat. *Immunology.* 1987;61:515–520.

[78]Lund B-O, Miller DM, Woods JS. Mercury induced H$_2$O$_2$ production and lipid peroxidation in vitro in rat kidney mitochondria. *Biochem Pharmacol.* 1991;42(suppl):S181–S187.

[79]Noelle RJ, Lawrence DA. Modulation of T-cell functions. II. Chemical basis for the involvement of cell surface thiol-reactive sites in control of T-cell proliferation. *Cell Immunol.* 1981;60:453–469.

[80]Mathieson PW. Mercury: God of Th2 cells? (ed) *Clin Exp Immunol.* 1995;102:229–230.

[81]Gillespie KM, Qasim Fj, Tibbats LM, *et al.* Interleukin-4 gene expression in mercury-induced autoimmunity. *Scand J Immunol.* 1995;41:268–272.

[82]Ochel M, Vohr HW, Pfeiffer C, *et al.* IL-4 is required for the IgE and IgG1 increase and IgG1 autoantibody formation in mice treated with mercuric chloride. *J Immunol.* 1991;146:3006–3011.

[83]Prigent P, Saoudi A, Pannetier C, *et al.* Mercuric chloride, a chemical responsible for T helper cell 2 mediated autoimmunity in Brown Norway rats, directly triggers T cells to produce interleukin-4. *J Clin Invest.* 1995;96:1484–1489.

[84]Van Vliet E, Urhberg M, Stein C, Gleichmann E. MHC control of IL-4 dependent enhancement of B cell Ia expression and Ig class switch in mice treated with mercuric chloride. *Int Arch Allergy Immunol.* 1993;101:392–401.

[85]Lockie LM, Smith DM. Forty-seven years experience with gold therapy in 1,019 rheumatoid arthritis patients. *Semin Arthritis Rheum.* 1985;14:238–246.

[86]Romagnoli P, Spinas GA, Sinigaglia F. Gold-specific T cells in rheumatoid arthritis patients treated with gold. *J Clin Invest.* 1992;89:254–258.

[87]Goebel C, Kubicka-Muranyi M, Tonn T, Gonzalez J, Gleichmann E. Phagocytes render chemicals immunogenic. Oxidation of gold (I) to the T-cell sensitizing gold (III) metabolite generated by mononuclear phagocytes. *Arch Toxicol.* 1995;69:450–459.

[88]Schuhmann D, Kubicka-Muranyi M, Mirtcheva J, Gunther J, Kind P, Gleichmann E. Adverse immune reactions to gold: Chronic treatment with an Au (I) drug sensitizes mouse T cells not to Au (I), but to Au (III) and induces autoantibody formation. *J Immunol.* 1990;145:2132–2139.

[89]Tournade H, Guery JC, Pasquier R, *et al.* Effect of the thiol group on experimental gold-induced autoimmunity. *Arthritis Rheum.* 1991;34:1594–1599.

[90]Tournade H, Guery JC, Pasquier R, *et al.* Experimental gold-induced autoimmunity. *Nephrol Dial Transplant.* 1991;6:621–630.

[91]Ueda Y, Wakashin M, Wakashin Y, *et al.* Experimental gold nephropathy in guinea pigs. Detection of autoantibodies to renal tubular antigens. *Kidney Int.* 1986;29:539–548.

[92]Quddus J, Johnson KJ, Gavalchin J, *et al.* Treating activated CD4+ T cells with either of two distinct DNA methyltransferase inhibitors, 5-azacytidine or procainamide, is sufficient to cause a lupus-like disease in syngeneic mice. *J Clin Invest.* 1993;92:38–53.

[93]Cedar H. DNA methylation and gene expression. In: Cedar, Razin, Riggs, eds. *DNA Methylation: Biochemistry and Biological Significance.* New York: Springer-Verlag, 1984;147–164.

[94]Veltman G, Lange CE, Juhe S, *et al.* Clinical manifestations and course of vinyl chloride disease. *Ann NY Acad Sci.* 1975;246:6–17.

[95]Haustein UF, Herrmann K. Environmental scleroderma. *Clin Dermatol.* 1994;12:467–473.

[96]Kahn MF, Bourgeois P, Aeschlimann A, *et al.* Mixed connective tissue disease after exposure to polyvinyl chloride. *J Rheumatol.* 1989;166:533–535.

[97]Magnavita N, Bergamaschi A, Garcovich A, Giulano G. Vasculitic purpura in vinyl chloride disease: A case report. *Angiology.* 1986;37:382–388.

[98]Black CM, Welsh KI, Walker AE, *et al.* Genetic susceptibility to scleroderma-like syndrome induced by vinyl chloride. *Lancet.* 1983;1:53–55.

[99]Ward A, Udnoon S, Watkins J, *et al.* Immunological mechanisms in the pathogenesis of vinyl chloride disease. *Br Med J.* 1976;936–938.

[100]Malinow MR, Bardana EJ Jr, Goodnight SH Jr. Pancytopenia during ingestion of alfalfa seeds. *Lancet.* 1981;1:615.

[101]Malinow MR, Bardana EJ Jr, Pirofsky B, Craig S, McLaughlin P. Systemic lupus erythematosus-like syndrome in monkeys fed alfalfa sprouts: Role of nonprotein amino acid. *Science.* 1982;216:415–417.

[102]Montanaro A, Bardana EJ Jr. Dietary amino acid-induced systemic lupus erythematosus. *Rheum Dis Clin North Am.* 1991;17:323–332.

[103]Roberts JL, Hayashi JA. Exacerbation of SLE associated with alfalfa ingestion. *N Engl J Med.* 1983;308:1361.

[104]Rosenthal GA. The biological effects and mode of action of L-canavanine, a structural analogue of L-arginine. *Q Rev Biol.* 1977;52:155–178.

[105]Alcocer-Varela J, Iglesias A, Llorente L, Alarcon-Segovia D. Effects of L-canavanine on T cells may explain the induction of systemic lupus erythematosus by alfalfa. *Arthritis Rheum.* 1985;28:52–57.

[106]Prete PE. Membrane surface properties of lymphocytes of normal (DBA/2) and autoimmune (NZB/NZW)F1 mice. Effects of L-canavanine and a proposed mechanism for diet-induced autoimmune disease. *Can J Physiol Pharmacol.* 1986;64:1189–1196.

[107]Felson DT, Anerson JJ, Meenan RT. The comparative efficacy and toxicity of second-line drugs in RA. Results of 2 metaanalyses. *Arthritis Rheum.* 1990;33:1449–1461.

[108]Nagata N, Hurtenbach U, Gleichmann E. Specific sensitization of Lyt-1+2−T cells to spleen cells modified by the drug D-penicillamine or a stereoisomer. *J Immunol.* 1986;136:136–142.

[109]Donker AJ, Venuto RC, Vladutiu AO, Brentjens JR, Andres GA. Effects of prolonged administration of D-penicillamine or captopril in various strains of rats. Brown Norway rats treated with D-penicillamine develop autoantibodies, circulating immune complexes, and disseminated intravascular coagulation. *Clin Immunol Immunopathol.* 1984;30:142–155.

4

Genetics of Environmentally Associated Rheumatic Disease

Frederick W. Miller

INTRODUCTION

The relative rarity and multifactorial etiologies of the rheumatic diseases have limited our understanding of their pathogenesis. Nonetheless, advances in the standardization of clinical evaluations and disease definitions, establishment of multicentered collaborations and registries, and the application of novel epidemiologic, serologic and molecular biologic methods have contributed to recent progress in understanding some of the causes of these enigmatic conditions. Findings from a variety of sources suggest that interactions of one or more environmental exposures and multiple gene products initiate and sustain pathologic immune activation and dysregulation that eventually result in rheumatic disorders. Because we do not yet know which specific exposures and genes are the primary risk factors for most rheumatic diseases, however, only those few cases in which temporal associations, evidence from dechallenge or rechallenge, strongly point to a specific environmental exposure as the causative trigger are currently labeled as environmentally associated rheumatic diseases (EARD). This chapter summarizes our current understanding of the role genetics plays in the development of EARD.

THE RHEUMATIC DISEASES: HETEROGENEOUS SYNDROMES COMPOSED OF MANY ELEMENTAL DISORDERS

An inherent difficulty in the study of rheumatic diseases is that because risk factors and pathogenetic mechanisms have not been well established, these diseases remain heterogeneous collections of clinical signs, symptoms and laboratory findings. Thus the definition and classification of the rheumatic diseases themselves, as well as the EARD, will likely remain unsatisfactory and controversial until the subgroups that comprise them, or what I refer to here as the "elemental disorders," are elucidated. An elemental disorder in this regard could be considered to be the minimal necessary and sufficient environmental exposure(s) and genes required to induce the pathology that results in a given sign-symptom complex. Unfortunately, we have not yet fully defined such a single elemental disorder.

The probability that multiple elemental disorders comprise each rheumatic disease (as defined by current clinicopathologic criteria) is a major potential confounder of all epidemiologic and therapeutic studies in this area. It is hoped that some of these definitions and classifications will become clearer as the currently blurred boundaries among the rheumatic disorders are dissected into their elemental disorders in the future.

EARD: COMPLEX (MULTIFACTORIAL) SYNDROMES WITHOUT VALIDATED DIAGNOSTIC CRITERIA

Most rheumatic diseases are rare, and EARD, as currently recognized, are even less common. For this reason it has been and likely will continue to be difficult to identify large enough populations to conduct classic population-based epidemiologic exposure/nonexposure studies with adequate power to ascertain environmental and genetic risk factors for these entities. This is discussed in detail in Chapter 1. Therefore, most studies of EARD have been case-control designs, collections of individual case reports or small case series. There are, however, no generally accepted criteria for the diagnosis of an EARD; thus one investigator may define a case quite differently from another, making comparisons of cases difficult.

In the absence of validated criteria for the definition of EARD, it has been suggested that a minimal set of conditions be present before considering a given case report as an EARD. These include the following:

1) The development of all signs, symptoms and laboratory abnormalities occurs after exposure to the environmental agent;

2) No other concomitant exposures in that patient have been associated with the syndrome;

3) Dechallenge (removal of the agent and its effects if possible) results in elimination of the syndrome or at least a decrease in the severity of its signs, symptoms and associated laboratory abnormalities;

4) Rechallenge (reexposure to the agent) results in reestablishment of the syndrome or an increase in the severity of signs, symptoms and laboratory abnormalities;

5) The syndrome occurs with a characteristic delay after the exposure (latency) or has other clinical and laboratory features previously associated with the environmental exposure in question;

6) The syndrome is characterized by atypical signs, symptoms, laboratory abnormalities, serologies, or genetic risk factors compared to classic idiopathic rheumatic diseases.

Although such criteria may bias against the recognition of new rheumatic-disease-inducing environmental agents, they offer much-needed consistency that is currently lacking in such studies. In order to enhance the quality of information available on these disorders, to permit more accurate comparisons among studies, and to perform valid meta-analyses, it is important for the reporting of individual cases or case series to contain as much information regarding the above as possible. It is also important that as thorough a study as feasible be undertaken in every subject with a putative EARD and that the information be collected in a standardized and uniform manner. It would also be useful to bank sera and cells from each patient for future studies and collaborative investigations. While these are only suggested guidelines at present, it is clear that the development and validation of criteria for EARD is critically needed for advancement of this field.

THE GENETIC BASIS FOR EARD

Evolutionary theory prescribes that we are products of our environments. And yet the environmental pressures that selected and shaped the human genome for millennia have changed significantly only in the last few centuries. First the industrial and now the postindustrial revolutions have completely altered the way humans live and interact with their environment. New emerging infectious agents and chemical compounds in the form of novel foods and dietary supplements, drugs, medical devices, occupational exposures and by-products of agricultural and industrial activities are added every year to the growing list of possible environmental dangers. Not only has there been an exponential increase in the

number of synthetic new chemical structures introduced into our environment, but also the concentrations and routes of exposure for many natural compounds have changed drastically.

Thus it should not be surprising that the prevalence of rheumatic and other immune-mediated diseases, thought for the most part to be the product of environmental triggers acting upon genetically susceptible individuals,[1] appears to be increasing. It is quite possible, for example, that human populations, whose genes have been selected primarily for their ability to evade or eliminate common natural toxins and infectious diseases,[2,3] are ill-equipped to metabolize or inactivate many of the present environmental agents and subsequently may respond to synthetic foreign structures with harmful immune effects.

Studies of idiopathic rheumatic or autoimmune diseases have clearly indicated that genetic factors are risks for their development.[4] The approaches used have included family studies that documented clustering of these diseases in blood relatives, and linkage analyses in animal models and humans that have identified from five[5] to more than a dozen[6] chromosomal regions as risk factors that may act in a threshold manner for the induction of disease. However, the genetics of autoimmunity remains relatively mysterious, except for the knowledge that it is highly complex and likely to be non-Mendelian in nature. Furthermore, none of the rheumatic and immune-mediated diseases that have been carefully investigated have demonstrated a concordance rate in monozygotic twins of more than 50%, strongly suggesting that environmental factors must also play an important role in the etiology of these diseases.

Many lines of evidence, from both clinical and animal model studies, also support a genetic basis for EARD.[7–11] They include major differences in pharmacokinetics and outcomes of environmental exposures in different animal strains or species; the relatively low attack rates of all known EARDs; the general difficulty of developing animal models for EARD; and associations of certain EARDs with specific genes or their products that often differ from the genetic risk factors seen in the similar idiopathic rheumatic diseases.

CONFOUNDERS AND APPROACHES TO OVERCOME THEM

As stated above, many aspects of EARDs make their study difficult. The lack of well-defined criteria and the possibility that multiple exposures may produce the same syndrome via a variety of pathogenetic mechanisms in different genetic backgrounds[4] are major reasons for the limited progress in this area to date. The polygenic nature of the genetic risks add to the difficulty of identifying single gene products as strong risk factors.[12] Linkage disequilibrium among the major histocompatibility complex (MHC) genes that are inherited as haplotypes and that differ in different racial and ethnic groups can also be a confounder.[4] Finally, the lack of a single gene product in any rheumatic disease or EARD that is not also present in the normal population makes it difficult to power studies appropriately to define weaker genetic risk factors.[4]

Several strategies have been used in an attempt to overcome these difficulties. First, the use of multiple appropriate control groups in a case-control design has been considered. In the analysis of methimazole-induced agranulocytosis in Japanese patients with Graves' disease, for example, controls from the general population were first racially matched to assess initial risk factors; this resulted in identification of a number of HLA genes as potential risk factors.[13] When these cases were matched by disease to overcome confounding

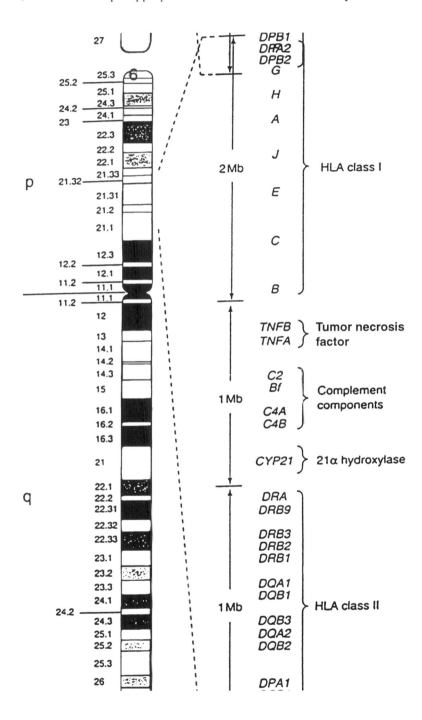

Fig. 4-1 Genes comprising the major histocompatibility (MHC) region on human chromosome 6 (From Tomlinson and Bodmer 1995).[71]

Table 4-1 Immunogenetic associations with selected immune-mediated environmentally associated rheumatic or autoimmune diseases

Environmental Exposure	Associated Disease	Immunogenetic Associations	Comments
Foods			
Toxic oil	Toxic oil syndrome	DR3, DR4	Weak association seen with chronic disease[42]
L-tryptophan	Eosinophilia myalgia syndrome	DR4	A trend in two small studies that did not reach statistical significance[43,44]
Drugs			
Gold salts	Proteinuria or thrombocytopenia	B8-DR3	In rheumatoid arthritis patients[45,46]
Gold salts	Skin reactions	B7	In rheumatoid arthritis patients[46]
Gold salts	Mucocutaneous lesions	B8-DR3, DR5	DR7 is protective; in RA patients[47]
Methimazole	Agranulocytosis	DRB1*08032	Odds ratio = 4.2 in Japanese Graves' disease[13]
Clozapine	Agranulocytosis	DRB1*0402, DQA1*0301, DQB1*0302	In Ashkenazi Jews[48]; separate HSP70 alleles were also identified as risk or protective factors[49]
Clozapine	Agranulocytosis	DR2, DQA1*0102, DQB1*0502	In non-Jewish subjects[48]
Hydralazine	Lupuslike illness	DR4	Also associated with slow acetylators[50,51]
Hydralazine	Lupuslike illness	C4 null alleles	The C4B null allele is linked with HLA DR4[52]
Procainamide	Lupuslike illness	DRw6	Seen in 18 of 34 (53%) compared to 17% of controls[53]
Venopyronum dragees	Lupuslike illness	DR4, DRw53, DQw3	Also noted GM 1;21 haplotype as a risk factor[54]
Penicillamine	Lupuslike illness	A11, B15	In RA patients[55]
Penicillamine	Myositis	DR2, DQw1	In Indian RA patients[56]
Penicillamine	Myositis	DR4	In white RA patients[57]
Medical Devices			
Silicone implants	Rheumatic symptoms	DQ2, DRw53	DRw53 highest with anti-B cell autoantibodies[58]
Silicone implants	Myositis	DQA1*0102	Relative risk = 7.8 compared to idiopathic myositis[59]
Occupational Chemicals			
Vinyl chloride	Sclerodermalike illness	DR3, DR5	Possible risk factors for severe disease[60]
Beryllium	Pulmonary disease	DPB1*0201, DPB1*0401	Associated with a glutamate at 69[61]
Silica, coal	Pneumoconiosis	DR8	DR1 was protective in coal miners[62]
Infectious Agents			
HIV	Sjögren's-like syndrome	DR5, DR6	With diffuse infiltration of CD8+ cells[63,64]
HIV	Thrombocytopenia-lymphadenopathy	DR5	In AIDS[64,65]
Borellia burgdorferi	Chronic Lyme arthritis	DR4, secondary DR2	Compared to Lyme patients without chronic arthritis[66]
Borellia burgdorferi	Chronic Lyme arthritis	DRB1*0404/08, DRw13, DPB1*0201, DPB1*1001	Compared to normal controls[67]
Leprosy	Uveitis	DRB1*1501	DRw53 was protective[68,69]
Group A streptococcus	Rheumatic fever	B883	A non-HLA B cell surface marker[9]
Group A streptococcus	Rheumatic fever	D8/17	May be the same marker as B883[70]

due to the genetic risks for Graves' disease, however, only HLA DRB1*08032 appeared as the major significant risk factor.

One approach to define which of several linked genes is the primary risk factor is to identify as many markers as possible along a given chromosomal region or haplotype, and then calculate the association of each marker with the given disorder.[14] The finding that autoimmune diseases are associated with ancestral MHC haplotypes that differ in various races and occasionally undergo recombination, can also allow for mapping of relevant genetic risk factors.[15] Because EARDs themselves may also be composed of several elemental disorders, dividing these syndromes into more homogeneous groups—on the basis of gender or demographic, ethnic, clinical and serologic features—may increase the chance of defining not only the strongest genetic risk factors but the weaker ones as well.[4] Recent investigations have used novel molecular genetic whole genome approaches to identify autoimmunity genes. These approaches may be applicable to the study of EARD as well.[16]

EVIDENCE FOR SPECIFIC GENETIC RISK FACTORS FOR EARD

Using the approaches outlined above, a number of genetic risk factors for EARD have been elucidated over the last several decades. These have been identified primarily as the polymorphic genes that regulate the rates and extent of metabolism of environmental chemicals (pharmacogenetic alleles) and those that determine the type and level of immune responses to them (immunogenetic alleles). Thus the pharmacogenetic and immunogenetic makeup of an individual, selected by forces very different from those seen in our environments today, appears to be central to determining whether or not a given environmental exposure will induce an EARD. It is also intriguing that the majority of EARDs, as is the case for most rheumatic diseases, affect women more often than men, suggesting a role for hormonal influences in the development of these disorders.[17,18]

The polymorphic enzyme systems that involve acetylation and those involving oxidation by myelocytes[19] and the cytochrome P450 systems[20] have been linked with one or more EARDs. Nonetheless, more genetic linkages have been noted in the MHC region on chromosome 6, in which the human leukocyte antigen (HLA) class I (HLA-A, -B, and -C) and class II (HLA-DR, -DQ, and -DP) regions reside. A map of this region is shown in Figure 4-1.

A wide range of environmental exposures, such as foods and dietary supplements, drugs and medical devices, chemicals used in occupations and infectious agents, has been linked to immune-mediated disorders via one or more immunogenetic risk factors (Table 4-1). Because of the difficulties in the study of EARD mentioned above, however, most investigations have found only weak associations of these disorders with single MHC alleles, resulting in rather low relative risks. In some cases there is disagreement among the results of these studies.[21] In fact, there is no example as yet where these data have been shown to be useful in screening populations prior to a given exposure to decrease the risk of the resulting disease. Of course, because it is likely that multiple genes are involved in risk for developing EARD, pharmacogenetic and immunogenetic loci, as well as possibly others, will need to be analyzed together to achieve a more accurate understanding of true relative risks. This is seldom done, partly because most studies cannot identify large enough EARD populations to allow the identification

of all genetic risk factors. For example, statistical estimates for the number of sibling pairs needed to assess the genetics of such complex diseases as rheumatoid arthritis or systemic lupus erythematosus are in the 200 to 300 range[22]—far more individuals than have been identified to date for any genetic study of an EARD.

MECHANISMS BY WHICH GENETIC RISK FACTORS MAY OPERATE IN EARD

Little data are available to support any detailed theory about the mechanisms by which EARDs occur. As is the case with idiopathic rheumatic diseases, however, it is likely that different mechanisms are operative in different EARDs. Current theories attempt to explain mechanisms within the conceptual framework that combinations of pharmacogenetic and immunogenetic alleles, and probably other genes, are necessary to be present together to form a composite genetic matrix in order for an adverse physiologic response to develop after a given environmental exposure, resulting in a specific EARD (Figure 4-2).

Several hypotheses have been proposed to explain the etiopathogenesis of EARD (Table 4-2). One possibility is that the associations of certain EARDs with specific genes relates to the capacity of an individual first to metabolize a given agent to toxic or highly reactive intermediates that may modify the structure of the self-protein, and then to bind and present the resulting altered structures with high affinity via HLA proteins encoded by MHC genes.[23] Another hypothesis relates to the finding that exposure to many environmental agents associated with EARD results in immunosuppression.[11] This raises the possibility that these agents may prevent the host from clearing prior infectious agents or from eliminating new ones.[24] In contrast, other environmental agents are directly immunostimulatory or act as adjuvants to increase the immune response to concurrent xenobiotics.[25,26] Yet other environmental chemicals are immunomodulatory, in the sense that they alter one or more regulatory networks that maintain the fine balance of the immune system, and thereby allow autoimmunity to develop.[11,27,28]

Some environmental agents and/or their metabolites are immunotoxins and directly induce cell death via apoptosis or cytotoxicity,[29] and yet it is also possible that they may induce defects in apoptotic processes, allowing for abnormally persistent or intensified immune responses.[30–32] Another proposed mechanism involves the concept of molecular mimicry. That is, the xenobiotic and the host share similar structures, so that an immune response to the environmental agent or one of its metabolites results in a cross-reactive autoimmune response to the similar self-structure.[11] Finally, the recent findings in the area of oxidative stress research have suggested other possible ways that chemicals may alter DNA and its repair mechanisms and lead to immunopathology.[29] Many xenobiotics induce oxidative stress via the pro-

Frederick W. Miller

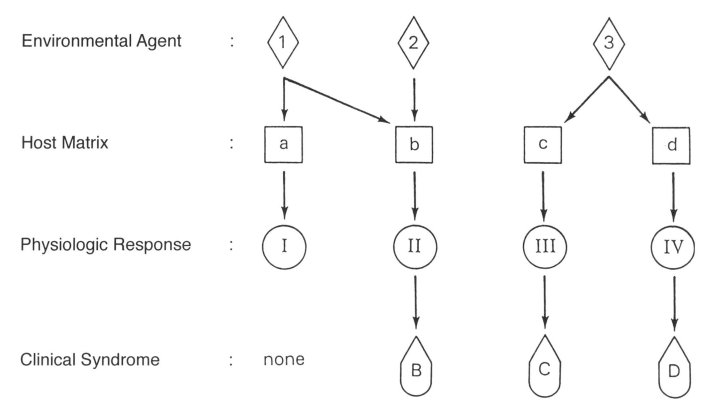

Fig. 4-2 Possible scenarios by which combinations of environmental agents and genetic risk factors may result in EARD. For example, an individual with a certain combination of pharmacogenetic/immunogenetic and other alleles (Host Matrix a) exposed to a chemical or infection (Environmental Agent 1) may develop an immune response or even autoantibodies (Physiologic Response I), but does not pass the threshold necessary to lead to development of pathology (Clinical Syndrome = none). Other persons with different genetic features (Host Matrix b) exposed to the same environmental agent, however, may develop a different response (Physiologic Response II) which results in EARD (Clinical Syndrome B).

It appears likely that, given the limited range of responses to environmental insults, and our current limited capacity to characterize them, different chemicals or infectious agents (represented as Environmental Agents 1 and 2) may result in what appears to be the same EARD (Clinical Syndrome B) on a given genetic background (Host Matrix b). In contrast, as is the case of patients with dissimilar HLA haplotypes developing different disorders following D-penicillamine therapy, the same material or infection (for example Environmental Agent 3) when given to different patients (Host Matrix c and d) can result in different physiologic responses (III and IV) that ultimately lead to different clinical syndromes (C or D respectively). Modified from Love and Miller 1993.[12]

Table 4-2 Possible etiopathogenetic mechanisms through which environmental agents may cause disease in genetically susceptible individuals

Mechanism	Possible Outcome
Altered self-protein	Results in an immune attack on altered self structures
Immunosuppression	Could allow infectious agents to reactivate or new ones successfully to infect the host
Immunostimulation	Either direct up-regulation or adjuvant activity to concurrent xenobiotic exposures
Immunotoxicity	Dysregulation of the immune network via imbalance or suppression
Molecular mimicry	Environmental agent shares structural similarity with host structures; cross-reactivity between agent and self structures results in autoimmunity
Oxidative stress	Alters DNA, resulting in new immune targets, impaired gene function or ineffective DNA repair mechanisms
Induction of apoptotic defects	Programmed cell death may not occur, resulting in novel immune targets or persistent immune responses

duction of reactive oxidative intermediates. Since some patients with inflammatory or autoimmune diseases have been shown to be more sensitive to genomic DNA damage and cytotoxic killing after oxidative stress,[33] and to have antibodies that recognize oxidized DNA bases,[34] it has been hypothesized that defects in oxidative repair mechanisms, increased oxidative stress, or both may play a role in the development of some of these conditions.[33,35,36]

FUTURE APPROACHES AND IMPLICATIONS

In order to sort out these etiopathogenetic possibilities for the development of EARD and perhaps avoid future occurrence, much additional clinical and laboratory research is needed. Approaches that seem promising include intensive and coordinated adverse event and EARD reporting by the many agencies and organizations involved in regulation and oversight of exposures to foods, drugs, biologics, medical devices, occupational and environmental toxins, and infectious agents; enhanced efforts to establish collaborative studies to develop and link registries and databases from the above sources to increase the power of epidemiologic studies and identify larger numbers of subjects for clinical research; new molecular genetic approaches using focused evaluations of multiple immunoregulatory genes (immunoprinting) combined with whole genome searches via microsatellite technology to assess genetic risks[16,37]; novel multigenic statistical linkage approaches[38]; and the development of more relevant animal models through the use of transgenic[39,40] or xenotransplantation technologies.[41]

The accurate identification of environmental risks in the context of individual genetic predispositions promises enormous potential for improving health care. For example, such information could identify individuals at risk with sufficient accuracy to support genetic screening in order to prevent disease in susceptible persons through avoidance of certain environmental exposures. On the other hand, since it is also likely that genetic backgrounds protective for the development of EARD will be found,[4] such information could enable the selection of subjects at reduced risk for an exposure that might decrease adverse events in early trials of new vaccines or therapeutic agents or in certain occupations. Finally, such information should result in better understanding "idiopathic" rheumatic and autoimmune diseases, and provide insight into pathogenesis that may suggest new approaches to therapy.

SUMMARY

Although the rarity, complexity and heterogeneity of the rheumatic disorders have limited our understanding of their pathogenesis, accumulating data suggest that most of the syndromes we recognize as rheumatic conditions are the result of one or more environmental exposures in genetically susceptible individuals. Thus it is useful to think of the rheumatic diseases as heterogeneous clinical-pathologic syndromes composed of many subgroups or elemental disorders, each of which may be defined by specific exposures and genes. Current limitations in defining environmental and genetic risk factors for these disorders result from the lack of validated diagnostic and classification criteria for environmentally associated diseases, poor coordination among government, academic and private organizations in collecting and sharing data needed for adequately powered studies, and increasing litigation coupled with decreasing resources for research. Despite these problems, certain metabolizer phenotypes and MHC alleles have been identified that appear to increase the risk for the development of a number of rheumatic and other immune-mediated diseases following exposures to selected dietary supplements, drugs, medical devices, occupational chemicals or infectious agents. These limited data suggest that important benefits could result from the more accurate identification of such genetic and environmental risks. These findings challenge us to overcome the above limitations and develop novel collaborations, epidemiologic approaches and laboratory methods to solve them.

REFERENCES

[1]Reveille JD. The interplay of nature versus nurture in predisposition to the rheumatic diseases. *Rheum Dis Clin North Am.* 1993;19:15–27.

[2]Hill AV, Allsopp CE, Kwiatkowski D, *et al.* Common west African HLA antigens are associated with protection from severe malaria. *Nature.* 1991;352:595–600.

[3]McLeod R, Buschman E, Arbuckle LD, Skamene E. Immunogenetics in the analysis of resistance to intracellular pathogens. *Curr Opin Immunol.* 1995;7:539–552.

[4]Miller FW. Genetics of autoimmune diseases. *Exp Clin Immunogenet.* 1995;12:182–190.

[5]Drake CG, Rozzo SJ, Vyse TJ, Palmer E, Kotzin BL. Genetic contributions to lupus-like disease in (NZB/NZW)F1 mice. *Immunol Rev.* 1995;144:51–74.

[6]Cordell HJ, Todd JA. Multifactorial inheritance in type 1 diabetes. *Trends Genet.* 1995;11:499–504.

[7]Hess EV, Farhey Y. Etiology, environmental relationships, epidemiology, and genetics of systemic lupus erythematosus. *Curr Opin Rheumatol.* 1995;7:371–375.

[8]Mongey AB, Hess EV. Drug and environmental effects on the induction of autoimmunity. *J Lab Clin Med.* 1993;122:652–657.

[9]Patarroyo ME, Winchester RJ, Vejerano A, *et al.* Association of a B-cell alloantigen with susceptibility to rheumatic fever. *Nature.* 1979;278:173–174.

[10]Hofstra AH, Uetrecht JP. Myeloperoxidase-mediated activation of xenobiotics by human leukocytes. *Toxicology.* 1993;82:221–242.

[11]Pelletier L, Bellon B, Tournade H, *et al.* Chemical-induced autoimmunity. *Immunol Ser.* 1991;55:315–353.

[12]Love LA, Miller FW. Noninfectious environmental agents associated with myopathies. *Curr Opin Rheumatol.* 1993;5:712–718.

[13]Tamai H, Sudo T, Kimura A, *et al.* Association between the DRB1 *08032 histocompatibility antigen and methimazole-induced agranulocytosis in Japanese patients with Graves' disease. *Ann Int Med.* 1996;124:490–494.

[14]Degli-Esposti MA, Abraham LJ, McCann V, Spies T, Christiansen FT, Dawkins RL. Ancestral haplotypes reveal the role of the central MHC in the immunogenetics of IDDM. *Immunogenetics.* 1992;36: 345–356.

[15]Degli-Esposti MA, Andreas A, Christiansen FT, Schalke B, Albert E, Dawkins RL. An approach to the localization of the susceptibility genes for generalized myasthenia gravis by mapping recombinant ancestral haplotypes. *Immunogenetics.* 1992;35:355–364.

[16]Todd JA. Genetic analysis of type 1 diabetes using whole genome approaches. *Proc Natl Acad Sci USA.* 1995;92:8560–8565.

[17]Holden RJ. The estrogen connection: The etiological relationship between diabetes, cancer, rheumatoid arthritis and psychiatric disorders. *Med Hypotheses.* 1995;45:169–189.

[18]Lahita RG. Sex hormones as immunomodulators of disease. *Ann NY Acad Sci.* 1993;685:278–287.

[19]Jiang X, Khursigara G, Rubin RL. Transformation of lupus-inducing drugs to cytotoxic products by activated neutrophils [see comments]. *Science.* 1994;266:810–813.

[20]Lennard MS. Genetically determined adverse drug reactions involving metabolism. *Drug Saf.* Vol 9, ISS 1, 1993;144.

[21]Adams LE, Mongey AB. Role of genetic factors in drug-related autoimmunity. *Lupus.* 1994;3:443–447.

[22]Risch N, Ghosh S, Todd JA. Statistical evaluation of multiple-locus linkage data in experimental species and its relevance to human studies: Application to nonobese diabetic (NOD) mouse and human insulin-dependent diabetes mellitus (IDDM). *Am J Hum Genet.* 1993;53:702–714.

[23]Thomas TJ, Seibold JR, Adams LE, Hess EV. Hydralazine induces Z-DNA conformation in a polynucleotide and elicits anti(Z-DNA) antibodies in treated patients. *Biochem J.* 1993;294: 419–425.

[24]Schattner A, Sthoeger Z, Geltner D. Effect of acute cytomegalovirus infection on drug-induced SLE. *Postgrad Med J.* 1994;70:738–740.

[25]Naim JO, Lanzafame RJ, van Oss CJ. The adjuvant effect of silicone-gel on antibody formation in rats. *Immunol Invest.* 1993;22:151–161.

[26]Potter M, Morrison S, Wiener F, Zhang XK, Miller FW. Induction of plasmacytomas with silicone gel in genetically susceptible strains of mice. *JNCI.* 1994;86:1058–1065.

[27]Vojdani A, Ghoneum M, Brautbar N. Immune alteration associated with exposure to toxic chemicals. *Toxicol Ind Health.* 1992;8:239–254.

[28]Campbell A, Brautbar N, Vojdani A. Suppressed natural killer cell activity in patients with silicone breast implants: Reversal upon explantation. *Toxicol Ind Health.* 1994;10:149–154.

[29]Revillard JP. The immune system as a target for chemical toxicity. *Eur Cytokine Netw.* 1991;2:81–87.

[30]Mountz JD, Wu J, Cheng J, Zhou T. Autoimmune disease. A problem of defective apoptosis. *Arthritis Rheum.* 1994;37:1415–1420.

[31]Bright J, Khar J, Khar A. Apoptosis: Programmed cell death in health and disease. *Biosci Rep.* 1994;14:67–81.

[32]Ray SK, Putterman C, Diamond B. Pathogenic autoantibodies are routinely generated during the response to foreign antigen: A paradigm for autoimmune disease. *Proc Natl Acad Sci USA.* 1996; 93:2019–2024.

[33]Bashir S, Harris G, Denman MA, Blake DR, Winyard PG. Oxidative DNA damage and cellular sensitivity to oxidative stress in human autoimmune diseases. *Ann Rheum Dis.* 1993;52:659–666.

[34]Frenkel K, Karkoszka J, Kim E, Taioli E. Recognition of oxidized DNA bases by sera of patients with inflammatory diseases. *Free Radic Biol Med.* 1993;14:483–494.

[35]Miesel R, Zuber M. Elevated levels of xanthine oxidase in serum of patients with inflammatory and autoimmune rheumatic diseases. *Inflammation.* 1993;17:551–561.

[36]Rubin RL. Role of xenobiotic oxidative metabolism. *Lupus.* 1994;3:479–482.

[37]Gomolka M, Menninger H, Saal JE, *et al.* Immunoprinting: Various genes are associated with increased risk to develop rheumatoid arthritis in different groups of adult patients. *J Mol Med.* 1995;73:19–29.

[38]Epplen JT, Buitkamp J, Bocker T, Epplen C. Indirect gene diagnoses for complex (multifactorial) diseases—a review. *Gene.* 1995;159:49–55.

[39]Taurog JD, Richardson JA, Croft JT, *et al.* The germfree state prevents development of gut and joint inflammatory disease in HLA-B27 transgenic rats. *J Exp Med.* 1994;180:2359–2364.

[40]Taurog JD, Maika SD, Simmons WA, Breban M, Hammer RE. Susceptibility to inflammatory disease in HLA-B27 transgenic rat lines correlates with the level of B27 expression. *J Immunol.* 1993;150:4168–4178.

[41]Elkon KB, Ashany D. The SCID mouse as a vehicle to study autoimmunity. *Br J Rheumatol.* 1993;32:4–12.

[42]Bell S, Brand K, Meurer M. Toxic oil syndrome—an example of an exogenously induced autoimmune disease [in German]. *Hautarzt.* 1992;43:339–343.

[43]Oursler JR, Farmer ER, Roubenoff R, Mogavero HS, Watson RM. Cutaneous manifestations of the eosinophilia-myalgia syndrome. *Br J Dermatol.* 1992;127:138–146.

[44]Kaufman LD, Gruber BL, Gregersen PK. Clinical follow-up and immunogenetic studies of 32 patients with eosinophilia-myalgia syndrome. *Lancet.* 1991;337:1071–1074.

[45]Singal DP, Reid B, Green D, D'Souza M, Bensen WG, Buchanan WW. Polymorphism of major histocompatibility complex extended haplotypes bearing HLA-DR3 in patients with rheumatoid arthritis with gold induced thrombocytopenia or proteinuria. *Ann Rheum Dis.* 1990;49:582–586.

[46]Scherak O, Smolen JS, Mayr WR, Mayrhofer F, Kolarz G, Thumb N. HLA antigens and side effects of gold and D-penicillamine in chronic polyarthritis [in German]. *Wien Klin Wochenschr Suppl.* 1984;156:51–52.

[47]Rodriguez-Perez M, Gonzalez-Dominguez J, Mataran L, Garcia-Perez S, Salvatierra D. Association of HLA-DR5 with mucocutaneous lesions in patients with rheumatoid arthritis receiving gold sodium thiomalate. *J Rheumatol.* 1994;21:41–43.

[48]Yunis JJ, Corzo D, Salazar M, Lieberman JA, Howard A, Yunis EJ. HLA associations in clozapine-induced agranulocytosis. *Blood.* 1995;86:1177–1183.

[49]Corzo D, Yunis JJ, Salazar M, *et al.* The major histocompatibility complex region marked by HSP70–1 and HSP70–2 variants is associated with clozapine-induced agranulocytosis in two different ethnic groups. *Blood.* 1995;86:3835–3840.

[50]Batchelor JR, Welsh KI, Tinoco RM, *et al.* Hydralazine-induced systemic lupus erythematosus: Influence of HLA-DR and sex on susceptibility. *Lancet.* 1980;1:1107–1109.

[51]Russell GI, Bing RF, Jones JA, Thurston H, Swales JD. Hydralazine sensitivity: Clinical features, autoantibody changes and HLA-DR phenotype. *Q J Med.* 1987;65:845–852.

[52]Speirs C, Fielder AH, Chapel H, Davey NJ, Batchelor JR. Complement system protein C4 and susceptibility to hydralazine-induced systemic lupus erythematosus. *Lancet.* 1989.1:922–924.

[53]Whiteside T, Mulhern L, Buckingham R, Luksock J. Procainamide induced lupus (PLE) is associated with an increased frequency of HLA-DR 6Y. *Arthritis Rheum.* 1982;25(suppl):S41 (Abstract).

[54]Grosse-Wilde H, Genth E, Grevesmuhl A, *et al.* HLA-DR4 and Gm 1;21 haplotypes are associated with pseudolupus induced by venopyronum dragees. *Arthritis Rheum.* 1987;30:878–883.

[55]Chalmers A, Thompson D, Stein HE, Reid G, Patterson AC. Systemic lupus erythematosus during penicillamine therapy for rheumatoid arthritis. *Ann Intern Med.* 1982;97:659–663.

[56]Taneja V, Mehra N, Singh YN, Kumar A, Malaviya A, Singh RR. HLA-D region genes and susceptibility to D-penicillamine-induced myositis [letter]. *Arthritis Rheum.* 1990;33:1445–1447.

[57]Carroll GJ, Will RK, Peter JB, Garlepp MJ, Dawkins RL. Penicillamine induced polymyositis and dermatomyositis. *J Rheumatol.* 1987;14:995–1001.

[58]Young VL, Nemecek JR, Schwartz BD, Phelan DL, Schorr MW. HLA typing in women with breast implants. *Plast Reconstr Surg.* 1995;96:1497–1519; discussion: 1520.

[59]Love LA, Weiner SR, Vasey FB, *et al.* Clinical and immunogenetic features of women who develop myositis after silicone implants. *Arthritis Rheum.* 1992;35:S46(abstract).

[60]Black CM, Welsh KI, Walker AE, *et al.* Genetic susceptibility to scleroderma-like syndrome induced by vinyl chloride. *Lancet.* 1983;1:53–55.

[61]Richeldi L, Sorrentino R, Saltini C. HLA-DPB1 glutamate 69: A genetic marker of beryllium disease. *Science.* 1993;262:242–244.

[62]Rihs HP, Lipps P, May-Taube K, *et al.* Immunogenetic studies on HLA-DR in German coal miners with and without coal worker's pneumoconiosis. *Lung.* 1994;172:347–354.

[63]Itescu S, Rose S, Dwyer E, Winchester R. Certain HLA-DR5 and -DR6 major histocompatibility complex class II alleles are associated with a CD8 lymphocytic host response to human immunodeficiency virus type 1 characterized by low lymphocyte viral strain heterogeneity and slow disease progression. *Proc Natl Acad Sci USA.* 1994;91:11472–11476.

[64]Haynes BF, Pantaleo G, Fauci AS. Toward an understanding of the correlates of protective immunity to HIV infection. *Science.* 1996;271:324–328.

[65]Raffoux C, David V, Couderc LD, *et al.* HLA-A, B and DR antigen frequencies in patients with AIDS-related persistent generalized lymphadenopathy (PGL) and thrombocytopenia. *Tissue Antigens.* 1987;29:60–62.

[66]Steere AC, Dwyer E, Winchester R. Association of chronic Lyme arthritis with HLA-DR4 and HLA-DR2 alleles. *N Engl J Med.* 1990;323:219–223.

[67]Ruberti G, Begovich AB, Steere AC, Klitz W, Erlich HA, Fathman CG. Molecular analysis of the role of the HLA class II genes DRB1, DQA1, DQB1, and DPB1 in susceptibility to Lyme arthritis. *Hum Immunol.* 1991;31:20–27.

[68]Joko S, Numaga J, Fujino Y, Masuda K, Hirata R, Maeda H. HLA and uveitis in leprosy [in Japanese]. *Nippon Ganka Gakkai Zasshi.* 1995;99:1181–1185.

[69]Joko S, Numaga J, Fujino Y, Masuda K, Hirata R, Maeda H. HLA-DR2 alleles and uveitis in leprosy [in Japanese]. *Nippon Rai Gakkai Zasshi.* 1995;64:112–118.

[70]Khanna AK, Buskirk DR, Williams RC Jr, *et al.* Presence of a non-HLA B cell antigen in rheumatic fever patients and their families as defined by a monoclonal antibody. *J Clin Invest.* 1989;83:1710–1716.

[71]Tomlinson IP, Bodmer WF. The HLA system and the analysis of multifactorial genetic disease. *Trends Genet.* 1995;11:493–498.

III

Fibrosing Disorders and the Environment

5

Toxic Oil Syndrome

Maravillas Izquierdo Martínez and Juan J. Gómez-Reino

INTRODUCTION

In May 1981, a new multisystemic epidemic disease appeared in Spain, affected more than 20,000 people and caused 350 deaths within the first year.[1] This condition was named toxic oil syndrome (TOS) late in March 1983.[2,3] Patients had an acute onset of fever, skin rashes, myalgia, eosinophilia and pleuropulmonary disease. These acute manifestations were gradually replaced by a chronic condition characterized by neuromuscular involvement, pulmonary arterial hypertension and sclerodermalike skin changes.[1–5]

An infectious cause was initially suspected and exhaustively investigated. However, this possibility was soon rejected. The clinical picture resembling an acute hypersensitivity syndrome, the lack of cases in groups at high risk for epidemic infection (for example, schoolchildren, military recruits), the high incidence of disease in lower socioeconomic groups, the failure to identify an infectious agent, and the occurrence of disease among multiple family members all suggested a food-borne illness. No cases were registered among children under six months of age. These findings led investigators to suggest the link between TOS and the consumption of an illegally manufactured cooking oil.[2] Subsequently, several case-control and case-series studies provided solid evidence of the association between the consumption of the toxic oil and the development of the disease.[3–7]

EPIDEMIOLOGY

The disease appeared in the vicinity of Madrid and spread over 14 provinces in central and northwestern Spain. More than 200 TOS cases per province were officially registered. The incidence rate was variable, the greatest being over 300 cases per 100,000 inhabitants at 18 months in some areas.[8] Studies carried out in two towns near Madrid found eosinophilia (over 500 cells/mm3) in close to 6% of the asymptomatic population, suggesting subclinical disease.

During May and June 1981, a total of 10,000 new cases were hospitalized. Many patients were seriously ill and required intensive care due to acute respiratory insufficiency. Six weeks after the outbreak of the epidemic, the association of the ingestion of oil with the disease was recognized and the implicated oil was withdrawn from the market. Subsequently there was a sharp drop in the incidence of new cases (Figure 5-1).

More than 20,000 individuals developed TOS. Seventy percent of the total cases occurred in Madrid. Up to December 1993, 1300 deaths were recorded, representing a 2.5% mortality rate during the acute phase of the disease. Survival studies revealed an excess of mortality between May 1 and December 31, 1981. The death rate in this period was 30.65 per 1000 person-years, fourfold higher than in the Spanish population in 1981 (7.77 per 1000 person-years).[9]

In the acute phase, there was a slight predominance of females affected over males (F/M:1.6/1). However, the difference became more pronounced during the chronic phase (F/M:5.6/1), particularly among the most seriously affected (F/M:10/1). The disease was evenly distributed over the 30 to 60 year age range. Twenty-two percent of the cases were in the pediatric age groups, but no cases were recorded among children under six months of age.[1–3]

TOXICOLOGY

The collection by the health authorities of large amounts of different types of illegally marketed consumable oils during the epidemic complicated identification of those associated with the disease. Nevertheless, batches of case-associated oils were available for analysis.

The implicated oil was denatured with aniline (2%) and had been imported from France for industrial use. The oil was refined to remove the aniline; it was combined with

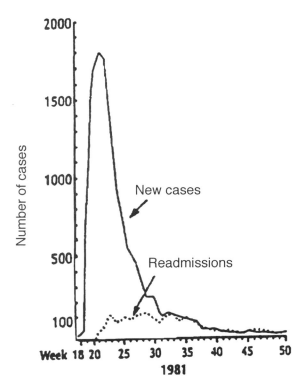

Fig. 5-1 Epidemic curve for new cases of TOS registered in 1981. Note that the numbers dropped sharply following the official announcement of the association with the ingestion of toxic oil in June 1981. Reproduced from Philen and Posada[47] with permission by W B Saunders Company, Orlando, Fla.

olive-residue oil, rapeseed oil, grapeseed oil, pig fat and sterified oil, and then illegally sold for human consumption.[10] An additional source of chemical contamination was the exposure of the oil to products in tanks used for transportation of petroleum products. Other than constituents related to aniline denaturation, TOS-related oils contained multiple trace contaminants.

Epidemiologic studies showed that high concentrations of oleyl anilide specifically identified the oils that contained the putative etiologic agent (case-related oils).[3,11–14] Further work showed high concentrations of 3-(N-phenylamino)-1,2-propanediol (PAP), the 3-oleyl ester of PAP (MEPAP), and the 1,2-di-oleyl ester of PAP (DEPAP) in case-associated oils; with odds ratios of 13.7 and 21.9, respectively. These findings support the hypothesis that one or more of the fatty acid esters of PAP was the etiologic agent for TOS.[15] PAP, MEPAP and DEPAP have also been found as microcontaminants in samples of L-tryptophan associated with eosinophilia myalgia syndrome (EMS), a disease sharing many clinical and pathological similarities with TOS.[16]

CLINICAL MANIFESTATIONS

TOS was a multisystemic disease. The evolution has shown several well-differentiated clinical phases (Table 5-1).[1,3–5,17,18]

In around 80% of affected individuals, the disease onset was an acute respiratory distress syndrome, with nonproductive cough, dyspnea and pleuritic pain, mild fever, nonscarring pruritic polymorphous rash of the extremities, neck and face, arthralgia, disabling myalgia, and muscle cramping. Less common were malaise or anorexia, diffuse abdominal pain with or without diarrhea, nausea or vomiting, and headache. Seldomly, hepatomegaly and enlarged lymph nodes were detected. Approximately 1% of patients had confusion and lethargy.[4,17]

Chest radiographs demonstrated a uni- or bilateral interstitial and alveolar pattern, similar to noncardiac pulmonary edema. Pleural and pericardial effusions were detected in one-sixth of patients.[3,4,17,19]

The most significant laboratory findings were a marked peripheral eosinophilia that frequently exceeded 3000 cells/mm³, and thrombocytopenia. Hypertrygliceridemia and mild elevations of hepatic enzymes were observed in nearly all hospitalized patients. Half of the patients had elevated IgE levels and antinuclear antibodies at low titers. The CD3 and CD8 peripheral blood lymphocyte subpopulations were decreased in over 75% in contrast to the CD4 subpopulation that remained within normal limits.[3,4,17,20]

Following the acute onset, TOS progressed to intermediate and chronic stages. The intermediate phase (July-August 1981) was distinguished by the association of variable degrees of neurological symptoms,[21] weight loss,[4,5,17] cutaneous nonpitting edema,[4,5,17] thromboembolic phenomena,[4,5,17] hepatopathy,[22] pulmonary hypertension[23,24] and arterial hypertension.[4,5] Severe myalgia and muscle weakness with hyporeflexia and superficial and deep sensory impairment defined the neurological disease. Electromyographic studies demonstrated a typical motor and sensory polyneuropathy. The cutaneous nonpitting edema gradually progressed to induration with or without patchy hyperpigmentation. Pulmonary and arterial hypertension were more frequent in children and young adults. A moderate to severe thrombocytopenia was common, but rare patients presented with thrombocytosis.[25] Other laboratory findings were hypoalbuminemia, hypertrigliceridemia and hypercholesterolemia. A few patients expired due to intestinal vascular occlusion.

Three months after the toxic oil exposure, the patients acquired a set of chronic signs and symptoms (summarized in Table 5-1). The neuromuscular syndrome was characterized by a diffuse symmetric peripheral neuropathy with progressive muscle atrophy (Figure 5-2). Sclerodermalike changes began to develop, and Raynaud's phenomenon accompanied the skin involvement.[4,26,27–32] Arthralgia and limitation of joint range of motion were common; nevertheless, arthritis was rare.

Nearly 15% of the patient population developed a more severe form of chronic TOS, most common in females. Case-control studies suggested the influence of certain isozymes of the cytochrome P450 and HLA class II haplotypes in the evolution toward severity and chronicity, respectively.[33–36]

Several treatments, including corticosteroids, plasma-

Table 5-1 Salient signs and symptoms in TOS patients

Acute Phase		Intermediate Phase		Early Chronic Phase		Late Chronic Phase	
May 1981 Clinical Manif.	June 1981 %	July 1981 Clinical Manif.	August 1981 %	Sept 1981 Clinical Manif.	May 1983 %	June 1983 Clinical Manif.	Dec 1994 %
Eosinophilia	86 (98)	Myalgia	49 (70)	Peripheral neuropathy	37 (80)	Fatigue	55 (80)
Pleuropulmonary	72 (80)	Weight loss	36 (80)	Muscle cramping	35	Sclerodermalike skin changes	35
Myalgia	71 (80)	Hepatopathy	21	Hepatopathy	32	Muscle cramping	35
Muscle cramping	60	Sicca syndrome	20 (70)	Sclerodermalike skin changes	22 (80)	Soft tissue tenderness	30 (80)
Arthralgia	50 (75)	Skin edema	14 (28)	Articular involvement	19 (75)	Psychiatric abnormalities	27 (75)
Fever	44 (76)	Sensory neuropathy	10 (20)	Dysphagia	15	Dyspnea on exertion	20
Rash	42 (62)	Alopecia	10 (47)	Pruritus	15	Headache	20
		Pulmonary hypertension	3	Sicca syndrome	15	Articular involvement	17
		Thromboembolism	1 (8)	Contracture	12	Sicca syndrome	15
				Pulmonary hypertension	10 (16)	Pruritus	15
				Arterial hypertension	4 (7)	Insomnia	14
				PFT abnormalities	6	Contracture	11
				Raynaud phenomenon	1 (4)	Hepatopathy	10
						Pulmonary hypertension	7
						Diabetes mellitus	7
						DLCO impairment	4
						Esophageal dysfunction	1
						Myocardial infarction	1
						Stroke	1

Percentage of clinical manifestations in outpatients and inpatients ().

DLCO—diffusing capacity for carbon monoxide

PFT—Pulmonary function tests

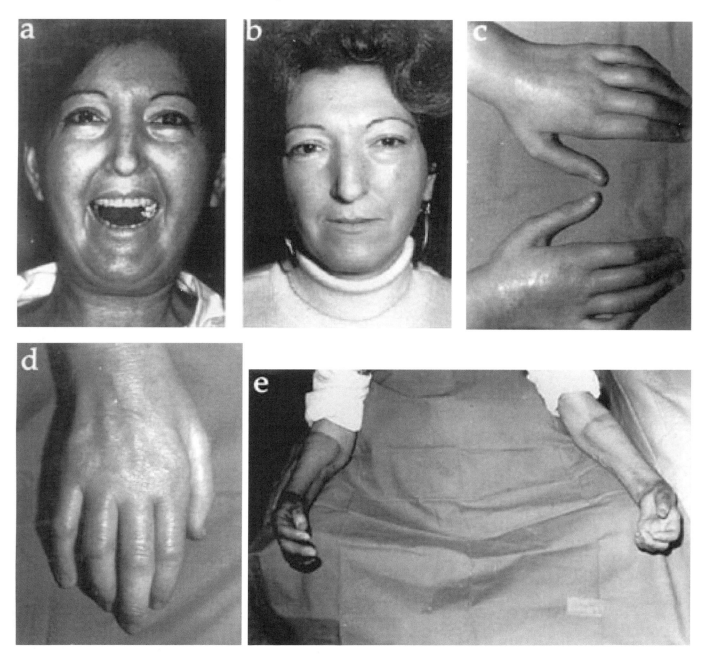

Fig. 5-2 Typical skin involvement and upper-limb deformities in TOS patients. Panels a and c show the infiltration of the skin in a patient during the intermediate stage. Note that the skin of the face and hands is thickened and shiny. Panels b and d show the same patient in the chronic phase. The skin is now retracted, although swelling of the fingers still persists. In panel e, the typical upper-limb deformity of the severe chronic phase can be appreciated. The arms are in pronation with flexion of the elbows. The hands have palmar retraction, extension of metacarpophalangeal joints and flexion of proximal and distal interphalangeal joints.

pheresis, D-penicillamine, colchicine, antioxidants, anticonvulsants, analgesics and many others were tried during the course of the disease. Glucocorticoids were effective in the control of acute respiratory involvement and eosinophilia, but did not prevent the progression to chronicity. Efficacy of diphenylhydantoin in the control of involuntary muscular movements was reported. Physiotherapy played an important role in functional recovery.[4,17,19]

EVOLUTION

Nearly one-third of individuals achieved remission in 1981. Long-term follow-up studies have demonstrated that a spectrum of features persisted among the remaining patients. These consisted of fatigue, myalgia, muscle cramping, neurocognitive complaints, liver dysfunction, pulmonary hypertension and sclerodermatous skin thickening.

To date, teratogenic effects in the newborn of mothers with TOS have not been detected.[37–39] The long-term incidence of potentially TOS-related malignant tumors, vascular-related conditions, and metabolic or immunological diseases is unknown. Lifelong follow-up of these patients will be required to resolve such issues.

PATHOLOGY

The salient pathological findings are outlined in Table 5-2. The most distinctive histological feature of TOS is the vascular lesion that involves vessels of every size and type.[4,40] Typically, vessels of the central nervous system are spared. The spectrum of endothelial damage ranges from swelling to cytoplasmic vacuolization and cellular necrosis.[4,40] Aggregates of fibrin and platelets over the endothelial cells are common. There are reduplication, thickening and fragmentation of basal lamina with proliferation of myointimal cells. Infiltration of the intima, perivascular areas and frequently media by mononuclear cells, eosinophils and scarce neutrophils appears early in the disease. In advanced stages, subintimal fibrosis may replace damaged endothelial cells and inflammatory infiltrates, producing luminal occlusion (Figure 5-3). Leukocytoclasia, fibrinoid necrosis and granuloma have not been seen.[4,40]

In the skin, during the acute phase, there are perivascular and interstitial mononuclear cell infiltrates.[4,26,27,40] These infiltrates are confined to the dermis, and extension to the fascia is rare. Late lesions include mucinosis and fibrosis of the superficial and deep dermis with encroachment of dermal appendages and atrophy. Fibroblasts have an activated appearance. *In situ* hybridization studies reveal cellular expression of type I and type III procollagen mRNA.[41]

The acute pulmonary lesions consist of septal edema, cuboidal metaplasia of type II pneumocytes, necrosis and desquamation of type I pneumocytes, and scarce interstitial mononuclear cell infiltrates.[4,23,24,40] In the chronic phase there is mild interstitial infiltration with mononuclear cells, and vascular intimal inflammation with or without fibrosis.[4,23,24,40] Interstitial fibrosis has not been seen.

The cardinal pathological finding in muscle during the acute phase is the inflammatory cell infiltration.[4,21,40,42] The infiltrates are comprised predominantly of mononuclear cells and involve epi- and perimysium. Muscle spindle capsules and the sheaths of nerves may be also inflamed. Denervation muscle atrophy and, in severe cases, endomysial fibrosis are characteristic of the chronic disease.[21,42]

The earliest anomaly in the peripheral nerve is a perivascular and interstitial round cell infiltration of peri-, epi- and endoneurium.[4,21,40,42] Fibroblast proliferation in the perineurium has been observed by electron microscopy. Focal perineural fibrosis, with a variable intensity, is present in the most advanced cases. In the nerve fascicles, there is axonal loss in parallel with the fibrosis.[40,42] Chromatolytic changes in the brain stem and in the motor neurons of the anterior horns of spinal cord have been seen at autopsy.[42,43]

Different laboratories have examined the participation of immune complexes, the eosinophil granule major basic protein (MBP) and fibrogenic growth factors in the pathogenesis of TOS. Immunofluorescence studies to identify immunoglobulins and complement in or around blood vessels are always negative.[40] In the acute phase, detection of intra- and extracellular MBP in lung, liver, skin and kidney tissues suggests a degranulation of eosinophils.[44] In the chronic phase, in the skin, there is a paucity of TGF-α in the epidermis and dermis but important amounts of EGF, FGF, PDGF (AA and BB) and IL-4 deposits in epidermis and periappendageal areas.[45]

THE PATHOGENESIS OF TOXIC OIL SYNDROME AND ITS RELEVANCE TO OTHER FIBROSING DISEASES

The pathogenesis of TOS remains uncertain.[46–48] The similarity of TOS to other rheumatic diseases suggests that the acute toxic damage triggered a chronic autoimmune mechanism that, in turn, sustained the disease. This chronic phase of TOS emerged when there was no further toxic exposure. No animal model could successfully test this hypothesis, in spite of the many efforts to reproduce the disease utilizing either case-related oils or some of their constituents.[46,47] Nevertheless, arguments in favor of a toxic-driven disease, other than the epidemiologic association, are many.

The acute interstitial pulmonary edema could originate from an increase in vascular permeability owing to the endothelial lesion. Radiation, nitrofurantoin and shock pro-

Table 5-2 Salient pathologic features of TOS

	Acute Phase	Chronic Phase
Blood vessel	Endothelial swelling	Proliferation of myointimal cells, perivascular, intimal cell infiltration and fibrosis
Skin	Perivascular and interstitial cell infiltration	Fibrosis and mucinosis of dermis
Lung	Septal edema cuboidal metaplasia	Mild interstitial cell infiltration
Muscle	Epi- and perimysium cell infiltration	Muscle atrophy and endomysial fibrosis
Nerve	Peri-, epi- and endoneurium cell infiltration	Fibrosis

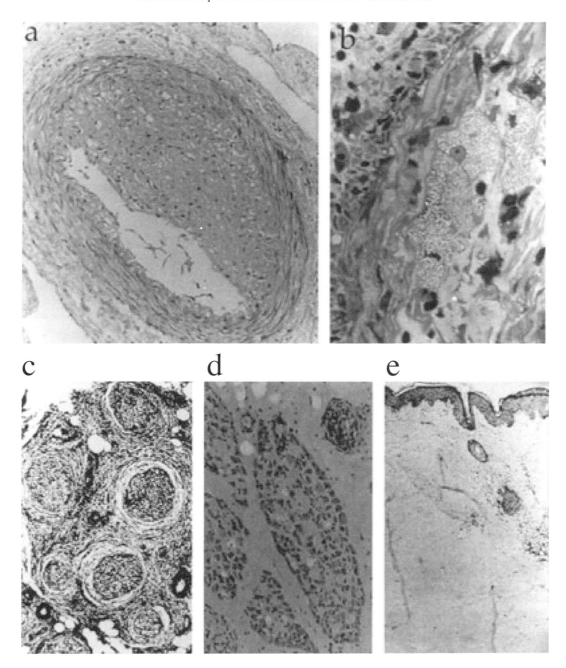

Fig. 5-3 Pathology of the most relevant lesions in TOS. Panels a and b show the typical vascular changes. Panel a: subintimal proliferation and mononuclear cell infiltration of a coronary artery. Panel b: an artery with intimal thickening caused by fibroblast proliferation. Panel c: a sural nerve with inflammatory cell infiltration and fibrosis of perineurium. Panel d: fascicular atrophy and fibrosis of a muscle. Panel e: profound dermal fibrosis with encroachment of appendages.

duce a similar picture.[4] In this regard, it is interesting to note the similarity of fatty acid anilides and nitrofurantoin. However, the disease produced in animals by anilides is not consistent with these observations.

The systemic inflammatory response syndrome (SIRS) is a condition characterized by widespread inflammation affecting the vascular endothelium.[49,50] In SIRS, the simultaneously occurring polymorphonuclear leukocytes and endothelial cell activation lead to leukothrombosis. The sub-

sequent local release of enzymes and oxygen radicals injures blood vessels. Mediators of this syndrome include TNF-α, IL-1, platelet activation factor, prostaglandins and complement components. There is up-regulation of adhesion molecules on polymorphonuclear leukocytes and endothelial cells.[50] Some acute manifestations of TOS (that is, acute interstitial lung disease and cerebral dysfunction) are indistinguishable from SIRS, yet the typical leukothrombosis in small blood vessels of the latter was never reported in the former. Furthermore, in TOS there was no proof of complement activation nor documentation favoring a mechanism similar to SIRS.

The blood vessel inflammation in TOS has stimulated investigation of prostaglandin and leukotriene synthesis by fatty acid anilides.[51–53] *In vitro*, oleoyl and, more vigorously, linoleoyl anilides bring about the generation of arachidonic acid by polymorphonuclear cells. In peritoneal macrophages from rodents, linoleoyl anilide enhances the production of prostaglandin 6-oxo-PGF1 and thromboxane. In other cell systems, it also increases the production of 12-hydroxy-eicosatetraenoic acid (12 HETE). Nevertheless, the large doses of oleoanilides used in these experiments argue against their *in vivo* relevance. The examination of other derivatives of aniline identified in the oil has also been the focus of investigation. It was argued that progoitrin (2-hydroxy-3-butenylglucosinolate) from rapeseed oil could react with aniline and generate 1-phenyl-5-vinyl-2-imidazolidinethione (IZT) or 5-vinyl-2-thiazolidinephenylamine (5-VTPA).[11,54] Both IZT and 5-VTPA feature the structure of phenytoin, which induces a reaction resembling graft-versus-host disease (GVHD).[55] Furthermore, IZT was used successfully in the popliteal lymph node assay,[56] an established method to screen chemicals capable of inducing GVHD. However, neither IZT nor 5-VTPA were detected in case-related oils.[57,58] Recently, aniline-derived PAP, MEPAP and DEPAP have been administered to rodents. None of the animals developed tissue damage comparable to TOS.[15,59]

Why some patients went on to a chronic condition is unknown. Female gender and HLA-DR3 and DR4 antigens are factors presumably involved in the progression.[35] These gender and genetic associations are reminiscent of what occurs in connective-tissue diseases resembling TOS. Chronic TOS, EMS, systemic sclerosis, GVHD, and eosinophilic fasciitis share common manifestations. The profound vascular damage suggests that constituents of the toxic oil induced an unidentified endothelial component. T helper lymphocytes could have recognized altered membrane antigens together with autologous MHC class II antigens and triggered the GVHD.[60] In animal models, GVHD has a chronic presentation and includes features of autoimmunity, sclerodermalike lesions and liver changes.[60] The initiation of the disease depends on the presence of susceptibility alleles at different loci and is under the influence of sex hormones and the metabolic pathway of the etiologic agent.[33,34,60]

In TOS, remarkable blood findings include high IgE levels, eosinophilia and presence of serum autoantibodies. Elevated IgE is also detected in nonatopic diseases associated with eosinophilia. In some studies, specific IgE against oleoyl anilides was encountered, suggesting an immediate hypersensitivity reaction.[61] The sera from patients with chronic TOS contain antibodies that recognized tumoral murine cell line proteins (unpublished observations). These autoantibodies may be merely disease markers or may be related to a distinctive pathogenetic mechanism.

As described above, fibrosis was a prominent pathologic finding in multiple organs. Fibroblast activation may be induced by cytokines derived from T lymphocytes and eosinophils.

TOS and, recently, EMS are examples of chemical-induced fibrosing diseases. Similarities among patients with TOS and EMS appear greater than differences. Furthermore, the overlap with other idiopathic fibrosing diseases may help to clarify their etiology and pathogenesis.

REFERENCES

[1]Villamor León J, Rodriguez Illera E, Pozo Rodriguez F, *et al.* Descripción clínica de la enfermedad en adultos (Clinical description of the illness in adults). In: *Simposium Nacional "Síndrome Tóxico"* (National Symposium on the Toxic Oil Syndrome). Madrid, 11–12 June 1982. Madrid: Ministry of Health and Consumer Affairs, 1982;47–73.

[2]Tabuenca JM. Toxic-allergic syndrome caused by ingestion of rapeseed oil denatured with aniline. *Lancet.* 1981;2:567–568.

[3]Kilbourne EM, Rigau-Perez JG, Heath CW, *et al.* Clinical epidemiology of toxic oil syndrome. Manifestations of a new illness. *N Eng J Med.* 1983;309:1408–1414.

[4]Toxic Epidemic Study Group. Toxic epidemic syndrome, Spain, 1981. *Lancet.* 1982;2:697–702.

[5]Serrano-Rios M, Faro V. Clinical and pathological features of TOS. In: Grandjean P, de Tarkovski S, eds. *Toxic Oil Syndrome. Mass Food Poisoning in Spain.* Copenhagen: WHO Regional Office for Europe, 1984;53–74.

[6]Posada de la Paz M, Abaitua Borda I, Kilbourne EM, *et al.* Late cases of toxic-oil syndrome: Evidence that the aetiological agent persisted in oil stored for up to one year. *Food and Chemical Toxicology.* 1989;8:517–521.

[7]Diaz de Rojas F, Castro Garcia M, Abaitua Borda I, *et al.* The association of oil ingestion with toxic oil syndrome in two convents. *Am J Epidemiol.* 1987;125:907–911.

[8]Kilbourne EM, Posada de la Paz M, Abaitua-Borda I. Eight epidemiological studies. In: World Health Organization Regional Office for Europe, ed. *Toxic Oil Syndrome: Current Knowledge and Future Perspectives.* Copenhagen: World Health Organization, 1992;5–25.

[9]Abaitua-Borda I, Kilbourne EM, Posada de la Paz M, Diez Ruiz-Navarro M, Gabriel-Sanchez R, Falk H. Mortality among people affected by toxic oil syndrome: Pilot study for retrospective followup of the cohort by mailed questionnaire. *Int J Epidemiol.* 1993;22:1077–1084.

[10]Guitart R, Gelpi E. Chemical composition of TOS-related oils. In: World Health Organization Regional Office for Europe, ed. *Toxic Oil Syndrome: Current Knowledge and Future Perspectives.* WHO Regional Publications. European Series, No. 42:99–142.

[11]Bernert JT, Pedregrast AH, Brandsma L, *et al.* Synthesis of N-(5-vinyl-1,3-thiazolidin-2-ylidene) phenylamine and analysis of oils implicated in the Spanish toxic oil syndrome for its presence. *Food Chem Toxicol.* 1989;27:159–164.

[12]Pestaña A, Muñoz E. Anilides and the Spanish toxic oil syndrome. *Nature.* 1982;298:608.

[13]Kilbourne EM, Bernert JT, Posada de la Paz M, *et al.* and the Tox-ico-Epidemiologic Study Group. Chemical correlates of patho-genicity of oils related to the toxic oil syndrome in Spain. *Am J Epi-demiol.* 1988;127:1210–1227.

[14]Posada de la Paz M, Philen RM, Abaitua Borda Y, *et al.* Factors associated with pathogenicity of oils related to the toxic oil syn-drome epidemic in Spain. *Epidemiology.* 1994;5:404–408.

[15]Hill RH Jr, Schurz HH, Posada de la Paz M, *et al.* Possible etio-logic agents for toxic oil syndrome: Fatty acid esters of 3-(N-phenylamino)-1,2-propanediol. *Arch Environ Contam Toxicol.* 1995;28:259–264.

[16]Mayeno AN, Belongia EA, Lin F, Lundy SK, Gleich GJ. 3-(phenylamino)alanine, a novel aniline-derived amino acid associ-ated with the eosinophilia-myalgia syndrome: A link to the toxic oil syndrome? *Mayo Clin Proc.* 1992;67:1134–1139.

[17]Abaitua Borda I, Posada de la Paz M. In: World Health Organiza-tion Regional Office for Europe, ed. *Toxic Oil Syndrome: Current Knowledge and Future Perspectives.* Copenhagen: World Health Organization, 1992;27–38.

[18]Alonso-Ruiz A, Calabozo M, Perez-Ruiz F, Mancebo L. Toxic oil syndrome: A long-term follow-up of a cohort of 332 patients. *Med-icine* (Baltimore). 1993;72:285–295.

[19]De la Cruz JL, Oteo LA, Sueiro A. Estudio evolutivo de la radi-ologia torácica en el síndrome tóxico. Análisis de la respuesta al tratamiento con corticoides. *Rev Clin Esp.* 1983;169:37–41.

[20]Bell SA, Du Clos TW, Khursigara G, Picazo JJ, Rubin RL. Autoantibodies to cryptic epitopes of C-reactive protein and other acute phase proteins in the toxic oil syndrome. *J Autoimmun.* 1995;8:293–303.

[21]Portera-Sanchez A, Franch O, del Ser T. Neuromuscular manifes-tations of the toxic oil syndrome: A recent outbreak in Spain. In: Battistin L, Hashim G, lajth A, eds. *Clinical and Biological Aspects of Peripheral Nerve Diseases.* New York: Alan S Riss, 1983;171–181.

[22]Solís Herruzo JA, Castellanos G, Colina F, *et al.* Hepatic injury in the toxic epidemic syndrome caused by ingestion of adulterated cooking oil (Spain 1981). *Hepatology.* 1984;4:131–139.

[23]Gomez-Sanchez MA, Mestre de Juan MJ, Gomez-Pajuelo C, Lopez JI, Diaz de Atauri MJ, Martinez-Tello FJ. Pulmonary hyper-tension due to toxic oil syndrome: A clinicopathologic study. *Chest.* 1989;95:325–331.

[24]Gomez-Sanchez MA, Saenz de la Calzada C, Gomez-Pajuelo C, Martinez-Tello FJ, Mestre de Juan MJ, James TN. Clinical and pathologic manifestations of pulmonary vascular disease in the toxic oil syndrome. *J Am Coll Cardiol.* 1991;18:1539–1545.

[25]Castro García M, Posada M, Díaz de Rojas F, Abaitua Borda I, Tabuenca Oliver JM. Hypercoagulable states and the toxic oil syn-drome. *Ann Intern Med.* 1986;104:730.

[26]Mateo IM, Izquierdo M, Fernandez-Dapica MP, Navas J, Cabello A, Gomez-Reino JJ. Toxic oil syndrome: Musculoskeletal manifes-tations. *J Rheumatol.* 1984;11:333–338.

[27]Alfonso-Ruiz A, Zea-Mendoza AC, Salazar-Vallinas JM, Rocamora-Ripoll A, Beltran-Gutierrez J. Toxic oil syndrome: A syndrome with features overlapping those of various forms of scle-roderma. *Semin Arthritis Rheum.* 1986;15:200–212.

[28]Oliva Aldamiz H. Patología de la glándula salival en el síndrome por aceite tóxico adulterado en España: una forma de síndrome de Sjögren secundario (Pathology of the labial salivary gland in the Spanish toxic oil syndrome: A form of secondary Sjögren's syn-drome). *Rev Clin Esp.* 1988;182:71–78.

[29]Olmedo Garzón FJ, Zea-Mendoza AC, Alonso-Ruiz A, *et al.* Epi-demic due to the ingestion of adulterated, toxic cooking oil: A new type of sclerodermatous syndrome. *Med Clin Barc.* 1982;79:1–8.

[30]Rush PJ, Bell MJ, Fam AG. Toxic oil syndrome (Spanish oil dis-ease) and chemically induced scleroderma-like conditions (editor-ial). *J Rheumatol.* 1984;11:262–264.

[31]Hernández Bronchud M. Toxic oil syndrome and vinyl chloride disease (letter). *Lancet.* 1984;2:931.

[32]Posada de la Paz M, Alonso Gordo JM, Castro García M, Díaz de Rojas F, Abaitua Borda I, Tabuenca Oliver JM. Toxic oil syndrome, scleroderma, and eosinophilic fasciitis (letter). *Arthritis Rheum.* 1984;27:120.

[33]Izquierdo Martínez M, Alvarez Castellanos F, de la Fuente Alvarez G. Determination of hydroxilator phenotype in TOS patients. An intrafamily pilot study. Research project WHO/FIS Ref. 88/2237.

[34]Ladona MG, Izquierdo Martínez M, Ampurdanés C, *et al.* Drug metabolism study in patients affected by Spanish toxic oil syn-drome: A molecular approach to detoxification-toxification mecha-nism involved. *Thérapie* (France). 1995;72:S.

[35]Vicario JL, Serrano-Rios M, San Andres F, Arnaiz-Villena A. HLA-DR3, DR4 increase in chronic stage of Spanish oil syndrome. *Lancet.* 1982;2:276.

[36]Díaz de Atauri MJ, Martín Escribano P, Arnaiz A, *et al.* HLA anti-gens in a sample of patients affected by Toxic Oil Syndrome (TOS). *Eur J Resp Dis.* 1993;S:P1947.

[37]Guerra Flecha JM, Aguarón de la Cruz A. Repercusiones del sín-drome tóxico sobre la gestación (Repercussiones of the toxic oil syndrome on gestation). *Rev Colomb Obstet Ginecol.* 1985;36:48–51.

[38]Tabuenca Oliver JM, Castro Garcia M, Ruiz Galiana J, *et al.* Span-ish toxic oil and congenital malformations. *Lancet.* 1983;1:181.

[39]Martínez Frías ML, Salvador J, Prieto L. Spanish toxic oil and congenital malformations. *Lancet.* 1982;2:1349.

[40]Martinez-Tello FJ, Navas-Palacios J, Ricoy JR, *et al.* Pathology of a new syndrome caused by ingestion of adulterated oil in Spain. *Vir-chows Arch Pathol Anat Histol.* 1982;397:261–285.

[41]Gomez-Reino JJ, Sanberg M, Carreira P, Vuorio E. Expression of types I, III and IV collagen genes in fibrotic skin and nerve lesions of toxic oil syndrome patients. *Clin Exp Immunol.* 1993;93:103–107.

[42]Ricoy JR, Cabello A, Rodriguez J, Tellez I. Neuropathological studies on the toxic syndrome related to adulterated rapeseed oil in Spain. *Brain.* 1983;106:817–835.

[43]Tellez I, Cabello A, Franch O, Ricoy JR. Cromatolytic changes in the central nervous system of patients with toxic oil syndrome. *Acta Neuropathol* (Berlin). 1987;74:354–361.

[44]Ten RM, Kephart GM, Posada de la Paz M, *et al.* Participation of eosinophils in the toxic oil syndrome. *Clin Exp Immunol.* 1990;82:313–317.

[45]Kaufman LD, Gomez-Reino JJ, Gruber B, Miller F. Fibrogenic growth factors in the eosinophilia myalgia syndrome and toxic oil syndrome. *Arch Dermatol.* 1994;130:41–47.

[46]World Health Organization, ed. Toxic oil syndrome and eosinophilia-myalgia syndrome. Pursuing parallels in pathogenesis. Report on a WHO meeting, Washington, DC, 8–10 May, 1991. World Health Organization Regional Office for Europe, 1991.

[47]Philen RM, Posada M. Toxic oil syndrome and eosinophilia myalgia syndrome: May 8–10, 1991, World Health Organization meeting report. *Semin Arthritis Rheum.* 1993;23:104–124.

[48]Gomez-Reino JJ. Immune system disorders associated with adulterated cooking oil. In: Berlin A, Dean J, Drapper MH, Smith EMB, Spreafico F, eds. *Immunotoxicology.* Dordrecht, the Netherlands: Martinus Nijhoff Publishers, 1987;376–388.

[49]Bone RC. Why new definitions of sepsis and organ failure are needed. *Am J Med.* 1993;95:348–350.

[50]Nogare D. Septic shock. *Am J Med Sci.* 1991;302:50–65.

[51]Aldridge WN: Experimental studies. In: World Health Organization Regional Office for Europe, ed. *Toxic Oil Syndrome: Current Knowledge and Future Perspectives.* Copenhagen: World Health Organization, 1992;67–97.

[52]Garcia Gil M. Cyclooxigenase of fatty acid anilides on the generation of arachidonic acid by human polymorphonuclear leucocytes. *FEBS Letters.* 1983;163:151–155.

[53]Ramis I, Bioque G, Rosello J, Bulbena O, Gelpi E. Cyclooxigenase products of metabolism of arachidonic acid of mouse macrophages exposed to N-phenilinoleamide from toxic oil samples. *Prostaglandins, Leukot Essent Fatty Acids.* 1990;39:147–149.

[54]Kammüller ME, Verhaar HJ, Verlius C, *et al.* 1-phenyl-5-vinyl-imidazolidinethione, a proposed causative agent of Spanish oil syndrome: Synthesis and identification in one of a group of case-associated oil samples. *Food Chem Toxicol.* 1988;2:119–127.

[55]Kammüller ME, Penninks AH, Seinen W. Spanish toxic oil syndrome and chemically induced graft-versus-host-like reactions. *Lancet.* 1984;2:805–806.

[56]Kammüller EM, Bloksman N, Seinen W. Chemical-induced autoimmune reactions and Spanish toxic oil syndrome. *J Toxicol Clin Toxicol.* 1988;26:157–174.

[57]Nomura GS, Ashley DL, Pendergrast AH, *et al.* Structural identification of a heterocyclic compound implicated in the Spanish toxic oil syndrome. *Food Chem Toxicol.* 1989;27:165–172.

[58]Verhaar HJM, Kammüller ME, Terlow JK, Brasma L, Seinen W. Spanish toxic oil syndrome: An isothiocyanate-derived compound cannot be substantiated as a causative agent. *Food Chem Toxicol.* 1989;27:205–207.

[59]Turner WE, Hill RH Jr, Hannon WH, Bernert JT, Kilbourne EM, Bayse DD. Bioassay screening for toxicants in oil samples from the toxic oil syndrome outbreak in Spain. *Arch Environ Contam Toxicol.* 1985;14:261–271.

[60]Gleichmann H, Gleichmann E. Mechanism of autoimmunity. In: Berlin A, Dean J, Drapper MH, Smith EMB, Spreafico F, eds. *Immunotoxicology.* Dordrecht, the Netherlands: Martinus Nijhoff Publishers, 1987.

[61]Lahoz C, Rose NR, Goter Robinson CJ. In: World Health Organization Regional Office for Europe, ed. *Toxic Oil Syndrome: Current Knowledge and Future Perspectives.* Copenhagen: World Health Organization, 1992;143–152.

6

Eosinophilia Myalgia Syndrome

Lee D. Kaufman and Gerald J. Gleich

Eosinophilia myalgia syndrome (EMS) is a new clinico-pathological entity that achieved worldwide recognition in 1989[1–7] as a systemic toxin-induced disorder with remarkable similarity to the previously described toxic oil syndrome (TOS) of Spain (1981),[8] idiopathic systemic sclerosis (SSc) and diffuse fasciitis with eosinophilia (DEF) (eosinophilic fasciitis or Shulman syndrome).[1,9–17] The spectrum of clinical and pathological features that distinguish EMS from similar conditions has been well characterized.

EPIDEMIOLOGY, ETIOLOGY AND PATHOGENESIS

L-Tryptophan as the Cause of EMS

Following recognition of EMS in 1989, attention was quickly directed to the question of causation. The first obvious candidate was L-tryptophan (LT) itself. Indeed, a patient had been described previously who developed scleroderma-like cutaneous changes while taking 5-hydroxytryptophan.[18] Moreover, other observations had related tryptophan to fibrosis, including the occurrence of a sclerodermalike disease and fibrosis in metastatic carcinoid syndrome[19,20] and retroperitoneal fibrosis associated with the 5-hydroxytryptamine (serotonin) antagonist methysergide.[21] Other candidates were suggested by reports that serotonin induced dermal fibrosis[22] and that serotonin, as well as indole, caused synovial fibrosis in laboratory animals.[23,24] Thus considerable literature exists suggesting that substances related to LT are associated with fibrosis.

Ingestion of LT itself is relatively safe. LT had been utilized by many patients as a hypnotic, with the underlying assumption that its effects were related to increased serotonin in the brain.[25] Although the Food and Drug Administration (FDA) cautioned against LT use[26] because of the concern that excessive LT ingestion might result in toxic levels of quinolinic acid (*vide infra*) in the central nervous system,[27] only occasional reactions following ingestion of LT were reported.[28,29] Thus, on balance, prior to the EMS epidemic, LT-containing products were considered to be safe. In fact, such products were recommended by physicians and the lay press. Once the EMS epidemic was recognized, efforts were made to uncover an etiological role for LT. Figure 6-1 shows the metabolic pathways of LT in humans.[30] The predominant metabolic pathway for LT is oxidation to formylkynurenine. After an additional series of metabolic transformations, quinolinic acid is produced. Quinolinic acid is a potent neurotoxin which has been implicated in the pathophysiology of several diseases, including Huntington's disease, hepatic encephalopathy, encephalopathy associated with human immunodeficiency virus infection, and Lyme disease.[31–33] Alterations in LT metabolism had also been related to diseases associated with fibrosis; serum levels of kynurenine were elevated in some patients with SSc and eosinophilic fasciitis.[34] Evaluation of LT metabolism in patients with EMS showed that untreated individuals had the greatest elevations in serum kynurenine,[35] and quinolinic acid was elevated in the cerebrospinal fluid of some individuals with acute EMS.[36] These observations suggested that quinolinic acid might be involved in the pathogenesis of neuropathy in EMS.

However, the hypothesis that LT metabolites were the cause of EMS is not supported by other considerations. For example, quinolinic acid is associated with an axon-sparing neurologic lesion distinct from that seen in EMS.[31] Furthermore, the rise in LT metabolites appears to be secondary to increased activity of the rate-limiting enzyme of LT metabolism, indoleamine-2,3-dioxygenase (IDO).[35] Increased activity of IDO is found in many inflammatory conditions[37] and therefore is not specific to EMS. Thus the hypothesis that LT itself might be implicated in the causation of EMS seems unlikely in view of its role as an essential amino acid and, most importantly, the paucity of reports of LT toxicity prior

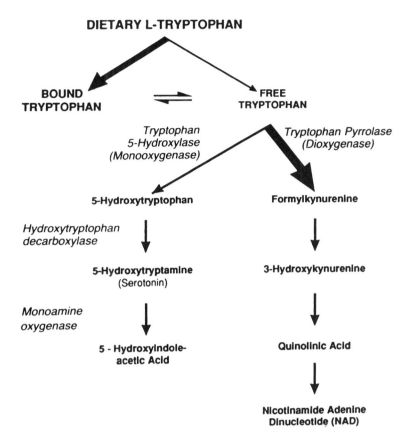

Fig. 6-1 Major metabolic pathways of L-tryptophan in humans. Important enzymes are indicated in italics. Reprinted with permission from Varga J, Uitto J, Jimenez SA. The cause and pathogenesis of the eosinophilia-myalgia syndrome. *Ann Intern Med.* 1992;116:140–147.

to 1989. Nonetheless, the possibility that LT metabolites are critical in the pathophysiology of EMS remains open. Most investigators suspected that a contaminant was a more likely etiological agent for EMS. This assumption was derived from initial clinical observations. For example, one of the initial individuals with EMS had ingested LT for two and a half years without adverse effect, but became ill in late August 1989.[38] Observations such as this suggested the hypothesis that a contaminant in LT was associated with EMS.

L-Tryptophan Contaminants as the Cause of EMS

Association between L-Tryptophan and EMS: Case-Control Studies

Following the recognition that patients ingesting LT developed EMS,[38] two case-control studies were performed to test the association between LT-containing products and EMS. The first, in New Mexico, defined EMS as unexplained peripheral blood eosinophilia (more than or equal to 2000/µl) and incapacitating myalgia. Review of white blood cell counts from regional medical laboratories revealed 11 cases.[39] These 11 cases were compared to 22 matched controls interviewed for information on symptoms and other clinical findings. All 11 cases (100%) had used LT-contain-

ing products, compared with only two of the controls (p < 0.00002). A second case-control study was performed in Minnesota.[40] Here, cases were identified by rheumatologists, who were asked by the Minnesota Department of Health to report patients with eosinophilia and either severe myalgia or muscle weakness, and by clinical pathologists and a pediatric neurologist (who was asked to identify patients with muscle biopsies showing eosinophilic perimyositis or perivasculitis). EMS was diagnosed using the criteria of an eosinophil count greater than 1000 cells/µl, myalgia or muscle weakness of sufficient severity to affect normal daily activities and a muscle biopsy (if performed) showing perimyositis, perivasculitis or fasciitis. Potential cases were excluded if the clinical and pathological features could have been caused by a predetermined list of diseases known to be associated with eosinophilia. The investigators had no prior knowledge of patients' use of LT-containing products. In this way, 12 cases were identified and compared to controls matched by age, sex and telephone exchange. All the case patients, but none of the controls, had ingested LT-containing products during the month before onset of illness and a similar time for the matched controls (odds ratio not calculable; p < 0.0008). These two case-control studies established an association between LT ingestion and the occurrence of EMS.

Once an association between EMS and LT had been established, inquiries turned to defining the extent of the epidemic and identifying factors which predisposed individuals to the development of EMS. To this end, case-control studies initially were performed in Minnesota and then in Oregon, yielding essentially comparable findings.[41,42] The Minnesota study also found a dramatic increase in the utilization of LT in the Minneapolis-St. Paul area during the period from 1984 to 1989.[42] Indeed, by 1989, it was estimated that approximately 2% of the population was ingesting LT (Figure 6-2).[42]

Association between L-Tryptophan Producers and EMS: Case-Control Studies

Associations between the six Japanese manufacturers of LT and the occurrence of EMS were sought using case-control studies. Case-control studies in Oregon,[41] Minnesota[42] and New York State[17] were performed comparing the sources of LT used by patients with EMS versus asymptomatic controls. In the Oregon study, controls were identified through a random telephone survey.[41] In the Minnesota study, controls were identified by a random-digit-dialing telephone survey of Minneapolis-St. Paul area households and from individuals who called the Minnesota Department of Health following public announcements.[42] In New York, controls were identified from a sample of LT users who called the New York State Department of Health hot line from November 13, 1989 through February 1, 1990. All three studies came to similar conclusions. In Oregon, 45 of 46 case patients (98%)

compared with three of 10 (30%) randomly selected controls and 15 of 31 (48%) volunteer controls had ingested LT produced by a single Japanese manufacturer. The odds of an EMS patient ingesting LT produced by that source were 23.4 times greater among case-associated lots than control lots (95% confidence interval, 2.8–1031). The Minnesota study revealed comparable information, with 29 of 30 case patients (97%) versus 21 of 35 controls (60%) having consumed LT manufactured by the same company (odds ratio, 19.3; 95% confidence interval, 2.5–844.9; $p < 0.001$). Strikingly similar results were obtained in the New York case-control study; of 113 case patients and 95 controls, all of the case patients and 69 (73%) of the controls used LT that was traced to the same source as in Oregon and Minnesota (odds ratio, infinite; 95% confidence limits, 10, infinite).[17]

Two studies, one performed in New York[17] and the other among patients of a psychiatric practice in South Carolina,[43] showed a relationship between dose of ingested LT and the occurrence of EMS. In the South Carolina study, 50% of patients (19 of 38) ingesting more than 4 g per day of implicated LT developed definite EMS, and 84% (32 of 38) developed either definite or possible EMS.[43] Increasing age also increased the risk for EMS; in contrast, gender, race and the use of other medications did not. The failure to find a gender or racial difference was especially striking because most of the reported series have shown increased occurrence in Caucasian females. The results from the South Carolina study suggest that this Caucasian female preponderance in most studies is due to greater exposure to LT than in other racial

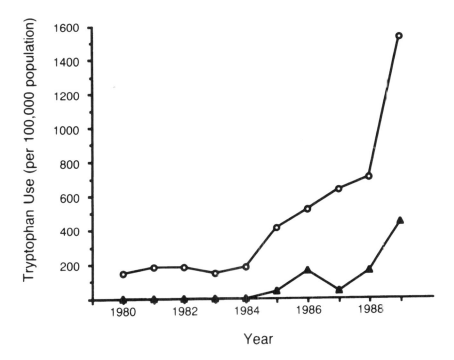

Fig. 6-2 Rates of tryptophan use among male (▲) and female (○) members of 2012 randomly selected households in metropolitan Minneapolis-St. Paul. Reprinted with permission from Belongia EA, Hedberg CW, Gleich GJ, *et al.* An investigation into the cause of the eosinophilia-myalgia syndrome associated with tryptophan use. *N Engl J Med.* 1990;323:357–365. Copyright 1990 Massachusetts Medical Society. All rights reserved.

groups or in men.[43] The South Carolina study also failed to find an association between EMS and various classes of medications; a similar result was found in the Minnesota case-control analysis.[42] In the New York study, a logistic regression model including dosage, indication for use and concurrent use of psychotropic medication showed that only increased dosage, older age and use of LT as a sleeping aid independently increased the risk of developing EMS.[17]

In Germany, all of the formulators of LT-containing products used raw materials exclusively from Japanese sources.[7] Cases of EMS were associated with LT from only two of the nine German companies. Both of these had used LT produced by the same source implicated for EMS in the United States. Thus the results seen in the United States were corroborated by findings in Germany.

L-Tryptophan Contaminants Associated with EMS

1,1'-Ethylidenebis(tryptophan)

The hypothesis that contaminants of LT were associated with EMS was tested by analyzing implicated and nonimplicated lots using high-performance liquid chromatography (HPLC).[42,44] These analyses took advantage of information that some lots of LT produced by the implicated Japanese manufacturer were involved in the causation of EMS, whereas others were not. A characteristic HPLC chromatographic pattern was associated with LT produced by that company, Showa Denko KK. Furthermore, the presence of a single peak was significantly associated with case lots (Figure 6-3).[42,45] This peak, referred to as peak E (for its associ-

ation with eosinophilia), was present in nine of 12 case lots (75%) and three of 11 control lots (27%) (odds ratio, 8.0; 95% CI. 0.92–76.6; p = 0.022). To determine whether the presence of peak E was related to manufacturing conditions employed by Showa Denko KK, the association between peak E and the use of *Bacillus amyloliquefaciens* strain 5, the use of 10 kg of powdered carbon per batch of LT and partial bypass of the reverse osmosis filter were examined.[42] The rationale for these tests comes from information regarding the manufacturing process employed by Showa Denko KK in which a genetically engineered strain of *B. amyloliquefaciens* (strain 5) that increased the synthesis of serine and 5-phosphoribosyl-1-pyrophosphate was introduced into the manufacturing process after December 25, 1988. Further, during the manufacturing process, the fermentation broth was subjected to several purification procedures, including exposure to powdered activated carbon and then to granular activated carbon. The quantities of powdered carbon employed in 1988 were generally equal to or greater than 20 kg per batch, whereas in 1989 the amount of powdered carbon in most batches was reduced to 10 kg. Also, from October 1988 to June 1989, a portion of some fermentation batches bypassed a filtration step employing a reverse-osmosis-membrane to remove chemicals with molecular weights of more than 1000. Initial analyses showed an association between development of EMS and the consumption of LT manufactured with 10 kg of powdered carbon per batch (p = 0.003), with *B. amyloliquefaciens* strain 5 (p = 0.003), and with partial bypassing of the reverse-osmosis filter (p = 0.001). Analyses of these conditions for their effect on peak E by stepwise multiple logistic regression demonstrated that the use of *B. amyloliquefaciens* strain 5 is the only variable

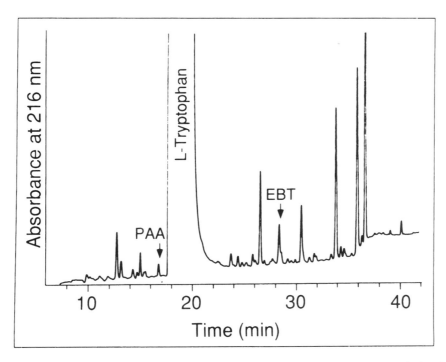

Fig. 6-3 High-performance liquid chromatography of EMS-associated L-tryptophan. Reprinted with permission from Mayeno AN, Gleich GJ. Eosinophilia-myalgia syndrome and tryptophan production: A cautionary tale. *TIBS Tech.* 1994;12:346–352.

significantly associated with the presence of peak E (p < 0.001). Here, the independent effects of bacterial strain and the amount of powdered carbon could not be distinguished because of their high correlations. Finally, HPLC analyses of LT consumed by the single patient with EMS who had consumed LT from a company other than Showa Denko KK (*vide supra*) demonstrated a chromatographic pattern that was characteristic of LT produced by Showa Denko KK, and peak E was also present. Thus it seems probable that the LT consumed by this patient was manufactured by Showa Denko KK.

The results of the Minnesota studies showed that implicated LT was produced by Showa Denko KK during the period from October 1988 to June 1989, and most patients had consumed lots produced during February 1989.[42] In Oregon, implicated lots of LT were produced from January through May 1989.[41] Subsequent analyses by Showa Denko KK itself showed that peak E levels increased to 300 parts per million in LT manufactured from January 1989 through April 1989 (Figure 6-4).[45] This finding suggests that some alteration in the manufacturing process occurred during this time, and that this was unrelated to strain 5. This conclusion seems reasonable because strain 5 was employed throughout 1989, and yet by September 1989 the concentration of peak E in LT lots was less than 25 parts per million. The precise changes which resulted in the remarkably increased concentration of peak E in lots produced in early 1989 remain obscure. It is noteworthy that peak E had been present in LT lots produced during 1988, but at maximal concentrations of approximately 50 parts per million and usually less than 25 parts per million (Figure 6-4).

The chemical structure of peak E revealed that it is 1,1'-ethylidenebis(tryptophan) (EBT) (Figure 6-5).[46] Although two reports initially suggested that the structure was 1-methyl-1,2,3,4-tetrahydro-β-carboline-3-carboxylic acid,[47,48] a test of the chemical linkage between the two tryptophans showed that the linkage was between the two indole nitrogens rather than the alpha amino groups.[46,49,50] It is worthy of mention that EBT hydrolyzes under acidic conditions, with a half-life of approximately 12 hours at pH 2 and 25°C. However, the half-life of gastric emptying following ingestion of water is approximately 10 minutes,[51] so it is likely that significant quantities of EBT would reach the small intestine and be available for absorption.

Phenylaminoalanine

The initial studies of the EMS-associated contaminants in LT by HPLC revealed EBT and also more than 60 minor contaminants.[52] Comparison of case-associated and nonimplicated LT showed the occurrence of two additional peaks, which were present in higher concentrations in implicated LT and not in control lots, namely peaks UV-5 and UV-28.[53] Peak UV-5 eluted before LT (Figure 6-3) and was determined to be 3-(phenylamino)alanine (PAA) (Figure 6-6).[54,55] Analyses of lots of LT consumed by patients with EMS and by control LT users showed that both PAA and EBT concentrations were considerably higher in the implicated lots compared to the control lots.[55] The median concentration of PAA was 89 ppm (range 35 to 160) in six retail lots consumed by patients and 31 ppm (range 11 to 88) in six retail lots consumed by control LT users (p = 0.055). The median concen-

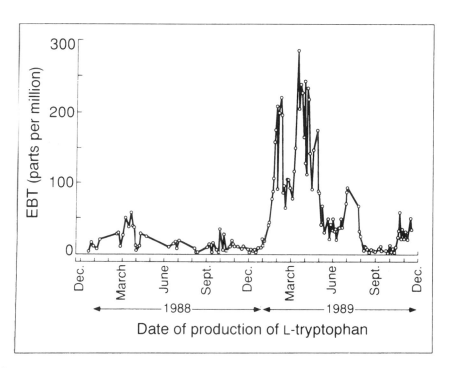

Fig. 6-4 Levels of 1,1'-ethylidenebis (L-tryptophan) (EBT) in lots of L-tryptophan produced by Showa Denko KK during 1988 and 1989. Reprinted with permission from Mayeno AN, Gleich GJ. Eosinophilia-myalgia syndrome and tryptophan production: A cautionary tale. *TIBS Tech.* 1994;12:346–352.

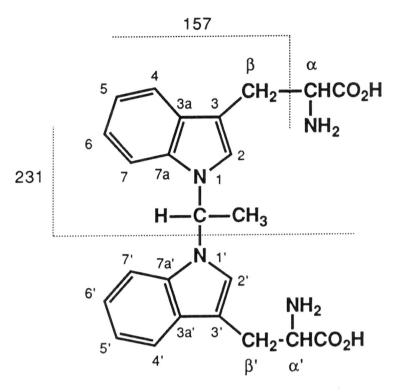

Fig. 6-5 The chemical structure of 1,1′-ethylidenebis (L-tryptophan). The numbering of the atoms in the tryptophan dimer is indicated, as are the massive fragments derived from fast atom bombardment-mass spectrometry. Reprinted with permission from Mayeno AN, Lin F, Foote CS, *et al.* Characterization of "Peak E", a novel aminoacid associated with the eosinophilia-myalgia syndrome. *Science.* 1990;250: 1707–1708. Copyright 1990 American Association for the Advancement of Science.

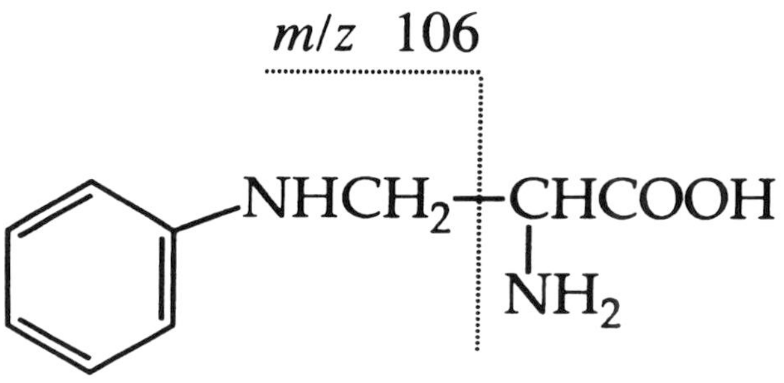

Fig. 6-6 The chemical structure of phenylaminoalanine. Fast atom bombardment-mass spectrometry gave a fragment with a peak at *M/z* 106. Reprinted with permission from Mayeno AN, Belongia EA, Lin F, Lundy SK, Gleich GJ. 3-(phenylamino)alanine, a novel aniline-derived amino acid associated with the eosinophilia-myalgia syndrome: A link to the toxic oil syndrome? *Mayo Clin Proc.* 1992;67:1134–1139.

tration of EBT was 114 ppm in the case lots (range 14 to 226) and 34 ppm in the control lots (range 8 to 75) (p = 0.025). These results indicate that the concentrations of both PAA and EBT were approximately threefold higher in EMS case lots than in control lots.

PAA is structurally similar to 3-phenylamino-1,2-propanediol (PAP), a substance isolated from samples of denatured oil implicated in the causation of TOS.[56] Because EMS and TOS share clinical and pathologic features, the discovery of chemically related contaminants raised the possibility of a common pathogenesis. Only two reactions, oxidation and transamination, are necessary to convert PAP to PAA (Figure 6-7).[55] Subsequent analyses showed that PAP can be transformed into PAA by both rat hepatocytes and human liver tissue.[57] However, the importance of this common link between EMS and TOS rests upon showing that these compounds cause disease, and, as will be discussed in detail

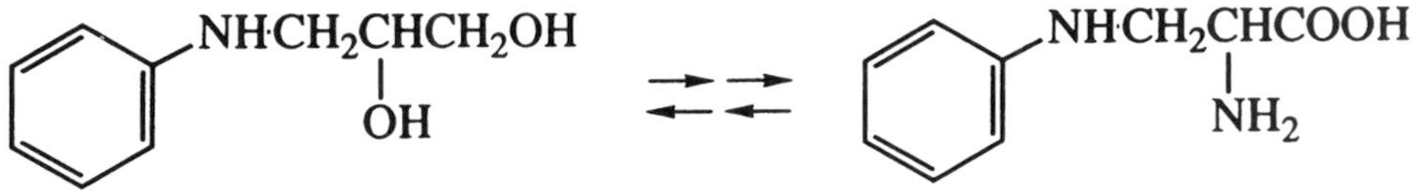

3-Phenylamino-1,2-propanediol   **3-(Phenylamino)alanine**

Fig. 6-7 Schema for conversion of 3-phenylamino-1,2-propanediol to PAA. Reprinted with permission; see Figure 6-6.

below, a robust animal model of these diseases remains elusive.

Other Contaminants

Continuing analyses of LT associated with EMS, utilizing case-associated LT lots from EMS patients who used only a single brand of LT, showed that six contaminants were associated with EMS.[52] The structures of three of these, namely EBT, PAA, and 2,3-indolylmethyl-L-tryptophan (peak 200) are known,[46,50,54,55,58] but the structures of the other three contaminants are currently unknown.[52] Furthermore, one contaminant, peak AAA, remained significantly associated with EMS even when the results were corrected with conditional logistic regression analysis stratified by time.[59] This adjustment for the strong sequential pattern over time among case and noncase lots showed that higher EBT levels are still associated with the lot's case status but that this association lacks statistical significance.[59] Application of this adjustment to the contaminants identified in priority case lots (defined as case lots taken by patients developing EMS with only brief exposure to a single LT brand, for example, use of only one bottle of LT or use of only one brand for 60 days or less) showed that only peak AAA is significantly associated with cases of EMS.[58] The other contaminant peaks, which were significant by other statistical tests, were not significant in the analyses using the time-dependence of LT production.

Finally, another report indicated that ingestion of L-5-hydroxytryptophan is associated with the occurrence of an EMS-related illness.[60] Analyses of the L-5-hydroxytryptophan in one of these cases showed an impurity eluting shortly after LT.[60] However, the nature of the impurity was not determined.

Biological Activities Associated with Implicated L-Tryptophan and L-Tryptophan Contaminants

Animal Models of EMS

The discovery of contaminants associated with EMS prompted a series of investigations to determine whether a bioassay or an animal model could be established. Establishment of either of these would permit a dissection of the LT contaminants to identify the critical contaminants. An early study[61] utilized Lewis rats as the model animal because of prior research indicating their sensitivity to various stimuli.[62] Implicated LT was administered by gavage to Lewis rats at doses comparable to those ingested by patients who developed EMS. Animals receiving implicated LT, but not those receiving USP grade LT or vehicle, developed histologic signs consistent with EMS. Peripheral blood eosinophilia was not observed.[51] Subsequent analyses in Lewis rats showed that case-associated LT, EBT and the "control" LT

(not implicated in the causation of EMS) induced increased fascial thickening compared with the vehicle-treated control animals.[63] Similarly, significant pancreatic pathology was noted in this study, and again this was seen both with implicated LT, EBT and "control" LT.[63] Analyses of immune activation showed that only animals treated with case-associated LT for six weeks showed increased frequencies of CD8, Ia and IL-2 receptor-positive cells in the peripheral blood. This study confirmed the pathological effects of EBT. But because persons ingesting "control" LT had not become ill during the EMS epidemic, the observation that "control" LT caused abnormalities in the Lewis rat raises questions about the validity of this animal model. In addition, Lewis rats treated with implicated LT showed increased perivascular inflammatory infiltrates enriched for degranulating mast cells, eosinophils and monocytes in the intestinal lamina propria.[64]

In female C57BL/6 mice, daily intraperitoneal administration of EBT stimulated inflammation and fibrosis in the dermis and subcutis, including the fascia and perimysial tissues.[65] In this model, inflammation was evident by day 6, but was more striking by day 21, as was fibrosis in the subcutis and dermis. Mast cells were also increased in the subcutis and dermis, especially during the first week of exposure. Quinolinic acid was initially lower in the plasma of animals exposed to EBT and subsequently, by day 21 and up to day 24, was significantly elevated. Continuing investigation of this model has shown enhanced expression of genes for types I, III and VI collagen in the dermis and subcutis of animals treated with EBT for three to 21 days.[66] However, these changes did not appear to achieve statistical significance, and although increased expression of TGF-β1 and of types I, III and VI collagen was observed, no quantitative analyses of these data were provided to ensure that the results differed among the various groups.

Attempts to demonstrate the toxicity of PAA in Wistar rats have shown that PAA is absorbed through the gastrointestinal tract, reaches peak blood levels approximately five hours after gastric gavage, and passes through the blood-brain barrier. Four metabolites of PAA were identified.[67] Lewis rats treated for six weeks by incorporation of PAA into their food pellets showed accumulation in tissues, and after 12 days on a PAA-free diet, levels of the drugs were still detectable in all tissues.[68] Administration of PAA to Sprague-Dawley rats for 13 consecutive weeks at dosages up to 100 ml per kg per day did not reveal any significant abnormalities to distinguish test animals from control animals.[69] Moreover, eosinophilia was not observed in any of these animals, and no thickening or inflammatory infiltrates occurred in the fascia.

Showa Denko KK also attempted to identify an animal model for EMS. In spite of tests on F-344 and Lewis rats and BALB/c mice, the administration of feed grade LT (presumably containing more impurities than that sold during the epidemic period in 1989), as well as EBT and 1-methyl-1,2,3,4-tetrahydro-β-carboline-3-carboxylic acid, no abnormalities characteristic of EMS were observed. Finally, in one report which tested the effects of intraperitoneal injection of EBT and unimplicated LT in Lewis rats, only sparse tissue eosinophilia was noted.[70]

A critique of all animal studies concluded that none was reproducible in the hands of other investigators.[71] Thus the present status of investigations of animal models is not satisfying. The absence of a robust animal model is a significant impediment to solving the riddle of which contaminant(s) in the implicated LT was responsible for disease causation.

Bioassays for L-Tryptophan and L-Tryptophan Contaminants Associated with EMS

As noted above, an animal model would be a valuable tool to dissect the pathophysiology of EMS as well as to identify the components in the contaminated LT causing disease. Because EMS patients developed striking eosinophilia, and since eosinophil maturation is under the control of cytokines such as IL-5, IL-3 and GM-CSF,[72] another approach to these questions would be the establishment of a bioassay for contaminants stimulating cytokine production by cells. This possibility is strengthened by a report that IL-5 activity was increased in the blood of patients with EMS[73] and another report that purified eosinophils degranulate when exposed to either EBT or implicated LT.[74] In the latter report, both implicated LT and peak E stimulated IL-5 receptor expression on eosinophils and production of IL-5 by splenic T cells. These results suggest that EBT is involved in the pathogenesis of EMS by activating eosinophils themselves and by causing IL-5 production by T cells.[74] However, neither eosinophil activation nor production of IL-5 by peripheral blood mononuclear cells by implicated LT or by the contaminants EBT and PAA could be demonstrated by other investigators (Kita H, Gleich GJ unpublished data). Another study tested the ability of LT contaminants to stimulate bone marrow cells and peripheral blood mononuclear cells and concluded that EBT or 1-methyl-1,2,3,4-tetrahydro-β-carboline-3-carboxylic acid, in conjunction with IL-2, induced eosinophil colonies from human bone marrow cultures.[75] Moreover, LT constituents plus IL-2 induced increased IL-6, but not IL-1β, in the peripheral blood mononuclear cells of normal individuals.[75]

The effects of EBT and two of its diastereoisomeric breakdown products were tested on spinal cord cultures derived from fetal mice.[76] Normally, about 30% of these immature spinal cord neuronal cells die in culture. In one-month-old spinal cord cultures (in which the numbers of neurons remain stable), one synthetic diastereoisomer, (-)-(1S,3S)-1-methyl-1,2,3,4-tetrahydro-β-carboline-3-carboxylic acid, (1S—βc), produced a 30% to 35% loss in the number of neurons; the R isomer of the same compound and EBT were not toxic, and neutralizing antiserum against the murine IL-1 receptor prevented the neuronal death associated with 1S—βc. In contrast to these results, 1S—βc in immature spinal

cord neuronal cultures prevented the 30% cell death which normally occurs in these cultures. These results, showing a stereospecificity for the EBT metabolites, were interpreted as supporting a role for the compounds in the pathophysiology of the neuropathic abnormalities associated with EMS.[76]

The possibility that EBT is incorporated into protein has also been explored.[77] First, competitive binding of LT and EBT to nuclear membranes was determined using ^{3}H tryptophan as the ligand. These results indicated that EBT has only a minimal inhibitory effect on the binding of radiolabeled LT to hepatic nuclear envelopes. Second, the possibility that EBT might be incorporated into protein was tested utilizing microsomes in a cell-free system. These results suggested that EBT might be incorporated into protein, as judged by inhibition of incorporation of radiolabeled LT compared to radiolabeled leucine. Third, radiolabeled EBT was incorporated into protein; this conclusion is strengthened by knowledge that the EBT was labeled in the ethylidene bridge and not in the LT residues. Although this result could be explained by hydrolysis of the LT to liberate a breakdown product, for example, acetaldehyde, this would not seem likely under the described conditions. Thus EBT might be incorporated into proteins and, hence, stimulate the immune system by formation of unnatural (antigenic) protein molecules.

Two studies concluded that EBT stimulates collagen production. In one,[78] EBT increased DNA synthesis in dermal fibroblasts up to fourfold in a concentration-dependent manner and caused a greater-than-threefold increase in alpha 1 (I) procollagen mRNA levels and collagenous protein. These results encourage belief that EBT stimulates fibroblasts to produce collagen and they are in keeping with the demonstration that fibroblast collagen synthesis is activated in biopsies from patients with EMS (*vide infra*). In the other study, EBT but not its hydrolysis product, MTCA, caused a concentration-dependent increase in collagen synthesis and in type I collagen mRNA levels independent of its effect on proliferation.[79] In contrast, expression of fibronectin mRNA was not altered. These results provide further support for EBT as a cause of fibrosis in EMS.

Finally, considering the importance of a bioassay both to dissect pathophysiology and to serve as a means of detecting specific contaminants within implicated LT, it is surprising that the bioassays noted above have not been used to identify the specific contaminants in implicated LT (other than EBT and PAA).

The Pathophysiology of EMS

Although EBT emerges as a strong contender for certain of the pathological manifestations of EMS, in particular the characteristic fibrosis which occurs in many patients, the pathogenic role of other contaminants is unknown. The possibility that the clinical and pathological sequelae were related to toxic products of LT metabolism has been investigated by measurement of plasma levels of LT, L-kynurenine and quinolinic acid in patients with EMS.[80] The results indicated that levels of LT in untreated EMS patients are lower than in glucocorticoid-treated EMS patients and in asymptomatic individuals consuming LT. Correspondingly, levels of L-kynurenine were increased in untreated EMS patients compared to normal controls and asymptomatic LT users, and plasma quinolinic acid was higher in untreated EMS patients compared to the controls. The levels of L-kynurenine and quinolinic acid in both treated and untreated EMS patients were strongly correlated ($r = +0.85$, $p < 0.01$). Significant correlations between eosinophil counts in the EMS patients and plasma L-kynurenine and quinolinic acid concentrations were also present ($r = 0.76$, $p < 0.001$ and $r = +0.67$, $p < 0.005$, respectively). Administration of an oral loading dose of LT led to reduced plasma levels of LT in untreated EMS patients and elevated L-kynurenine and quinolinic acids in these patients compared to normal controls and to glucocorticoid-treated EMS patients.[80] Glucocorticoid therapy of patients with EMS resulted in reductions in their plasma levels of L-kynurenine and quinolinic acid. Further, both L-kynurenine and quinolinic acid were elevated in the cerebrospinal fluids of patients with EMS compared to normal controls. To investigate the possible role of interferon (IFN)-γ, a potent inducer of indoleamine-2,3-dioxygenase and the rate-limiting enzyme in the kynurenine pathway,[81–83] four patients with scleroderma were given IFN-γ, and LT metabolites were measured both before and after IFN-γ administration.[80] This administration resulted in striking elevations of LT metabolites in serum, but statistical significance was not achieved ($p = 0.06$). The authors interpreted their data as consistent with the hypothesis that LT metabolites, especially quinolinic acid (which has direct neurotoxic effects[84] at concentrations sometimes comparable to those in EMS patients), played a significant role in the pathogenesis of the disease.

However, the reason that LT administration with its associated contaminants causes the elevations in LT metabolites is unknown.[35] The possibility that IFN-γ might drive these abnormalities has been tested. Only two of 20 sera from patients with EMS contained levels of IFN-γ above the normal range.[85] Nonetheless, serum levels may not reflect tissue concentrations, so this finding cannot be taken as evidence that IFN-γ has no effect, but rather that IFN-γ concentrations were not so great as to be reflected in the peripheral circulation. Furthermore, neopterin, a marker of macrophage activation induced by IFN-γ,[86] was elevated in the serum of patients with TOS but not in patients with EMS, whether or not the EMS patients had received glucocorticoids.[87] Thus, these studies of LT metabolism demonstrate that a toxic metabolite, quinolinic acid, is elevated, and may be partially responsible for the pathophysiological manifestations of EMS. These abnormalities suggest that an LT contaminant(s) altered the functioning of the immune system in such a manner as to induce IFN-γ, increase indoleamine-2,3-dioxygenase activity and increase the production of quinolinic acid.

Evidence for immune activation comes from studies of infiltrating leukocytes in affected tissues of patients with EMS. Analyses of patients with EMS did not show abnormalities in levels of T cells nor activation of T cells in the peripheral blood (Gleich GJ, unpublished data). However, investigation of tissues showed a predominant T cell infiltrate with CD8+ cells outnumbering CD4+ cells by sixfold to twentyfold.[88] Between 60% and 80% of the T cells in this study were activated. In contrast, B cells and eosinophils were relatively sparse (accounting for less than 3% of inflammatory cells), very few cells expressed the γΔ T cell receptor or natural killer-cell markers, and the microvascular complement membrane attack complex was absent.[88] The authors interpreted these findings to indicate the existence of a cellular immune response directed against a connective tissue component in EMS. Another report demonstrated that inflammatory cells in tissue consist predominantly of CD8+ T cells, accounting for $45 \pm 8.9\%$ of infiltrating cells, compared with $36 \pm 10\%$ CD4 cells and $19 \pm 12\%$ macrophages.[89] Mean numbers of fibroblasts in the fascia, perimysial connective tissue and the spindle capsule were increased in EMS patients' specimens compared to patients with chronic inflammatory myopathies or dystrophies ($p < 0.01$). Thirty percent of fibroblasts in EMS muscle biopsy specimens expressed HLA-DR antigen, whereas none of the control samples expressed this antigen. These authors also concluded that the T cells were the predominant cell among the infiltrates. They also showed that the number of eosinophils was small, comprising less than 1% of the total cell infiltrates, and they did not detect widespread deposition of eosinophil granule major basic protein (MBP) in these samples. They concluded that the fibroblast may be the target cell in EMS. That is, proinflammatory cytokines could induce HLA-DR expression on tissue fibroblasts which, in turn, could result in activation of T cells, culminating in a cellular autoimmune attack against the fibroblasts and extracellular matrix.

Evidence for eosinophil involvement in EMS comes from initial observations showing increases in peripheral blood eosinophils,[38] as well as increases in eosinophil degranulation shown by strikingly elevated levels of two eosinophil granule proteins, namely MBP and the eosinophil-derived neurotoxin (EDN) in both serum and urine of affected patients. Serum levels of MBP and EDN were approximately tenfold greater than normal values, urine levels of MBP were up to sixtyfold greater, and EDN up to a thousandfold greater than in normal individuals.[38] Histologic localization of eosinophils and eosinophil degranulation by staining for eosinophil granule MBP showed striking eosinophil degranulation in tissues of some patients, whereas others were less impressive.[12]

Investigation of EMS patients with cutaneous fibrosis has demonstrated thickening of the fascia with deep dermal fibrosis and accumulation of mononuclear cells and eosinophils.[90] Affected skin biopsy specimens from four patients with EMS and fibrosis examined by *in situ* hybridization for type I procollagen gene expression showed increased hybridization signals in the deep dermis and fascia.[90] These results point to a causal relationship between stimulation of fibroblasts, collagen gene expression and dermal and fascial fibrosis. A subsequent analysis of cutaneous fibrotic lesions from seven patients with EMS and six patients with TOS demonstrated significantly more staining in skin biopsy specimens with antibody to TGF-β (p < 0.05) and platelet-derived growth factor (p < 0.05) in EMS compared with TOS.[91] These reports suggest that the pathophysiology of tissue fibrosis may differ in EMS and TOS.

Finally, tissue eosinophilia and eosinophil degranulation are associated with fibrosis. For example, while eosinophilia in lymph nodes is frequent in patients with Hodgkin's disease, only the nodular sclerosing variant has striking extracellular deposition of the granule MBP.[92] Furthermore, eosinophil infiltration and degranulation are increased in inflammatory fibrotic conditions such as retroperitoneal fibrosis, sclerosing mediastinitis, sclerosing cholangitis and pulmonary fibrosis, whereas noninflammatory fibrotic lesions, such as keloids, scars, Dupuytren's contracture and fibrosclerosis, showed neither eosinophil infiltration nor degranulation.[93] Similarly, two other syndromes associated with fibrosis and inflammation, namely orbital pseudotumor[94] and Riedel's invasive fibrous thyroiditis,[95] both show striking tissue eosinophilia and eosinophil degranulation; whereas other thyroid diseases, including multinodular goiter, Graves' disease and Hashimoto's disease, and normal thyroid tissue do not demonstrate these abnormalities.[95] The mechanisms by which the eosinophil might cause fibrosis remain largely undefined, although eosinophil-conditioned tissue culture media stimulated fibroblast proliferation and collagen production,[96] and the granule protein, eosinophil-derived neurotoxin, stimulated fibroblast proliferation.[97] Also, eosinophils express transforming growth factor-β (TGF-β_1)[98] and tissue eosinophils expressing TGF-β_1 have been related to fibrosis in asthma.[99]

Spectrum of Organ-Specific Disease

The onset of EMS is protean, with generalized myalgia and fatigue often accompanied by fever, a diffuse erythematous macular (occasionally urticarial) skin rash, prominent peripheral edema and weight loss.[100] Approximately 20% of individuals develop pulmonary infiltrates, resembling the Löffler syndrome (pulmonary infiltrates with eosinophilia). Over two to six months, the evolution of disease is typified by hyperesthesia, neuropathy, myopathy, alopecia, xerostomia, polyarthralgia (less frequently synovitis), distinct muscle spasm and fibrosing skin disease.[100] The progression of disease is variable. Although a benign course may occur,[101] most individuals who come to medical attention and are fol-

lowed up at referral centers have chronic morbidity related to muscle cramping, neuropathy, musculoskeletal soft tissue pain syndromes, cutaneous scarring with hyperpigmentation, profound fatigue and cognitive impairment.[102,103] EMS is potentially fatal, with a mortality of 2.7% during the first year[104] ascribed most commonly to severe ascending paralysis[104] and less often to sequelae of pulmonary hypertension,[12] myocarditis[12] and possible arrythmia due to cardioneuropathy.[104,105] Furthermore, in view of a strict case definition established by the Centers for Disease Control (CDC) for surveillance purposes and passive reporting, the total number of deaths is likely to be even greater.[106]

The evolution of EMS occurs over acute, intermediate and chronic stages (Table 6-1).[107] However, these are arbitrary subdivisions and should be considered part of a continuum. Despite the characteristic clinical findings of EMS, there has been no consensus regarding diagnostic criteria. The lack of a uniform case definition, variability of sampling time and likely differences in the populations studied have all contributed to a broad fluctuation in prevalence for some of the clinical findings displayed in Table 6-2.

Skin

Sclerodermatous skin thickening that mimics SSc or DEF is the most notable cutaneous manifestation of

Table 6-1 Clinical stages of EMS

Acute (≤ 2 mo)	Intermediate (2–6 mo)	Chronic (> 6 mo)
Myalgia	Myalgia	Myalgia
Arthralgia[a]	Arthralgia	Arthralgia[a]
Fever/fatigue	Fatigue	Fatigue
Diffuse erythematous rash	Sclerodermalike skin thickening[b]	Sclerodermalike skin thickening[b]
Hyperesthesia	Neuropathy[c]	Neuropathy[d]
Dyspnea/cough[e]	Dyspnea[f]	Dyspnea[g]
Diarrhea	Myopathy	Myopathy
Myocarditis	Muscle cramps	Muscle cramps[h]
	Alopecia	Cutaneous hyperpigmentation
	Xerostomia	Cognitive impairment
		Tremor[i]
		Myokymia

[a]Occasional synovitis.

[b]Peau d'orange (eosinophilic fasciitis) and/or induration resembling systemic sclerosis (diffuse, limited or localized).

[c]Sensory or sensorimotor (occasionally with ascending Guillain-Barré-like paralysis).

[d]Sensory or sensorimotor > mononeuritis multiplex.

[e]Parenchymal or interstitial infiltrates > pulmonary hypertension.

[f]Interstitial lung disease; pulmonary hypertension.

[g]Respiratory muscle fatigue > interstitial lung disease; pulmonary hypertension.

[h]In some patients associated with myoclonus.

[i]Effort and posture related.

Reprinted with permission from reference 107.

Table 6-2 Prevalence of selected chronic features in EMS*

Manifestation	Percentage
Fatigue	35–95
Myalgia	50–91
Neuropathy	30–91
Muscle cramps	43–90
Subjective cognitive impairment	33–86
Sclerodermatous skin change	44–82
Arthralgia	41–77
Myopathy	40–75
Dyspnea	8–50
Hyperpigmentation	25–42

*Summary of follow-up data ranging from 12 to 36 months
Reprinted with permission from reference 107.

EMS.[35,90,108–117] Skin induration may be diffuse,[35,90,108–112,117] limited[35,90,108–112,117] or localized (morpheaform and linear)[108,115] in distribution. Fibrosing skin changes are often associated with papular mucinosis[9,118–120] and parallel the deposition of mucin in SSc.[121] Hyperpigmentation, a late feature of EMS, may occur with or without skin thickening.[103,122] Patients with EMS do not develop acral sclerosis, Raynaud phenomenon, digital ischemic lesions or tendon friction rubs,[10,16,115,123–125] all hallmarks of diffuse SSc.

EMS is a clinically more severe disease than idiopathic DEF.[115,124–126] Histopathologically, it can be distinguished from DEF by the presence of pancutaneous and subcutaneous inflammation, whereas in DEF inflammation is localized to the subcutis.[127] Furthermore, perineural inflammatory lesions are found in EMS and are rare in DEF.[127] Tissue eosinophilia does not differentiate EMS from DEF.[124,127] In fact, it is not uncommon to find a paucity of tissue eosinophilia in both DEF[128] and EMS.[88,89,117,129–132]

Neuromuscular Manifestations

Incapacitating myalgia is considered among the defining features of EMS. Severe and distinctive muscle cramping is common throughout all stages of illness, occurring predominantly in the jaw, lower extremities, abdominal wall and subcostal muscles. The report of a dental fracture[16] underscores the force of this muscle spasm, which in some individuals has been shown to be the consequence of myoclonus.[133]

Proximal muscle weakness[10,13,14,16,123,134] resembling the idiopathic inflammatory myopathies is common during the initial several months of disease. However, in contradistinction to the pathologic changes of polymyositis, the inflammatory lesion of EMS is perimysial[88,129–132,135] and rarely associated with myonecrosis.[12,129,135,136] Although a microangiopathy with arterial or arteriolar lymphocytic infiltrates by light microscopy and capillary or arteriolar endothelial thickening by electron microscopy have been described,[137] necrotizing vasculitis is absent.[12,129,130,132,135] This important feature distinguishes EMS from the Churg-Strauss variant of systemic necrotizing vasculitis.

Neurologic involvement usually manifests as an axonal sensorimotor peripheral neuropathy,[9,10,16,36,138] at times complicated by an ascending paralytic course.[16,139,140] The pathology of peripheral nerve involvement is a perineurial inflammatory infiltrate with axonal sparing and parallels the sparing of myofibers of muscle. Sensory neuropathy on examination may be discordant from electrophysiologic studies,[103] most likely related to the insensitivity of standard nerve conduction velocities to detect the perineuritis of small dermal nerves.[14,127,137,141] Additional manifestations of peripheral nerve disease include mononeuritis multiplex,[142] demyelinating neuropathy,[143,144] tremor,[133] myokymia[133] and myoclonus.[133] Acute central nervous system disease with white matter lesions on magnetic resonance imaging has been rarely noted.[12,145–148]

Fatigue and Cognitive Impairment

Fatigue, depressive symptoms and cognitive deficits are common disabling features of EMS. Fatigue severity correlates with pain intensity and depressive symptoms. Some patients have had diffuse pain syndromes consistent with fibromyalgia[149] which may be analogous to soft tissue and chronic fatigue syndromes following infectious triggers.[150,151]

Impairment of memory, concentration and word finding were reported to be present in 42% to 63% of individuals with EMS who were surveyed by questionnaire one to two years after disease onset.[152] Preliminary studies of cognitive function demonstrated that 15 of 24 (62%) patients with subjective cognitive complaints had impairment on tests of verbal and visual memory, conceptual reasoning and motor speed when compared with age- and education-matched controls.[153] One-year follow-up studies in 11 patients from this group of 24 revealed no change or worsening in those individuals with impairment.[154] Furthermore, EMS patients score worse in these same cognitive areas when compared to controls matched for level of depressive symptoms, indicating that depression does not fully explain cognitive deficits.

Articular Involvement

Polyarthralgia occurs in up to 50% of patients with EMS and most often affect the knees, elbows and shoulders.[1,9,10,13,17,155] Synovitis has occasionally been observed as part of the acute[9] and chronic[103] manifestations of EMS. Joint contractures of the upper and lower extremities commonly occur in association with sclerodermatous skin thickening.[156]

Pulmonary Manifestations

Dyspnea and/or cough were reported in up to two-thirds of patients with acute disease and were accompanied by interstitial or alveolar pulmonary infiltrates and/or pleural effusion in 10% to 50% of these individuals.[1,9,10,14,16,155,157] Pleural effusions were characterized as both sterile exudates[9,158,159] as well as transudates,[160] and occasionally manifested increased numbers of eosinophils.[161]

Lung biopsies have demonstrated interstitial and alveolar collections of lymphocytes, macrophages, occasional plasma cells and variable numbers of eosinophils.[159,161,162] Immunophenotyping of cells in lung biopsy specimens[163] and bronchoalveolar lavage (BAL) fluid[161] from a small number of patients demonstrated the primary effector cell to be a CD8+ lymphocyte. Prominent perivascular and vessel wall infiltrates producing a nonnecrotizing vasculitis have also been noted.[159,160,162,164] This "vasculitic" lesion was noted more often in the pulmonary than the systemic circulation. The presence of inflammatory pulmonary disease in EMS is distinctly different from the noninflammatory lesion characteristic of early lung involvement in TOS.[165]

Acute and chronic pulmonary hypertension has been observed in EMS[161,162,166,167] as well as TOS.[165,168,169]

Many patients with EMS have respiratory complaints that are unexplained by pulmonary vascular and/or interstitial lung disease. These symptoms may be related to respiratory muscle dysfunction as determined by maximal static inspiratory and expiratory pressures.[170]

Cardiac Manifestations

Clinically documented cardiac abnormalities considered to be directly related to EMS include sinus tachycardia,[9,14] myocarditis,[12,155] coronary vasospasm[171] and right ventricular dysfunction secondary to pulmonary hypertension.[10,12]

Detailed pathological studies of the heart have revealed vascular and neural abnormalities consisting of small vessel coronary artery fibromuscular dysplasia, endarteritis and panarteritis affecting the sinus node, atrioventricular node and His bundle.[105] A unique inflammatory and/or fibrosing cardioneuropathy was also seen throughout the conduction system and in the coronary chemoreceptors. Furthermore, an obliterative periarterial fibrosis within the sinus node (similar to that occurring in SSc) was reported. Similar though less inflammatory lesions have also been observed in the hearts of patients dying of TOS.[172]

It is likely that the postmortem cardiac findings affecting the conduction system contributed to the sudden death of many patients with EMS. In that regard, cardiac manifestations prior to death were documented in 23 (64%) of patients whose deaths were reported to the CDC.[104] Furthermore, 15 (57%) of these individuals had an arrythmia and 12 (52%) had evidence of cardiac dysfunction or myocarditis.

Gastrointestinal Manifestations

Symptoms related to the gut during the acute epidemic of EMS were often omitted from clinical descriptions and were presumably underestimated or considered insignificant. Diarrhea was the most common manifestation recorded and in one series was present in 24% of 119 patients surveyed.[17] One report described abdominal bloating with diarrhea and hemorrhagic stools as the principal presenting features of two patients.[158] In another patient with malabsorption, a small bowel biopsy revealed deep mucosal eosinophil and mast cell infiltrates.[173] Similar findings were seen in the colonic mucosa of Lewis rats developing fasciitis and perimyositis following ingestion of implicated LT.[64]

Hepatomegaly, and at least one liver chemistry abnormality were present in 5% and 43%, respectively, of 1075 patients surveyed by the CDC.[1] In addition, 64% of the EMS patients whose deaths were reported to the CDC had clinical or pathological evidence of hepatic or pancreatic disease.[104] These figures are in contradistinction to the paucity of hepatobiliary[10,12] and pancreatic[174] involvement observed in clinical case series.

Little information has been accumulated concerning upper gastrointestinal complaints. Nevertheless, esophageal dysmotility was reported in six of nine patients undergoing radiographic or manometric evaluation.[10]

DIAGNOSIS OF EMS

Formal clinical and/or laboratory criteria for the diagnosis of EMS have not been established. The initial diagnostic guidelines formulated in 1989 by the CDC for national surveillance may have underestimated the number of individuals who developed EMS by approximately two- to threefold.[106] Peripheral blood eosinophilia may be absent in patients who otherwise demonstrate many clinical and/or pathological features of EMS. This may be critical for the diagnosis of sporadic cases of EMS and in differentiating EMS from related conditions. During acute/subacute disease, the constellation of myalgia, sclerodermalike skin changes (most often resembling eosinophilic fasciitis), paresthesia, alopecia and typical muscle cramping (frequently with trismus and subcostal involvement) are highly suggestive, if not characteristic, of EMS. The pathological finding of perimyositis and epineuritis on muscle and nerve biopsies helps to confirm the clinical suspicion.

Unfortunately, there is no single diagnostic test for EMS. An elevated serum aldolase (usually with a normal or low creatine kinase) in association with the clinical and biopsy findings outlined above helps to distinguish EMS from other myopathic or eosinophilic diseases.

In patients with chronic EMS initial symptoms may be nonspecific, and a suspected diagnosis is dependent upon data collected retrospectively. The muscle biopsy findings of late-stage EMS are not well delineated. Moreover, the late manifestations of EMS must be carefully differentiated from the protean features of idiopathic connective diseases, chronic fatigue syndrome, soft tissue rheumatic syndromes (such as fibromyalgia) and unrelated neuromuscular disorders.

THERAPY

Reports on therapy consist of anecdotal observations only. This is due to the highly epidemic nature in which EMS occurred, the distribution of a relatively small number of cases over a large geographical area and the lack of previous experience with this disease. No specific therapy has been demonstrated to alter the natural history of EMS. Recommendations should be individualized depending upon the needs and clinical findings of each patient.[175]

The abrupt onset of multisystem disease and inflammatory infiltrative lesions of skin, muscle and nerve initially led most clinicians to extrapolate therapy from experience with idiopathic connective-tissue diseases. Various immunomodulating agents were employed with disappointing results. Contrary to previous experience with most acute diseases associated with peripheral blood or tissue eosinophilia, corticosteroids have been of little benefit for the early or late manifestations of EMS. The most impressive impact of these agents appeared to be on the resolution of acute pulmonary infiltrates, with a modest decrease in myalgia and peripheral edema. Nevertheless, retrospective epidemiologic surveys and five years of prospective clinical observations indicate that corticosteroids do not appear to influence the development of cutaneous, neuropathic or chronic cardiopulmonary disease and cannot be advocated for these purposes. A short course of moderate- to high-dose prednisone therapy (40 to 60 mg per day for two to four weeks with subsequent tapering over an additional one to two months) would be appropriate to assess individual response during acute disease.

Chronic therapy in doses over 5 mg of prednisone per day is not indicated in EMS.

Antiinflammatory, immunosuppressive or immunomodulatory antirheumatic agents such as cyclophosphamide, azathioprine, hydroxyurea or cyclosporine have not demonstrated therapeutic efficacy. In one study, methotrexate (7.5 to 10 mg per week) was evaluated prospectively in seven EMS patients over a mean of 4.5 months. A significant (p < .05) increase in functional class and reductions in skin thickening (assessed by total skin score) and edema were reported. These findings are encouraging; however, in the absence of a control group or data confirming these results from other centers, it is difficult to assess the measured improvement as related to therapy or secondary to natural history. Plasmapheresis and intravenous gammaglobulin have also been utilized with reports of subjective improvement in some individuals. Unfortunately, these potentially toxic and/or expensive interventions cannot be recommended due to a paucity of data demonstrating efficacy. Plaquenil, D-penicillamine, colchicine, isotretinoin and flavonoids have been advocated in small numbers of patients. As with other isolated reports of benefit, measurement of improvement or resolution was not clearly defined.

In view of these findings, most clinicians experienced in the care of EMS patients have concluded that immunosuppressive agents are not recommended for the cutaneous, neuromuscular or constitutional manifestations of the disease. The optimal management of late EMS will most likely include a multidisciplinary approach based upon neurological, rheumatological, neuropsychological, psychiatric and

Table 6-3 Recommended pharmacologic therapy for common symptoms of chronic EMS

	Agent	Dosage
Muscle Cramping	Amitriptyline (Elavil)	10–50 mg/day
	Baclofen (Lioresal)	10–80 mg/day
	Dantrolene (Dantrium)*	25–150 mg/day
	Cyclobenzaprine (Flexeril)	10–40 mg/day
	Benzodiazepines[†]	
Depression	Amitriptyline (Elavil)	10–200 mg/day
	Fluoxetine (Prozac)	20–60 mg/day
	Sertraline (Zoloft)	50–200 mg/day
Insomnia	Amitriptyline (Elavil)	10–100 mg/day
	Trazodone (Desyrel)	25–100 mg/day
	Benzodiazepines[†]	
Fatigue	Pemoline (Cylert)	18.75–112.5 mg/day
	Amantadine (Symmetrel)	200 mg/day
	Methylphenidate (Ritalin)[†]	2.5–20 mg/day
	Fluoxetine (Prozac)	20 mg/day
Neuropathy	Amitriptyline (Elavil)	10–100 mg/day
	Nortriptyline (Pamelor)	10–75 mg/day

*Potential for significant hepatotoxicity.
[†]In selected patients.
Reprinted with permission from reference 107.

rehabilitative evaluations. The approach to selected clinical problems in this setting is outlined in Table 6-3.

REFERENCES

[1]Swygert LA, Maes EF, Sewell LE, Miller L, Falk H, Kilbourne EM. Eosinophilia-myalgia syndrome: Results of national surveillance. *JAMA.* 1990;264:1698–1703.

[2]Amor B, Rajzbaum G, Poiraudeau S, Haas C, Kahan A. Eosinophilia-myalgia linked with L-tryptophan (letter). *Lancet.* 1990;335:420.

[3]Centers for Disease Control. Eosinophilia-myalgia syndrome—Canada. *MMWR.* 1990;39:2–3.

[4]Walker KG, Eastmond CJ, Best PV, Matthews K. Eosinophilia-myalgia syndrome associated with prescribed L-tryptophan (letter). *Lancet.* 1990;336:695–696.

[5]Farinelli S, Mariani A, Grimaldi A, Mariani M, Iannessi A, DeRosa F. Eosinophilia-myalgia syndrome associated with 5-OH-tryptophan: Description of a case. *Rec Prog Med.* 1991;82:381–384.

[6]Mizutani T, Mizutani H, Hashimoto K, *et al.* Simultaneous development of two cases of eosinophilia-myalgia syndrome with the same lot of L-tryptophan in Japan. *J Am Acad Dermatol.* 1991;25:512–517.

[7]Carr L, Ruther E, Berg PA, Lehnert H. Eosinophilia-myalgia syndrome in Germany: An epidemiologic review. *Mayo Clin Proc.* 1994;69:620–625.

[8]Kaufman LD, Izquierdo Martinez M, Gomez Reino JJ. Toxic oil syndrome and eosinophilia myalgia syndrome: Similar, different or the same disorder? (editorial). *J Rheumatol.* 1994;21:2177–2178.

[9]Kaufman LD, Seidman RJ, Gruber BL. L-tryptophan associated eosinophilic perimyositis, neuritis, and fasciitis: A clinicopathologic and laboratory study of 25 patients. *Medicine* (Baltimore). 1990;69:187–199.

[10]Varga J, Heiman-Patterson TD, Emery DL, *et al.* Clinical spectrum of the systemic manifestations of the eosinophilia-myalgia syndrome. *Semin Arthritis Rheum.* 1990;19:313–328.

[11]Clauw DJ, Nashel DJ, Umhau A, Katz P. Tryptophan-associated eosinophilic connective-tissue disease: A new clinical entity? *JAMA.* 1990;263:1502–1506.

[12]Martin RW, Duffy J, Engel AG, *et al.* The clinical spectrum of the eosinophilia-myalgia syndrome associated with L-tryptophan ingestion: Clinical features in 20 patients and aspects of pathophysiology. *Ann Intern Med.* 1990;113:124–134.

[13]Chartash EK, Given WP, Vishnubhakat SM, *et al.* L-tryptophan induced eosinophilia-myalgia syndrome. *J Rheumatol.* 1990;17:1527–1533.

[14]Glickstein SL, Gertner E, Smith SA, *et al.* Eosinophilia-myalgia syndrome associated with L-tryptophan. *J Rheumatol.* 1990;17:1534–1543.

[15]Philen RM, Eidson M, Kilbourne EM, *et al.* Eosinophilia-myalgia syndrome: A clinical case series of 21 patients. *Arch Intern Med.* 1991;151:533–537.

[16]Thacker HL. Eosinophilia-myalgia syndrome: The Cleveland clinic experience. *Cleve Clin J Med.* 1991;58:400–408.

[17]Back EE, Henning KJ, Kallenbach LR, Brix KA, Gunn RA, Melius JM. Risk factors for developing eosinophilia myalgia syndrome among L-tryptophan users in New York. *J Rheumatol.* 1993;20:666–672.

[18]Sternberg EM, Van Woert MH, Young SN, *et al.* Development of a scleroderma-like illness during therapy with L-5-hydroxytryptophan and carbidopa. *N Engl J Med.* 1980;303:782–787.

[19]Freeze JF, Lindgren JA, Bull JM. Scleroderma-like lesions in the carcinoid syndrome. *Arch Intern Med.* 1973;131:550–553.

[20]Zarafonetis CJD, Lorber SH, Hanson SM. Association of functioning carcinoid syndrome and scleroderma. I. Case report. *Am J Med Sci.* 1958;236:1–14.

[21]Utz DC, Rooke ED, Spittell JA Jr, Bartholomew LG. Retroperitoneal fibrosis in patients taking methysergide. *JAMA.* 1965;191:983–985.

[22]MacDonald RA, Robbins SL, Mallory GK. Dermal fibrosis following subcutaneous injections of serotonin creatinine sulfate. *Proc Soc Exp Biol Med.* 1958;97:334–337.

[23]Gum OB, Smyth CJ, Hamilton PK Jr, Moens C. Effect of intra-articular serotonin and other amines on connective tissue proliferation of rabbit joints. *Arthritis Rheum.* 1960;3:447–448.

[24]Nakoneczna I, Forbes JC, Rogers KS. The arthritogenic effect of indole, skatole and other tryptophan metabolites in rabbits. *Am J Pathol.* 1969;57:523–538.

[25]Young SN, Teff KL. Tryptophan availability, 5-HT synthesis and 5-HT function. *Prog Neuropsychopharmacol Biol Psychiatry.* 1989;13:373–379.

[26]Ballentine C. The essential guide to amino acids. *FDA Consumer.* 1985;19:23–25.

[27]Freese A, Schwartz KJ, During M. Potential neurotoxicity of tryptophan (letter). *Ann Intern Med.* 1988;108:312–313.

[28]Steiner W, Fontaine R. Toxic reaction following the combined administration of fluoxetine and L-tryptophan: Five case reports. *Biol Psychiatry.* 1986;21:1067–1071.

[29]Baloh RW, Deitz J, Spooner JW. Myoclonus and ocular oscillations induced by L-tryptophan. *Ann Neurology.* 1982;11:95–97.

[30]Varga J, Uitto J, Jimenez SA. The cause and pathogenesis of the eosinophilia-myalgia syndrome. *Ann Intern Med.* 1992;116:140–147.

[31]Schwarcz R, Whetsell WO Jr, Mangano RM. Quinolinic acid: An endogenous metabolite that produces axon-sparing lesions in rat brain. *Science.* 1983;219:316–318.

[32]Heyes MP, Brew BJ, Martin A, *et al.* Quinolinic acid in cerebrospinal fluid and serum in HIV-1 infection—relationship to clinical and neurological status. *Ann Neurol.* 1991;29:202–209.

[33]Halperin JJ, Heyes MP. Neuroactive kynurenines in Lyme borreliosis. *Neurology.* 1992;42:43–50.

[34]Stachow A, Jablonska S, Skiendzielewska A. 5-hydroxytryptamine and tryptamine pathways in scleroderma. *Br J Dermatol.* 1977;97:147–154.

[35]Silver RM, Heyes MP, Maize JC, Quearry B, Vionnet-Fuasset M, Sternberg EM. Scleroderma, fasciitis, and eosinophilia associated with the ingestion of tryptophan. *N Engl J Med.* 1990;322:874–881.

[36]Heiman-Patterson TD, Bird SJ, Parry GJ, *et al.* Peripheral neuropathy associated with eosinophilia-myalgia syndrome. *Ann Neurol.* 1990;28:522–528.

[37]Lehrer S, Brown RR, Lee CM, *et al.* Tryptophan metabolism in women with breast cancer (letter). *Int J Cancer.* 1988;42:137.

[38]Hertzman PA, Blevins WL, Mayer J, Greenfield B, Ting M, Gleich GJ. Association of the eosinophilia-myalgia syndrome with the ingestion of tryptophan. *N Engl J Med.* 1990;322:869–873.

[39]Eidson M, Philen RM, Sewell CM, Voorhees R, Kilbourne EM. L-tryptophan and eosinophilia-myalgia syndrome in New Mexico. *Lancet.* 1990;335:645–648.

[40]Centers for Disease Control. Eosinophilia-myalgia syndrome and L-tryptophan-containing products—New Mexico, Minnesota, Oregon, and New York, 1989. *MMWR.* 1989;38:785–788.

[41]Slutsker L, Hoesly FC, Miller L, Williams LP, Watson JC, Fleming DW. Eosinophilia-myalgia syndrome associated with exposure to tryptophan from a single manufacturer. *JAMA.* 1990;264:213–217.

[42]Belongia EA, Hedberg CW, Gleich GJ, *et al.* An investigation into the cause of the eosinophilia-myalgia syndrome associated with tryptophan use. *N Engl J Med.* 1990;323:357–365.

[43]Kamb ML, Murphy JJ, Jones JL, *et al.* Eosinophilia-myalgia syndrome in L-tryptophan-exposed patients. *JAMA.* 1992;267:77–82.

[44]Trucksess MW. Separation and isolation of trace impurities in L-tryptophan by high-performance liquid chromatography. *J Chromatography.* 1993;630:147–150.

[45]Mayeno AN, Gleich GJ. Eosinophilia-myalgia syndrome and tryptophan production: A cautionary tale. *TIBS Tech.* 1994;12:346–352.

[46]Mayeno AN, Lin F, Foote CS, *et al.* Characterization of "Peak E," a novel amino acid associated with the eosinophilia-myalgia syndrome. *Science.* 1990;250:1707–1708.

[47]Sakimoto K. The cause of the eosinophilia-myalgia syndrome associated with tryptophan use (letter). *N Engl J Med.* 1990;323:992–993.

[48]Centers for Disease Control. Analysis of L-tryptophan for the etiology of the eosinophilia-myalgia syndrome. *MMWR.* 1990;39:589–591.

[49]Centers for Disease Control. Update: Analysis of L-tryptophan for the etiology of the eosinophilia-myalgia syndrome. *MMWR.* 1990;39:789–790.

[50]Smith MJ, Mazzola EP, Farrell TJ, *et al.* 1,1'-ethylidenebis (L-tryptophan) structure determination of contaminant "97"—implicated in the eosinophilia-myalgia syndrome (EMS). *Tetrahedron Lett.* 1991;32:991–994.

[51]Hunt JN, Knox MT. Regulation of gastric emptying. In: Code CF, ed. *Handbook of Physiology.* Washington, DC: American Physiology Society, 1968;1917–1935.

[52]Hill RH Jr, Caudill SP, Philen RM, *et al.* Contaminants in L-tryptophan associated with eosinophilia-myalgia syndrome. *Arch Environ Contam Toxicol.* 1993;25:134–142.

[53]Toyo'oka T, Yamazaki T, Tanimoto T, *et al.* Characterization of contaminants in EMS-associated L-tryptophan samples by high-performance liquid chromatography. *Chem Pharm Bull* (Japan). 1991;39:820–822.

[54]Goda Y, Suzuki J, Maitani T, Yoshihira K, Takeda M, Uchiyama M. 3-anilino-L-alanine, structural determination of UV-5, a contaminant in EMS-associated L-tryptophan samples. *Chem Pharm Bull* (Japan). 1992;40:2236–2238.

[55]Mayeno AN, Belongia EA, Lin F, Lundy SK, Gleich GJ. 3-(phenylamino)alanine, a novel aniline-derived amino acid associated with the eosinophilia-myalgia syndrome: A link to the toxic oil syndrome? *Mayo Clin Proc.* 1992;67:1134–1139.

[56]Vázquez Roncero A, Janer del Valle C, Maestro Durán R, Graciani Constante E. New aniline derivatives in cooking oils associated with the toxic oil syndrome (letter). *Lancet.* 1983;2:1024–1025.

[57]Mayeno A, Benson L, Naylor S, Colberg-Beers M, Puchalski J, Gleich G. Biotransformation of 3-(phenylamino)-1,2-propanediol to 3-(phenylamino)alanine: A chemical link between toxic oil syndrome and eosinophilia-myalgia syndrome. *Chem Res Toxicol.* 1995;8:911–916.

[58]Müller A, Busker E, Günther K, Hoppe B. Characterization of byproducts in L-tryptophan. *Bioforum.* 1991;14:350–354.

[59]Philen RM, Hill RH Jr, Flanders WD, *et al.* Tryptophan contaminants associated with eosinophilia-myalgia syndrome. *Am J Epidemiol.* 1993;138:154–159.

[60]Michelson D, Page SW, Casey R, *et al.* An eosinophilia-myalgia syndrome related disorder associated with exposure to L-5-hydroxytryptophan. *J Rheumatol.* 1994;21:2261–2265.

[61]Crofford LJ, Rader JI, Dalakas MC, *et al.* L-tryptophan implicated in human eosinophilia-myalgia syndrome causes fasciitis and perimyositis in the Lewis rat. *J Clin Invest.* 1990;86:1757–1763.

[62]Sternberg EM, Hill JM, Chrousos GP, *et al.* Inflammatory mediator-induced hypothalamic-pituitary-adrenal axis activation is defective in streptococcal cell wall arthritis-susceptible Lewis rats. *Proc Natl Acad Sci USA.* 1989;86:2374–2378.

[63]Love LA, Rader JI, Crofford LJ, *et al.* Pathological and immunological effects of ingesting L-tryptophan and 1,1'-ethylidenebis (L-tryptophan) in Lewis rats. *J Clin Invest.* 1993;91:804–811.

[64]DeSchryver-Kecskemeti K, Gramlich TL, Crofford LJ, *et al.* Mast cell and eosinophil infiltration in intestinal mucosa of Lewis rats treated with L-tryptophan implicated in human eosinophilia myalgia syndrome. *Mod Pathol.* 1991;4:354–357.

[65]Silver RM, Ludwicka A, Hampton M, *et al.* A murine model of the eosinophilia-myalgia syndrome induced by 1,1'-ethylidenebis (L-tryptophan). *J Clin Invest.* 1994;93:1473–1480.

[66]Suzuki S, Tourkina E, Ludwicka A, *et al.* A contaminant of L-tryptophan enhances expression of dermal collagen in a murine model of eosinophilia myalgia syndrome. *Proc Assoc Amer Phys.* 1996;108:1–9.

[67]Adachi J, Mio T, Ueno Y, *et al.* Identification of four metabolites of 3-(phenylamino)alanine, a constituent in L-tryptophan products implicated in eosinophilia-myalgia syndrome, in rats. *Arch Toxicol.* 1994;68:500–505.

[68]Adachi J, Gomez M, Smith C, Sternberg E. Accumulation of 3-(phenylamino)alanine, a constituent in L-tryptophan products implicated in eosinophilia-myalgia syndrome, blood and organs of Lewis rats. *Arch Toxicol.* 1995;69:266–270.

[69]Sato M, Hagiwara Y, Kawase Y. Subchronic toxicity of 3-phenylamino alanine, an impurity in L-tryptophan reported to be associ-

ated with the eosinophilia-myalgia syndrome. *Arch Toxicol.* 1995;69:444–449.

70Emslie-Smith AM, Mayeno AN, Nakano S, Gleich GJ, Engel AG. 1,1'-ethylidenebis(tryptophan) induces pathologic alterations in muscle similar to those observed in the eosinophilia-myalgia syndrome. *Neurology.* 1994;44:2390–2392.

71Clauw DJ. Animal models of the eosinophilia myalgia syndrome. *J Rheumatol.* 1996;23(suppl 46):93–98.

72Gleich GJ, Kita H, Adolphson CR. Eosinophils. In: Frank MM, Austen KF, Claman HN, Unanue ER, eds. *Samter's Immunologic Diseases.* Boston: Little, Brown and Company, 1995;205–206.

73Owen WF Jr, Petersen J, Sheff DM, *et al.* Hypodense eosinophils and interleukin 5 activity in the blood of patients with the eosinophilia-myalgia syndrome. *Proc Natl Acad Sci USA.* 1990; 87:8647–8651.

74Yamaoka K, Miyasaka N, Inuo G, *et al.* 1,1'-ethylidene(tryptophan) (peak E) induces functional activation of human eosinophils and interleukin 5 production from T lymphocytes: Association of eosinophilia-myalgia syndrome with an L-tryptophan contaminant. *J Clin Immunol.* 1994;14:50–60.

75Yamaguchi Y, Tsunoda J, Suda T, Miura Y, Shioiri-Nakano K, Kasahara T. Effect of synthesized constituents in the L-tryptophan product on the differentiation of eosinophils and the induction of IL-6: A possible cause of eosinophilia-myalgia syndrome. *Biochem Biophys Res Commun.* 1991;178:1008–1013.

76Brenneman DE, Page SW, Schultzberg M, *et al.* A decomposition product of a contaminant implicated in L-tryptophan eosinophilia myalgia syndrome affects spinal cord neuronal cell death and survival through stereospecific, maturation and partly interleukin-1-dependent mechanisms. *J Pharmacol Exp Ther.* 1993;266:1029–1035.

77Sidransky H, Verney E, Cosgrove JW, Latham PS, Mayeno AN. Studies with 1,1'-ethylidenebis(tryptophan), a contaminant associated with L-tryptophan implicated in the eosinophilia-myalgia syndrome. *Toxicol Appl Pharmacol.* 1994;126:108–113.

78Tagaki H, Ochoa MS, Zhou L, Helfman T, Murata H, Falanga V. Enhanced collagen synthesis and transcription by peak E, a contaminant of L-tryptophan preparations associated with the eosinophilia-myalgia syndrome epidemic. *J Clin Invest.* 1995;96:2120–2125.

79Zangrilli JG, Mayeno AN, Vining V, Varga J. 1,1'-ethylidenebis(L-tryptophan), an impurity in L-tryptophan associated with eosinophilia-myalgia syndrome, stimulates type I collagen gene expression in human fibroblasts in vitro. *Biochem Mol Biol Int.* 1995;37:925–933.

80Silver RM, McKinley K, Smith EA, *et al.* Tryptophan metabolism via the kynurenine pathway in patients with the eosinophilia-myalgia syndrome. *Arthritis Rheum.* 1992;35:1097–1105.

81Ozaki Y, Edelstein MP, Duch DS. The actions of interferon and anti-inflammatory agents on induction of indoleamine 2,3-dioxygenase in human peripheral blood monocytes. *Biochem Biophys Res Commun.* 1987;144:1147–1153.

82Pfefferkorn ER, Rebhun S, Eckel M. Characterization of an indoleamine 2,3-dioxygenase induced by gamma-interferon in cultured human fibroblasts. *J Interferon Res.* 1986;6:267–279.

83Schiller J, Storer B, Paulnock D, Brown R, Borden E. A direct comparison of biological response modulation and clinical side effects by interferon-beta ser, interferon-gamma, or the combination of inteferons-beta ser and gamma in humans. *J Clin Invest.* 1990;86:1211–1221.

84Whetsell WO, Schwarcz R. Prolonged exposure to submicromolar concentrations of quinolinic acid causes excitotoxic damage and organotypic cultures of rat corticospinal systems. *Neurosci Lett.* 1989;97:271–275.

85Clauw DJ, Zackrison LH, Katz P. Serum cytokines and the eosinophilia myalgia syndrome (letter). *Ann Intern Med.* 1992; 117:344–345.

86Huber C, Batchelor JR, Fuchs D, *et al.* Immune response-associated production of neopterin. *J Exp Med.* 1984;160:310–316.

87Silver RM, Sutherland SE, Carreira P, Heyes MP. Alterations in tryptophan metabolism in the toxic oil syndrome and in the eosinophilia-myalgia syndrome. *J Rheumatol.* 1992;19:69–73.

88Emslie-Smith AM, Engel AG, Duffy J, Bowles CA. Eosinophilia myalgia syndrome: I. Immunocytochemical evidence for a T-cell-mediated immune effector response. *Ann Neurol.* 1991;29:524–528.

89Illa I, Dinsmore S, Dalakas MC. Immune-mediated mechanisms and immune activation of fibroblasts in the pathogenesis of eosinophilia-myalgia syndrome induced by L-tryptophan. *Hum Pathol.* 1993;24:702–709.

90Varga J, Peltonen J, Uitto J, Jimenez S. Development of diffuse fasciitis with eosinophilia during L-tryptophan treatment: Demonstration of elevated type I collagen gene expression in affected tissues: A clinicopathologic study of four patients. *Ann Intern Med.* 1990;112:344–351.

91Kaufman LD, Gomez-Reino JJ, Gruber BL, Miller F. Fibrogenic growth factors in the eosinophilia myalgia syndrome and the toxic oil syndrome. *Arch Dermatol.* 1994;130:41–47.

92Butterfield JH, Kephart GM, Banks PM, Gleich GJ. Extracellular deposition of eosinophil granule major basic protein in lymph nodes of patients with Hodgkin's disease. *Blood.* 1986;68:1250–1256.

93Noguchi H, Kephart GM, Colby TV, Gleich GJ. Tissue eosinophilia and eosinophil degranulation in syndromes associated with fibrosis. *Am J Pathol.* 1992;140:521–528.

94Noguchi H, Kephart GM, Campbell RJ, *et al.* Tissue eosinophilia and eosinophil degranulation in orbital pseudotumor. *Ophthalmology.* 1991;98:928–932.

95Heufelder AE, Goellner JR, Bahn RS, Gleich GJ, Hay ID. Tissue eosinophilia and eosinophil degranulation in Riedel's invasive fibrous thyroiditis. *J Clin Endocrinol Metab.* 1996;81:977–984.

96Birkland TP, Cheavens MD, Pincus SH. Human eosinophils stimulate DNA synthesis and matrix production in dermal fibroblasts. *Arch Dermatol Res.* 1994;286:312–318.

97Noguchi H, Hoerl BJ, Gleich GJ. Eosinophil-derived neurotoxin (EDN) stimulates fibroblast proliferation. *FASEB.* 1990;4:A1943.

98Wong DTW, Elovic A, Matossian K, *et al.* Eosinophils from patients with blood eosinophilia express transforming growth factor beta 1. *Blood.* 1991;78:2702–2707.

99Ohno I, Nitta Y, Yamauchi K, *et al.* Transforming growth factor β1 (TGF-β1) gene expression by eosinophils in asthmatic airway inflammation. *Am J Respir Cell Mol Biol.* 1996;15:404–409.

100 Kaufman LD. The evolving spectrum of eosinophilia myalgia syndrome. *Rheum Dis Clin North Am.* 1994;20:973–994.

101 Hertzman PA, Clauw DJ, Kaufman LD, *et al.* Eosinophilia myalgia syndrome: Status of 205 patients and results of treatment two years after onset. *Ann Intern Med.* 1995;122:851–855.

102 Kaufman LD. Eosinophilia-myalgia syndrome: Morbidity and mortality (editorial). *J. Rheumatol.* 1993;20:1644–1646.

103 Kaufman LD. Chronicity of the eosinophilia-myalgia syndrome (EMS): A reassessment after 3 years. *Arthritis Rheum.* 1994;37:84–87.

104 Swygert LA, Back EE, Auerbach SB, Sewell LE, Falk H. Eosinophilia-myalgia syndrome: Mortality data from the U.S. national surveillance system. *J Rheumatol.* 1993;20:1711–1717.

105 James TN, Kamb ML, Sandberg GA, Silver RM, Kilbourne EM. Postmortem studies of the heart in three fatal cases of the eosinophilia-myalgia syndrome. *Ann Intern Med.* 1991;115:102–110.

106 Kaufman LD, Philen RM. Tryptophan: Current status and future trends for oral administration. *Drug Safety.* 1993;8:89–98.

107 Kaufman LD, Krupp LB. Eosinophilia-myalgia syndrome associated with L-tryptophan ingestion. In: Lichtenstein LM, Fauci AS, eds. *Current Therapy in Allergy, Immunology and Rheumatology.* Philadelphia: Mosby, 1996;336–340.

108 Kaufman LD, Seidman RJ, Phillips ME, Gruber BL. Cutaneous manifestations of the L-tryptophan associated eosinophilia-myalgia syndrome: A spectrum of sclerodermatous skin disease. *J Am Acad Dermatol.* 1990;23:1063–1069.

109 Bulpitt KJ, Verity MA, Clements PJ, Paulus HE. Association of L-tryptophan and an illness resembling eosinophilic fasciitis: Clinical and histopathologic findings in four patients with eosinophilia-myalgic syndrome. *Arthritis Rheum.* 1990;33:918–929.

110 Freundlich B, Werth VP, Rook AH, *et al.* L-tryptophan ingestion associated with eosinophilic fasciitis but not progressive systemic sclerosis. *Ann Intern Med.* 1990;112:758–762.

111 Jaffe I, Kopelman R, Baird R, Grossman M, Hays A. Eosinophilic fasciitis associated with the eosinophilia-myalgia syndrome. *Am J Med.* 1990;88:542–546.

112 Connolly SM, Quimby SR, Griffing WL, Winkelmann RK. Scleroderma and L-tryptophan—a possible explanation of the eosinophilia-myalgia syndrome. *J Am Acad Dermatol.* 1990;23:451–457.

113 Case Records of the Massachusetts General Hospital; Case 4–1990. *N Engl J Med.* 1990;322:252–261.

114 Gorn A. Case 4–1990: Eosinophilic fasciitis. *N Engl J Med.* 1990;322:931.

115 Blauvelt A, Falanga V. Idiopathic and L-tryptophan-associated eosinophilic fasciitis before and after L-tryptophan contamination. *Arch Dermatol.* 1991;127:1159–1166.

116 Gordon ML, Lebwohl MG, Phelps RG, Cohen SR, Fleischmajer R. Eosinophilic fasciitis associated with tryptophan ingestion: A manifestation of eosinophilia-myalgia syndrome. *Arch Dermatol.* 1991;127:217–220.

117 Oursler JR, Farmer ER, Roubenoff R, Mogavero HS, Watson RM. Cutaneous manifestations of the eosinophilia-myalgia syndrome. *Br J Dermatol.* 1992;127:138–146.

118 Dubin DB, Kwan TH, Morse MO, Case DC. Cutaneous mucinosis in a patient with eosinophilia-myalgia syndrome associated with L-tryptophan ingestion. *Arch Dermatol.* 1990;126:1517–1518.

119 Farmer KL, Hebert AA, Rapini RP, Jordan RE. Dermal mucinosis in the eosinophilia-myalgia syndrome. *Arch Dermatol.* 1990;126:1518–1520.

120 Valicenti JMK, Fleming MG, Pearson RW, Budz JP, Gendleman MD. Papular mucinosis in L-tryptophan-induced eosinophilia-myalgia syndrome. *J Am Acad Dermatol.* 1991;25:54–58.

121 Fleischmajer R, Perlish JS. Glycosaminoglycans in scleroderma and scleredema. *J Invest Derm.* 1972;58:129–132.

122 Duffy J, Bowles C, Martin R. Eosinophilia-myalgia syndrome (EMS) 3 years later (abstract). *Arthritis Rheum.* 1993;36:R15.

123 Kaufman LD, Gruber BL, Gregersen PK. Clinical follow-up and immunogenetic studies of 32 patients with the eosinophilia-myalgia syndrome. *Lancet.* 1991;337:1071–1074.

124 Martin RW, Duffy J, Lie JT. Eosinophilic fasciitis associated with use of L-tryptophan: A case control study and comparison of clinical and histopathologic features. *Mayo Clin Proc.* 1991;66:892–898.

125 Hibbs JR, Mittleman B, Hill P, Medsger TA Jr. L-tryptophan-associated eosinophilic fasciitis prior to the 1989 eosinophilia-myalgia syndrome outbreak. *Arthritis Rheum.* 1992;35:299–303.

126 Varga J, Griffin R, Newman JH, Jimenez SA. Eosinophilic fasciitis is clinically distinguishable from the eosinophilia-myalgia syndrome and is not associated with L-tryptophan use. *J Rheumatol.* 1991;18:259–263.

127 Feldman SR, Silver RM, Maize JC. A histopathologic comparison of Shulman's syndrome (diffuse fasciitis with eosinophilia) and the fasciitis associated with the eosinophilia-myalgia syndrome. *J Am Acad Dermatol.* 1992;26:95–100.

128 Barnes L, Rodnan GP, Medsger TAJ, Short D. Eosinophilic fasciitis: A pathologic study of twenty cases. *Am J Pathol.* 1979;96:493–507.

129 Seidman RJ, Kaufman LD, Sokoloff L, Miller F, Iliya A, Peress NS. Neuromuscular pathology of the eosinophilia-myalgia syndrome. *J Neuropathol Exp Neurol.* 1991;50:49–62.

130 Verity MA, Bulpitt KJ, Paulus HE. Neuromuscular manifestations of L-tryptophan-associated eosinophilia-myalgia syndrome—a histomorphologic analysis of 14 patients. *Hum Pathol.* 1991;22:3–11.

131 Hollander D, Adelman LS. Eosinophilia-myalgia syndrome associated with ingestion of L-tryptophan: Muscle biopsy findings in 4 patients. *Neurology.* 1991;41:319–321.

132 Lin JD, Phelps RG, Gordon ML, *et al.* Pathological manifestations of the eosinophilia myalgia syndrome: Analysis of 11 cases. *Hum Pathol.* 1992;23:429–437.

133 Kaufman LD, Kaufman MA, Krupp LB. Movement disorders in the eosinophilia myalgia syndrome: Tremor, myoclonus, and myokymia. *J Rheumatol.* 1995;22:157–160.

134 Sagman DL, Melamed JC. L-tryptophan-induced eosinophilia-myalgia syndrome and myopathy. *Neurology.* 1990;40:1629–1630.

135 Herrick MK, Chang Y, Horoupian DS, Lombard CM, Adornato BT. L-tryptophan and the eosinophilia-myalgia syndrome—pathologic findings in eight patients. *Hum Pathol.* 1991;22:12–21.

[136]Estrada CA, Harrington DW, Glasberg MR. Eosinophilic myositis an expression of L-tryptophan toxicity? *J Rheumatol.* 1990; 17:1554–1556.

[137]Smith SA, Roelofs RI, Gertner E. Microangiopathy in the eosinophilia-myalgia syndrome. *J Rheumatol.* 1990;17:1544–1550.

[138]Smith BE, Dyck PJ. Peripheral neuropathy in the eosinophilia-myalgia syndrome associated with L-tryptophan ingestion. *Neurology.* 1990;40:1035–1040.

[139]Kaufman LD, Finn AF Jr, Seidman RJ, *et al.* Eosinophilic neuritis, perimyositis and vasculitis associated with ingestion of L-tryptophan. *J Rheumatol.* 1990;17:795–800.

[140]Nolfo E, Wright-Browne V, Therrien M, Ardolino A, Macinski Z. Plasmapheresis in a case of eosinophilia-myalgia syndrome with ascending polyneuropathy. *Chest.* 1991;100:584.

[141]Kaufman LD, Seidman RJ. L-tryptophan-associated eosinophilia-myalgia syndrome: Perspective of a new illness. *Rheum Dis Clin North Am.* 1991;17:427–441.

[142]Selwa JF, Feldman EL, Blaivas M. Mononeuropathy multiplex in tryptophan-associated eosinophilia-myalgia syndrome. *Neurology.* 1990;40:1632–1633.

[143]Donofrio PD, Stanton C, Miller VS, *et al.* Demyelinating polyneuropathy in eosinophilia-myalgia syndrome. *Musc Nerv.* 1992; 15:796–805.

[144]Freimer ML, Glass JD, Chaudry V, *et al.* Chronic demyelinating polyneuropathy associated with eosinophilia-myalgia syndrome. *J Neurol Neurosurg Psychiatry.* 1992;55:352–358.

[145]Tolander LM, Bamford CR, Yoshino MT, Downing S, Bryan G. Neurologic complications of the tryptophan-associated eosinophilia-myalgia syndrome. *Arch Neurol.* 1991;48:436–438.

[146]Lynn J, Rammohan KW, Bornstein RA, Kissel JT. Central nervous system involvement in the eosinophilia-myalgia syndrome. *Arch Neurol.* 1992;49:1082–1085.

[147]Adair JC, Rose JW, Digre KB, Balbierz JM. Acute encephalopathy associated with the eosinophilia-myalgia syndrome. *Neurology.* 1992;42:461–462.

[148]Greenfield BM, Mayer JW, Sibbitt RR. The eosinophilia myalgia syndrome and the brain (letter). *Ann Intern Med.* 1991;115:159–160.

[149]Zackrison LH, Blank CA, Katz P, Clauw DJ. Fibromyalgia and the eosinophilia myalgia syndrome (abstract). *Arthritis Rheum.* 1993;36:R27.

[150]Dinerman H, Steere AC. Lyme disease associated with fibromyalgia. *Ann Intern Med.* 1992;117:281–285.

[151]Krupp LB, Mendelson WB, Friedman R. An overview of chronic fatigue syndrome. *J Clin Psychiatry.* 1991;52:403–410.

[152]Centers for Disease Control. Eosinophilia-myalgia syndrome: Follow-up survey of patients—New York, 1990–1991. *MMWR.* 1991;40:401–403.

[153]Krupp LB, Masur DM, Kaufman LD. Neurocognitive dysfunction in the eosinophilia-myalgia syndrome. *Neurology.* 1993;43: 931–936.

[154]Gaudino E, O'Loughlin T, Kaufman LD, Masur DM, Krupp LB. A longitudinal study of cognitive functioning in the eosinophilia myalgia syndrome (abstract). *Ann Neurol.* 1993;34:248.

[155]Centers for Disease Control. Clinical spectrum of eosinophilia-myalgia syndrome—California. *MMWR.* 1990;39:89–91.

[156]Hertzman PA, Falk H, Kilbourne EM, Page S, Shulman LE. The eosinophilia-myalgia syndrome: The Los Alamos conference. *J Rheumatol.* 1991;18:867–873.

[157]Williamson MR, Eidson M, Rosenberg RD, Williamson S. Eosinophilia-myalgia syndrome: Findings on chest radiographs in 18 patients. *Radiology.* 1991;180:849–852.

[158]Strongwater SL, Woda BA, Yood RA, *et al.* Eosinophilia-myalgia syndrome associated with L-tryptophan ingestion—analysis of four patients and implications for differential diagnosis and pathogenesis. *Arch Intern Med.* 1990;150:2178–2186.

[159]Strumpf IJ, Drucker RD, Anders KH, Cohen S, Fajolu O. Acute eosinophilic pulmonary disease associated with the ingestion of L-tryptophan-containing products. *Chest.* 1991;99:8–13.

[160]Banner AS, Borochovitz D. Acute respiratory failure caused by pulmonary vasculitis after L-tryptophan ingestion. *Am Rev Respir Dis.* 1991;143:661–664.

[161]Campagna AC, Blanc PD, Criswell LA, *et al.* Pulmonary manifestations of the eosinophilia-myalgia syndrome associated with tryptophan ingestion. *Chest.* 1992;101:1274–1281.

[162]Tazelaar HD, Myers JL, Drage CW, King TF, Aguayo S, Colby TV. Pulmonary disease associated with L-tryptophan-induced eosinophilic myalgia syndrome: Clinical and pathological features. *Chest.* 1990;97:1032–1036.

[163]Tazelaar HD, Myers JL, Strickler JG, Colby TV, Duffy J. Tryptophan-induced lung disease: An immunophenotypic, immunofluorescent, and electron microscopic study. *Mod Pathol.* 1993;6:56–60.

[164]Travis WD, Kalafer ME, Robin HS, Luibel FJ. Hypersensitivity pneumonitis and pulmonary vasculitis with eosinophilia in a patient taking an L-tryptophan preparation. *Ann Intern Med.* 1990;112: 301–303.

[165]Toxic Epidemic Syndrome Study Group. Toxic epidemic syndrome, Spain, 1981. *Lancet.* 1982;2:697–702.

[166]Catton CK, Elmer JC, Whitehouse AC, Clode JB, Hustrulid RI. Pulmonary involvement in the eosinophilia-myalgia syndrome. *Chest.* 1991;99:327–329.

[167]Yakovlevitch M, Siegel M, Hoch DH, Rutlen DL. Pulmonary hypertension in a patient with tryptophan-induced eosinophilia-myalgia syndrome. *Am J Med.* 1991;90;272–273.

[168]Gomez-Sanchez MA, Mestre de Juan MJ, Gomez-Pajuelo C, Lopez JI, Diaz de Atauri MJ, Martinez-Tello FJ. Pulmonary hypertension due to toxic oil syndrome: A clinicopathologic study. *Chest.* 1989;95:325–331.

[169]Gomez-Sanchez MA, Saenz de la Calzada C, Gomez-Pajuelo C, Martinez-Tello FJ, Mestre de Juan MJ, James TN. Clinical and pathologic manifestations of pulmonary vascular disease in the toxic oil syndrome. *J Am Coll Cardiol.* 1991;18:1539–1545.

[170]Read CA, Clauw D, Weir C, Taveira Da Silva A, Katz P. Dyspnea and pulmonary function in the L-tryptophan-associated eosinophilia-myalgia syndrome. *Chest.* 1992;101:1282–1286.

[171]Hertzman PA, Maddoux GL, Sternberg EM, *et al.* Repeated coronary artery spasm in a young woman with the eosinophilia-myalgia syndrome. *JAMA.* 1992;267:2932–2934.

[172]James TN, Posada de la Paz M, Abaitua-Borda I, Gomez-Sanchez A, Martinez-Tello FJ, Soldevilla LB. Histologic abnormalities of large and small coronary arteries, neural structures, and

the conduction system of the heart found in postmortem studies of individuals dying from the toxic oil syndrome. *Am Heart J.* 1991;121:803–815.

[173]DeSchryver-Kecskemeti K, Bennert KW, Cooper GS, Yang P. Gastrointestinal involvement in L-tryptophan (L-Trp) associated eosinophilia-myalgia syndrome (EMS). *Dig Dis Sci.* 1992;37: 697–701.

[174]Chiba S, Miyagawa K, Tanaka T, *et al.* Tryptophan-associated eosinophilia-myalgia syndrome and pancreatitis (letter). *Lancet.* 1990;336:121.

[175]Hertzman PA, Kaufman LD, Love LA, *et al.* The eosinophilia myalgia syndrome—guidelines for patient care. *J Rheumatol.* 1995;22:161–163.

7

Fibrosing Conditions Associated with Organic Solvents and Drugs

Carlo L. Mainardi and Snezana Trajkovic

Diseases characterized by fibrosis, such as hepatic cirrhosis, pulmonary fibrosis, systemic sclerosis and related conditions, have been associated with occupational exposures. The purpose of this chapter is to review the relationship between fibrosis and certain organic compounds and drugs.

SYSTEMIC SCLEROSIS (SSC) AND SSC-LIKE SYNDROMES ASSOCIATED WITH ORGANIC COMPOUNDS

SSc is characterized by Raynaud's phenomenon and fibrosis of skin and visceral organs. The disease occurs at least three times more frequently in women than in men.[1] Pathogenetic mechanisms contributing to the syndrome include abnormalities in the immune response, with autoantibody formation, vascular injury and vasospasm, and the overproduction of connective-tissue components by fibroblasts.

The role of occupational and environmental exposures in the pathogenesis of SSc has received a great deal of attention in the medical literature as well as the lay press. Occupational exposure is thought to be a significant risk factor in SSc among middle-aged men.[2] A variety of agents have been implicated in these syndromes (see Table 7-1).

Vinyl Chloride (VC)

Vinyl chloride is a halogenated form of ethylene, such as trichloroethylene and perchloroethylene. It is the monomer which is polymerized to the ubiquitous polyvinylchloride (PVC). Unlike the other halogenated aliphatic compounds listed in Table 7-1, VC is a gaseous substance. Some workers in the PVC industry who are exposed to the VC monomer (such as those who clean the reactors) are susceptible to a disease which resembles SSc.[3–5]

Classically, VC-associated disease presents with a triad of symptoms and signs's. Raynaud's phenomenon, acro-osteolysis and sclerodermalike skin lesions. Subtle differences distinguish VC-associated disease from SSc. Typically, the bony lesions of SSc are limited to resorption of the distal phalangeal tufts associated with tapered fingertips. In contrast, VC-associated disease involves the mid-shaft of the distal phalanges with the appearance of "bullet holes."[4] The digits are shortened and widened presenting as "pseudoclubbing." Furthermore, in VC-associated disease, bony erosions can be seen at other sites such as the sacroiliac joints, carpal bones and the long bones of the arms and legs. (See Table 7-2).

Skin lesions in VC-associated disease are clinically and microscopically indistinguishable from those of SSc. However, the lesions of VC-associated disease tend to be patchy, are frequently found on the extensor surfaces of the hands and wrists, and tend to spare the face and trunk. Nailbed capillary abnormalities, similar to but not as severe as those found in SSc, are also seen.[4]

Systemic symptoms and visceral involvement also occur. These include fatigue, paresthesia, arthralgia, myalgia, loss of libido, impotence, emotional instability, pulmonary fibrosis and esophageal dysfunction. Unlike SSc, VC-associated disease may be associated with thrombocytopenia, hepatic fibrosis and splenic fibrosis.[6] The hepatic lesion can progress to angiosarcoma.[6] Results of laboratory investigations often yield nonspecific findings. Circulating immune complexes have been reported, yet autoantibodies are not present.[7] It is believed that genetic factors predispose individuals to this condition. This is supported by the observation that less than 5% of those workers exposed to VC are affected.[8] Cessation of exposure to VC results in amelioration of the symptoms and signs. Attention to VC exposure in the workplace has resulted in an apparent reduction in the frequency of VC disease.

Trichloroethylene

Trichloroethylene (TCE) is a halogenated aliphatic organic compound which is chemically similar to VC. It is a

Table 7-1 Occupational and environmental agents associated with SSc-like syndromes

Silica
Silicone Breast Implants
Contaminated Rapeseed Oil
Vinyl Chloride
Organic Solvents
   Aliphatic
      Trichloroethylene
      Perchloroethylene
   Aromatic
      Toluene
      Benzene
Biogenic Amines
   [bis(4-amino-3-methyl-cyclohexyl)methane](BAMM)
   meta-phenylaminediamine
Paraffin Breast Injections
Drugs
   Pentazocine
   Bleomycin
   Cocaine
Agents associated with eosinophilia myalgia syndrome/toxic oil
   syndrome

colorless solvent which is used extensively to degrease metals, to strip paint, and in the dry cleaning industry. It was previously used as an anesthetic. The vapor of TCE is absorbed by inhalation. Acute toxicity causes euphoria, dizziness, drowsiness, confusion, nausea and loss of consciousness. It is also absorbed through the skin and can produce a contact dermatitis as well as exfoliative dermatitis. TCE can penetrate protective clothing including rubber gloves. Prolonged contact with TCE has been associated with variety of manifestations including skin blistering, neuropathy, headache, emotional instability and alcohol intolerance which is char-

acterized by flushing of the face and neck, known as "degreaser's flush."

SSc-like syndrome in workers exposed to TCE was first reported in 1978.[9] Subsequent reports have confirmed this association.[10–12] The clinical manifestations are similar to SSc and VC-associated disease, although certain findings are uncommon for both conditions. All patients with TCE disease have either sclerodactyly, Raynaud's phenomenon, or both. Other manifestations include pigmentary changes, gynecomastia, peripheral neuropathy, impotence and malabsorption. Hepatic involvement does not appear to be as prevalent as in VC-associated disease. Autoantibodies have been detected. Acute systemic disease may also occur. For example, a 47-year-old woman was reported who developed fatal disease after a single 2.5-hour dermal exposure to TCE in an electronic plant. The patient succumbed with proximal skin thickening, microangiopathic hemolytic anemia, restrictive pulmonary disease, reflux esophagitis, pericardial effusion and renal insufficiency with severe hypertension.[12] A similar syndrome has been reported after exposure to another closely related halogenated aliphatic hydrocarbon, perchloroethylene (which is tetrachloroethylene).[13] Figure 8-1 displays the molecular structure of these halogenated aliphatic hydrocarbons.

Recently, two patients were described with biopsy-proven fasciitis following exposure to TCE.[14] Neither patient exhibited sclerodactyly nor presented with Raynaud's phenomenon. Visceral manifestations and immune abnormalities suggestive of SSc were absent. It is of interest that one of these patients was exposed to TCE by ingestion of contaminated well water and her symptoms improved with the use of bottled water.

Generalized morphea due to exposure to TCE in laundry workers, carpenters, laboratory personnel and painters has been reported.[15] Some of these patients were exposed to other solvents which may have contributed to the clinical

Table 7-2 Contrasting features of vinyl chloride-associated disease and SSc

Manifestation	VC Disease	SSc
Raynaud's phenomenon	Yes	Yes
Sclerodactyly	Yes	Yes
Acro-osteolysis	Midshaft of distal phalanx "Bullet hole" appearance	Resorption of distal tuft of distal phalanx
Skin induration	Patchy distribution Extensor surfaces of limbs Spares face and trunk	Involves extremities, face and trunk
Visceral involvement	Pulmonary fibrosis Esophageal dysfunction Liver fibrosis Splenic fibrosis Thrombocytopenia Spares kidneys	Pulmonary fibrosis Esophageal dysfunction Spares liver and spleen Renal involvement

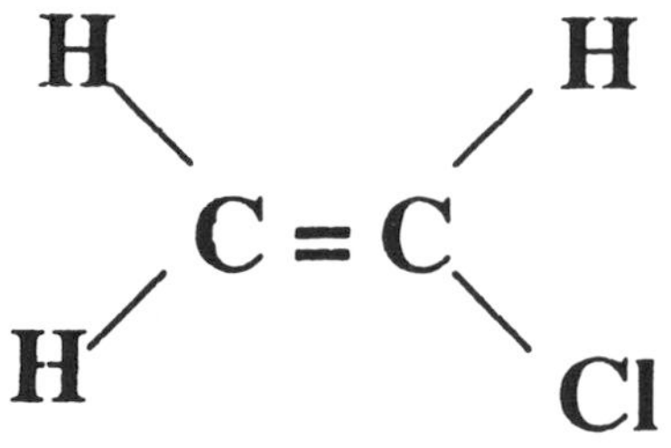

Figure 7-1 Halogenated hydrocarbons which have been implicated in SSc-like conditions through occupational exposure.

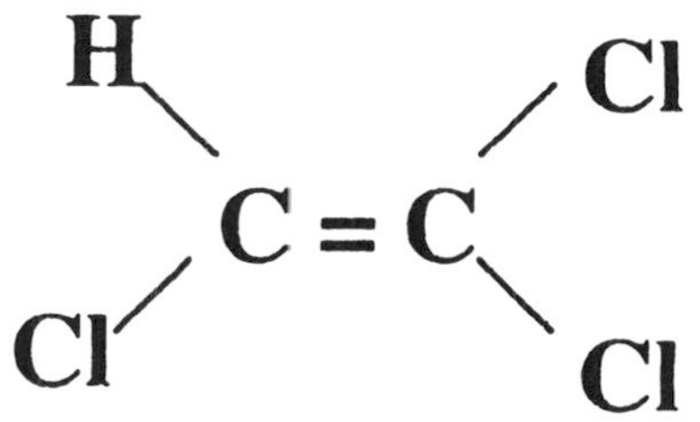

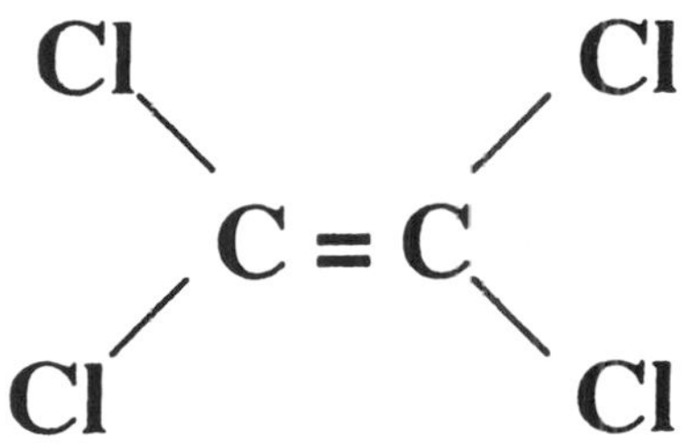

findings. Esophageal dysfunction and/or pulmonary fibrosis were present in some of these individuals.

Amine Compounds

A scleroderma-like disorder has been described in men engaged in the polymerization of epoxy resins.[16] Although these workers were exposed to several organic compounds, circumstantial and laboratory evidence strongly suggested that exposure to the vapor of a cyclohexamine, bis(4-amino-3-methyl-cyclohexyl)methane (BAMM) was responsible for the clinical syndrome. The patients complained of fatigue, muscle weakness and weight loss. Other systemic findings and Raynaud's phenomenon were absent. Skin involvement was striking, with diffuse erythema, induration, diffuse pruritus, pigmentary changes, and loss of body hair. Induration of the skin involved all extremities, both distally and proximally. Histological examination of the skin revealed changes similar to those seen in SSc.

Another report included two cases of SSc related to occupational amine exposure.[17] Both of these patients had Raynaud's phenomenon, skin induration and restrictive pulmonary disease. In one patient, the disease appeared to be related to exposure to meta-phenylaminediamine. Although the second patient had occupational exposure to other agents, the onset of disease also correlated with exposure to meta-phenylaminediamine.

The association of occupational exposure to BAMM is of relevance to understanding the role of other amine compounds in fibrosing conditions. The carcinoid syndrome, in which metabolites of tryptophan accumulate, has been associated with sclerosis of the heart valves, retroperitoneal fibrosis and sclerodermalike lesions.[18–20] Methysergide, a serotoninlike compound, has also been associated with a fibrotic condition.[21] A sclerodermalike illness was also described in a patient receiving L-5-hydroxytryptophan and carbidopa for intention myoclonus.[22] The eosinophilia myalgia syndrome (discussed in Chapter 6) was also associated with an amine compound (1,1'-ethylidenebis [tryptophan]) contaminating commercially available tryptophan.[23] Figure 8-2 illustrates the structures of aromatic amines implicated in SSc-like syndromes.)

Other Organic Compounds

Individuals who are exposed to organic solvents usually work with a variety of potentially noxious agents, making it difficult to implicate a single agent. In a study of 56 men with SSc in the United Kingdom, exposure to compounds reported to be associated with sclerodermatous syndromes was evaluated. Exposure only to organic solvents was reported to any extent.[24]

Aromatic solvents, especially benzene,[25,26] have been associated with a syndrome restricted to skin fibrosis. In addi-

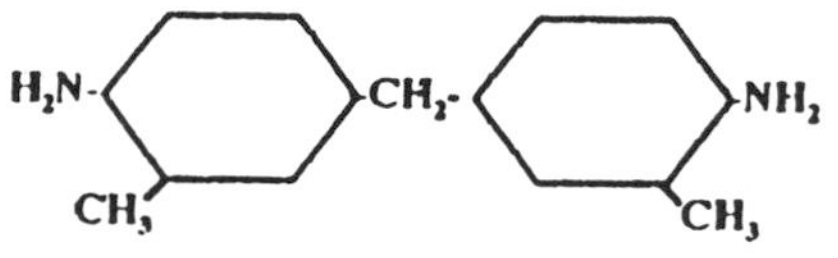

Figure 7-2   Aromatic amines which have been implicated in SSc-like syndromes.

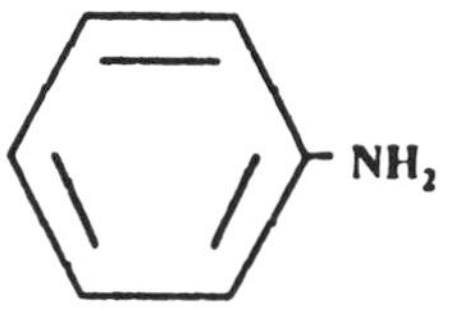

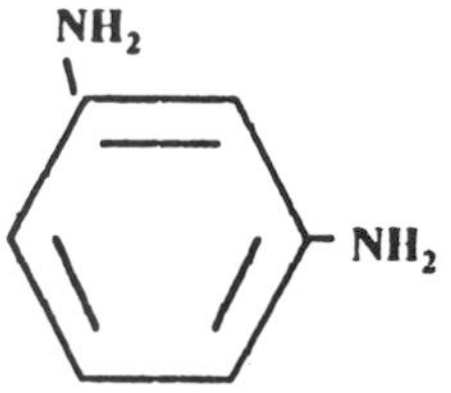

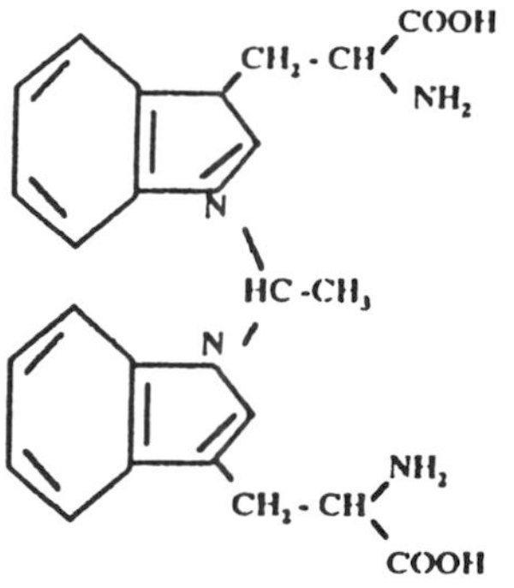

tion, a case of a man with a systemic disease similar to SSc who was exposed to a variety of organic solvents including benzene, toluenes, toluidines, xylenes, aniline and ethanolamine has been reported.[27]

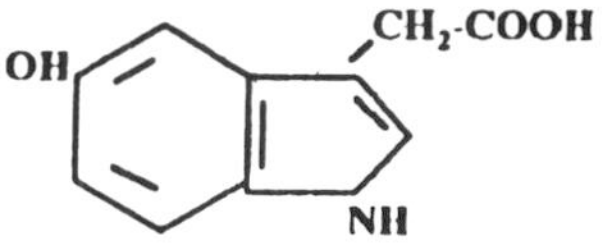

An SSc-like syndrome was reported in a man with recent exposure to herbicides, specifically to aminotriazole, bromouracil and diuron.[28] This patient had skin thickening with involvement of the hands, arms, face and trunk, myopathy and esophageal dysfunction. Raynaud's phenomenon was not described. Some improvement occurred with corticosteroid therapy.

SSC-LIKE SYNDROMES ASSOCIATED WITH DRUGS

Drug therapy has been implicated in fibrotic conditions. Bleomycin is used extensively in cancer chemotherapy and has skin and pulmonary toxicity. Pulmonary toxicity generally presents as interstitial fibrosis and can be fatal. Cutaneous involvement is characterized by a variety of pigmentary changes, ulceration, erythema and induration. Raynaud's phenomenon does not occur and the skin changes are reversible with withdrawal of bleomycin.[29,30]

Skin induration resembling SSc is seen in pentazocine (Talwin) abuse. This occurs in individuals who use injectable pentazocine, and induration is found around the injection sites. Areas of induration coalesce and may ulcerate. A per-

sonal or family history of diabetes mellitus is common among these patients. Vasospastic and visceral manifestations of SSc are absent.[31]

The association of cocaine abuse and SSc remains controversial. Reports of SSc occurring in cocaine abusers have appeared in the literature.[32,33] The vasospastic effect of large doses of cocaine is well-recognized and has been implicated in renal crisis in a patient with SSc.[34] Nevertheless, the etiologic relationship between cocaine abuse and SSc remains clouded by the potential of contaminating substances and the fact that only few cases have been reported despite widespread cocaine abuse.

OTHER FIBROSING CONDITIONS ASSOCIATED WITH ORGANIC COMPOUNDS

Hydrocarbon (including gasoline) inhalation can cause acute pneumonitis, especially in children. This syndrome is generally reversible; however, pulmonary fibrosis has been reported in cable plant workers.[35] Exposure to mist and vapor of petroleum distillates was implicated in the lung injury and fibrosis.[35] The herbicide paraquat is a potent inducer of pulmonary fibrosis. The agent, concentrated in the cells of the lower respiratory tract, causes severe alveolitis with subsequent fibrosis.[36]

The liver is also susceptible to fibrosis from occupational exposure. Liver fibrosis due to organic solvents can progress to malignant neoplasms, as with vinyl chloride exposure. Benzene, which has been implicated in SSc and in the induction of leukemia, has also been reported to cause myelofibrosis.[37]

OTHER FIBROSING CONDITIONS AND DRUGS

Drugs known to induce pulmonary fibrosis include cytotoxic drugs (methotrexate, cyclophosphamide, chlorambucil), gold salts and D-penicillamine. This often develops within the first six months of therapy and is characterized by a severe respiratory disorder with dyspnea and nonproductive cough. Resolution of symptoms usually follows cessation of the responsible agent, but fibrosis may result.[38,39] Amiodarone, nitrofurantoin, hydralazine and procainamide can also cause pulmonary fibrosis.

The most common example of drug-induced fibrosis is alcoholic liver disease but other drugs cause hepatic fibrosis. These include methotrexate in the doses used to treat nonmalignant conditions such as rheumatoid arthritis and psoriasis.[40] Careful monitoring of liver function during methotrexate therapy may reduce the incidence of these complications. Other drugs which induce hepatic fibrosis include isoniazid, methyldopa and amiodarone.

Retroperitoneal fibrosis is an uncommon disorder in which the retroperitoneal fat is replaced by fibrotic tissue which follows an inflammatory reaction. Systemic symptoms are common and include fever, weight loss and malaise. However, the most disabling manifestation is generally related to ureteral obstruction by the fibrotic mass. Although the majority of cases of retroperitoneal fibrosis are idiopathic, the syndrome has been reported in association with drugs, notably ergot alkaloids and bromocriptine.[41]

REFERENCES

[1]Silman AJ. Epidemiology of scleroderma. *Ann Rheum Dis.* 1991; 50:846–853.

[2]Yamakage A, Ishikawa H. Generalized morphea-like scleroderma occurring in people exposed to organic solvents. *Dermatologica.* 1982;165:186–193.

[3]Lebach WK, Marstellar HJ. Vinyl chloride-associated disease. *Adv Int Med Ped.* 1981;47:1–110.

[4]Maricq HR. Vinyl chloride disease. In: Black CM, Myers AR, eds. *Current Topics in Rheumatology. Systemic Sclerosis.* London: Gower Medical Publishing Ltd., 1985;105–113.

[5]Haufstein UF, Ziegler V. Environmentally induced systemic sclerosis-like disorders. *Int J Dermatol.* 1985;24:147–151.

[6]Jones DB, Smith PM. Progression of vinyl chloride induced hepatic fibrosis to angiosarcoma of the liver. *Br J Indust Med.* 1982;39:306–307.

[7]Milford WA. Evidence of an immune complex disorder in vinyl chloride workers. *Proc R Soc Med.* 1976;69:289.

[8]Black C, Pereira S, McWhirter A, Welsh K, Laurent R. Genetic susceptibility to scleroderma-like syndrome in symptomatic and asymptomatic workers exposed to vinyl chloride. *J Rheumatol.* 1986;13:1059–1072.

[9]Saihan EM, Burton JL, Heaton KW. A new syndrome with pigmentation, scleroderma, gynaecomastia, Raynaud's phenomenon, and peripheral neuropathy. *Br J Dermatol.* 1978;99:437–440.

[10]Flindt-Hansen H, Isager X. Scleroderma after occupational exposure to trichloroethylene and trichloroethane. *Acta Dermatol Venerol* (Stockholm). 1987;67:263–263.

[11]Czirjak L, Schlammadinger J, Szegedi G. Systemic sclerosis and exposure to trichloroethylene. *Dermatologica.* 1993:186:236.

[12]Lockey JE, Kelly CR, Cannon GW, Colby TV, Aldrich V, Livingstone GK. Progressive systemic sclerosis associated with exposure to trichloroethylene. *J Occup Med.* 1987;29:493–496.

[13]Sparrow GA. A connective tissue disorder similar to vinyl chloride disease in a patient exposed to perchloroethylene. *Clin Exp Dermatol.* 1977;2:17–22.

[14]Waller PA, Clauw D, Cupps T, Metcalf JS, Silver RM, LeRoy EC. Fasciitis (not scleroderma) following prolonged exposure to an organic solvent (trichloroethylene). *J Rheumatol.* 1994;21:1567–1570.

[15]Yamakage A, Ishikawa H. Generalized morphea-like scleroderma occurring in people exposed to organic solvents. *Dermatologica.* 1982;165:186–193.

[16]Yamakage A, Ishikawa H, Saito Y, Hattori A. Occupational scleroderma-like disorder occurring in men engaged in the polymerization of epoxy resins. *Dermatologica.* 1980;161:33–44.

[17]Owens GR, Medsger TA. Systemic sclerosis secondary to occupational exposure. *Am J Med.* 1988;85:114–116.

[18]Sjoerdsma A, Roberts WC. The cardiac disease associated with the carcinoid syndrome (carcinoid heart disease). *Am J Med.* 1964; 36:5–14.

[19]Morin LJ, Zuerner RT. Retroperitoneal fibrosis and carcinoid tumor. *JAMA.* 1971;216:1647–1650.

[20]Fries JF, Lindgren JA, Bull JM. Scleroderma-like lesions and the carcinoid syndrome. *Arch Int Med.* 1973;131:550–554.

[21]Graham JR. Cardiac and pulmonary fibrosis during methysergide therapy for headache. *Am J Med Sci.* 1967;254:1–11.

[22]Sternberg EM, Van Woert MH, Young SN, *et al.* Development of a scleroderma-like illness during therapy with L-5-hydroxytryptophan and carbidopa. *N Engl J Med.* 1980;303:782–787.

[23]Mayeno AN, Lin F, Foote CS, *et al.* Characterization of "Peak E," a novel amino acid associated with eosinophilia-myalgia syndrome. *Science.* 1990;250:1707–1710.

[24]Silman AJ, Jones S. What is the contribution of occupational environmental factors to the occurrence of scleroderma in men? *Ann Rheum Dis.* 1992;51:1322–1324.

[25]Czirjak L, Szegedi G. Benzene exposure and systemic sclerosis (letter). *N Engl J Med.* 1987;107:118.

[26]Walder B. Do solvents cause scleroderma? *Int J Dermatol.* 1983; 22:157–158.

[27]Bottomly WW, Sheehan-Dare RA, Hughes P, Cunliffe WJ. A sclerodermatous syndrome with unusual features following prolonged occupational exposure to organic solvents. *Br J Dermatol.* 1993; 128:203–206.

[28]Dunnill MGS, Black MM. Sclerodermatous syndrome after occupational exposure to herbicides—response to systemic steroids. *Clin Exp Dermatol.* 1994;19:518–520.

[29]Cohen I, Mosher M, O'Keefe E, *et al.* Cutaneous toxicity of bleomycin therapy. *Arch Dermatol.* 1972;107:553–555.

[30]Finch WR, Buckingham RB, Rodnan GP, Prince RK, Winkelstein A. Scleroderma induced by bleomycin. In: Black CM, Myers AR, eds., *Current Topics in Rheumatology. Systemic Sclerosis.* London: Gower Medical Publishing Ltd., 1985;114–121.

[31]Palestine RF, Millns JL, Sigel GT, *et al.* Skin manifestations of pentazocine abuse. *J Acad Dermatol.* 1980;2:47–55.

[32]Kerr HD. Cocaine and scleroderma. *South Med J.* 1989;82:1275–1276.

[33]Trozak DJ, Gould WM. Cocaine abuse and connective tissue disease. *J Am Acad Dermatol.* 1984;10:532.

[34]Lam M, Ballou SP. Reversible scleroderma renal crisis after cocaine use (letter). *N Engl J Med.* 1992;326:1435.

[35]Skyberg K, Ronneberg A, Kamoy J-I, Dale K, Borgersen A. Pulmonary fibrosis in cable plant workers exposed to mist and vapor of petroleum distillates. *Environ Res.* 1986;40:261–273.

[36]Thurlbeck WM, Thurlbeck SM. Pulmonary effects of paraquat poisoning. *Chest.* 1976;69:276–280.

[37]Hu H. Benzene-associated myelofibrosis (letter). *Ann Int Med.* 1987;106:171–172.

[38]Podell JE, Klinenberg JR, Kramer LS, Brown HV. Pulmonary toxicity with gold therapy. *Arthritis Rheum.* 1980;23:347–354.

[39]White DA, Rankin JA, Stover DE, *et al.* Methotrexate pneumonitis. Bronchoalveolar lavage findings suggest an immunologic disorder. *Am Rev Resp Dis.* 1989;139:18–26.

[40]Weinblatt ME. Methotrexate. In: Kelley WN, *et al.,* eds. *Textbook of Rheumatology.* Philadelphia: Saunders and Co., 1993;767–776.

[41]Larrieu AJ, Weiner I, Abston S, Warren MM. Retroperitoneal fibrosis. *Surg Gynecol Obst.* 1980;150:699–709.

IV

Rheumatic Syndromes Related to Medication and Other Potential Environmental Exposures

8

Environmentally Induced Systemic Lupus Erythematosus

Robert L. Rubin

INTRODUCTION

The report of Hoffman 1945[1] describing a 19-year-old army recruit who developed cutaneous, hematologic and renal disease with features of systemic lupus erythematosus (SLE) after treatment with topical and oral sulfadiazine is often cited as the first description of drug-induced lupus (DIL). In retrospect, this patient appeared to have had a hypersensitivity-like reaction to sulfadiazine associated with exacerbation or onset of SLE. Despite the widespread use of oral sulfa drugs, only one other report of lupus associated with these antibiotics has appeared.[2] This false signature case of DIL exemplifies the confusion in the literature regarding the complex relationships among environmental factors and lupuslike symptoms.

The association between environmental agents and symptoms of lupus can be organized into three major categories:

1) Drug exposure that is temporally related to a syndrome that resembles SLE in the majority of cases. This category encompasses DIL and drug-associated exacerbation of SLE or initiation of SLE flares. The latter group involves cases of preexisting SLE which persists or recurs after withdrawal of the implicated medication, while bona fide DIL usually occurs in the setting of a previously normal immune system and disappears after discontinuation of the medication.

2) Drugs or environmental agents associated with autoimmune disease displaying some lupuslike symptoms or signs. This category includes drug-induced hemolytic anemia, eosinophilia myalgia syndrome (EMS) associated with L-tryptophan (Chapter 6), toxic oil syndrome associated with aniline-adulterated cooking oil (Chapter 5), "adjuvant disease" associated with silicone breast implants (Chapter 7), silicosis associated with silica or asbestos dust (Chapter 7), and autoimmunity associated with vinyl chloride exposure (Chapter 8).

3) Environmental agents suspected of causing lupuslike disease based solely on studies in experimental animals. The principal examples in this category are the lupuslike syndrome associated with alfalfa sprouts (L-canavanine) in monkeys, and sclerodermalike autoimmunity associated with heavy metals in rats and mice.

DRUG-INDUCED LUPUS

Historical Perspective

The first report of a drug-related late-onset "collagen disease" resembling SLE, published in 1952, described 17 out of 211 hydralazine-treated patients who developed lupuslike symptoms.[3] However, because the treatment regimen of these patients was combined with hexamethonium chloride, the first unambiguous association between hydralazine and lupuslike disease should be attributed to Dustan and her colleagues at the Cleveland Clinic.[4] In this report, 13 out of 139 patients became ill after receiving 400 to 800 milligrams of hydralazine per day for an average of 12 months. In their follow-up paper in 1954, Perry and Schroeder[5] demonstrated that hexamethonium ion was not implicated in the lupuslike reaction in their prior publication because patients fully recovered after discontinuation of only hydralazine. Although procainamide was introduced for the treatment of cardiac arrhythmia at about the same time, it was not until 1962 that Ladd reported a patient who developed lupuslike features after six months of procainamide therapy.[6] During the next three years, another 11 cases of procainamide-induced lupus were reported.[7] By 1966 a scattering of cases of lupuslike disease as a side effect of therapy with isoniazid (INH), diphenylhydantoin, sulphamethoxypyridazine (a long-acting sulfonamide no longer in use), primidone and tetracycline appeared. Since these initial reports, it has become widely appreciated that patients treated with a diverse array of drugs can develop autoantibodies and clinical features similar to those seen in patients with idiopathic SLE. Reports of autoimmune features appearing after treatment with biologic materials such as recombinant cytokines (Chapter 13) suggest that the spectrum of drugs with the capacity to induce lupus will continue to increase.

Medications Associated with Drug-Induced Lupus

Drugs reported to be associated with a lupuslike syndrome are listed in Table 8-1. Generally, drugs that induce lupus also, with a much higher frequency, induce autoantibodies, but patients often remain asymptomatic, a condition termed drug-induced autoimmunity. Excluded from this list are drugs implicated only in the exacerbation of SLE; this situation is considered a separate and distinct phenomenon which is discussed in "Drugs Associated with Exacerbation of SLE or Initiation of SLE Flares" below. Also excluded are drugs whose initially reported association with a lupuslike syndrome has not been confirmed, despite many decades of use in countless patients. Eight drugs in Table 8-1 are enclosed in brackets because they are no longer in use; associations with some of these drugs were limited to single case reports. Thus, 38 drugs currently in use have a propensity for inducing autoantibodies and occasionally a lupuslike syndrome. Table 8-1 divides these drugs into therapeutic classes and indicates their approximate risk levels based on the number of reports. By far the highest-risk drugs are procainamide and hydralazine, with approximately 20% incidence for pro-

Table 8-1 Drugs documented to induce lupuslike disease in previously asymptomatic subjects

Agent*	Risk**	Agent*	Risk**
Antiarrhythmics		**Antithyroidals**	
Procainamide (Pronestyl)	High	Propylthiouracil (Propyl-thyracil)	Low
Quinidine (Quinaglute)	Moderate	[Thionamide]	N.A.
Disopyramide (Norpace)	Very low	[Methylthiouracil]	N.A.
Propafenone (Rythmol)	Very low		
		Antibiotics	
Antihypertensives		Isoniazid (INH)	Low
Hydralazine (Apresoline)	High	Nitrofurantoin (Macrodantin)	Very low
Methyldopa (Aldomet)	Low	Minocycline (Minocin)	Very low
Captopril (Capoten)	Low	[Sulfamethoxypyridazine]	N.A.
Acebutolol (Sectral)	Low		
Enalapril (Vasotec)	Very low	**Anti-Inflammatories**	
Clonidine (Catapres)	Very low	D-penicillamine (Cuprimine)	Low
Atenolol (Tenormin)	Very low	Sulfasalazine (Azulfidine)	Low
Labetalol (Normodyne, Trandate)	Very low	Phenylbutazone (Butazolidin)	Very low
Pindolol (Visken)	Very low		
Minoxidil (Loniten)	Very low	**Diuretics**	
Prazosin (Minipress)	Very low	Chlorthalidone (Hygroton)	Very low
[Practolol]	N.A.	Hydrochlorothiazide (Diuchlor H)	Very low
Antipsychotics		**Miscellaneous**	
Chlorpromazine (Thorazine)	Low	Lovastatin (Mevacor)	Very low
Perphenazine (Trilafon)	Very low	Levodopa (Dopar)	Very low
Phenelzine (Nardil)	Very low	Aminoglutethimide (Cytadren)	Very low
Chlorprothixene (Taractan)	Very low	Alpha-interferon (Wellferon)	Very low
Lithium carbonate (Eskalith)	Very low	Timolol eye drops (Timoptic)	Very low
		[Psoralen]	N.A.
Anticonvulsants		[Nomifensine]	N.A.
Phenytoin (Dilantin)	Very Low	[Phenopyrazone	N.A.
Carbamazepine (Tegretol)	Low	(in Venopyronum/Venocuran)]	
Trimethadione (Tridone)	Very low		
Primidone (Mysoline)	Very low		
Ethosuximide (Zarontin)	Very low		
[Phenylethyacetylurea]	N.A.		

*Commonly used brand names are enclosed in parentheses. Bracketed drugs are no longer in use and their risk is indicated as nonapplicable (N.A.).
**Risk refers to likelihood for lupuslike disease, not autoantibody induction, which is usually much more common. For references, see.[247]

cainamide and 5% to 8% for hydralazine during one year of therapy at currently used doses. The risk for developing lupuslike diseases for the remainder of the drugs is less than 1% of treated patients. Quinidine can be considered to be of moderate risk, while sulfasalazine, chlorpromazine, penicillamine, methyldopa, carbamazepine, acebutalol, INH, captopril and propylthiouracil are relatively low-risk. The remaining 27 drugs should be considered very low-risk based on the paucity of case reports in the literature. Obviously, the perception of risk is not rigorous since it depends on dose and frequency of prescriptions as well as occasion to publish case reports, and should not be equated with a fundamental, lupus-inducing propensity. Some drugs of very low risk may be falsely implicated or are currently of negligible risk because customary treatment doses have been decreased. Nevertheless, most reports of DIL are convincing because cessation of therapy usually results in prompt resolution of symptoms and eventually autoantibodies. It should be appreciated that criteria for a diagnosis of DIL-like disease are not as rigorous as those for diagnosis of SLE, as discussed in "Diagnostic Criteria for Drug-Induced Lupus" below.

As early as 1957, it was recognized that anticonvulsants can induce lupuslike features.[8] However, because manifestations of convulsive disorders may precede a diagnosis of SLE by many years, some of these patients may have had SLE rather than DIL. Furthermore, many of these patients are treated with more than one drug, making it difficult to identify the responsible medication. DIL associated with the use of phenytoin (diphenylhydantoin) and carbamezepine is well documented.

As with anticonvulsant therapy, patients who develop DIL or autoantibodies associated with antituberculous drugs use more than one medication. Triple therapy with INH, para-aminosalicylic acid (PAS), and streptomycin was once standard practice. The best evidence, however, points to INH as the drug most likely to induce autoimmunity.[9] The major manifestation of autoimmunity in patients on INH appears to be the development of low-titer antinuclear antibodies (ANA), and clinically diagnosed DIL is rare.[10] Interestingly, antihistone antibodies in these patients are predominantly IgA, suggestive of the involvement of the mucosal immune system in INH-induced autoimmunity.[11]

A broad variety of therapeutic indications is encompassed by lupus-inducing drugs listed in Table 8-1. Consequently, the structures of these drugs show wide disparity, reflected in their diverse biochemical action. Although some of these drugs are aromatic amines (procainamide, practolol and sulfpyridine, a metabolite of sulfasalazine) or aromatic hydrazines (hydralazine, INH), there is no common denominator of a pharmacologic, therapeutic or chemical nature that links the drugs with their capacity to induce lupuslike disease. Nevertheless, the remarkable similarity in clinical features and laboratory findings in lupus induced by this collection of drugs strongly suggests that the same mechanism underlies the process regardless of the inciting agent. The relationship of this process to drug chemistry is discussed in "Oxidative Metabolism of Lupus-Inducing Drugs" below.

Diagnostic Criteria For Drug-Induced Lupus

Specific criteria for the diagnosis of DIL have not been formally established. Although some of the criteria for the classification of SLE are applicable to DIL, the requirement for four manifestations, as established by the American College of Rheumatology,[12] is overly rigid for DIL. Furthermore, these criteria are obviously not useful for distinguishing between drug-induced and idiopathic SLE. Patients frequently present with mild or few lupuslike symptoms, so that they could readily be underdiagnosed if SLE criteria are strictly applied. The following are general guidelines for identifying DIL:

1) Continuous treatment with a known lupus-inducing drug for at least one month and usually much longer. DIL usually occurs after several months or years of continuous therapy and should not be confused with the short-term toxic side effects that are often associated with pharmaceuticals. The latency period for onset of lupuslike symptoms varies greatly—for procainamide, a median of ten months was calculated, although in a study of 50 patients, one-fourth did not develop symptoms until two or more years of therapy.[13] For hydralazine, the majority of patients require six months to two years exposure,[14] but it is not uncommon for a patient to be treated for greater than three years before symptoms manifest. This variation is largely due to differences in drug dosage required to maintain therapeutic control, resulting in different steady-state plasma drug concentration. However, genetic factors may also be involved, as discussed in "Genetic Factors in Drug-Induced Lupus" below.

2) Common presenting symptoms are arthralgia, myalgia, malaise, fever, serositis (pleuropericarditis, especially with procainamide) and polyarthritis (especially with quinidine). Rash or other dermatologic problems, or glomerulonephritis typical of SLE, are rare in DIL. In some patients, symptoms appear gradually and worsen over the course of many months of treatment with the implicated drug. In others, symptom onset is rapid, but symptoms do not necessarily worsen.

3) A common laboratory abnormality is the presence of antinuclear antibodies (ANA) which are due to antihistone antibodies, especially IgG anti-[(H2A-H2B)-DNA]. Antihistone antibodies are particularly useful for distinguishing asymptomatic drug-treated patients who develop benign ANA (that is, drug-induced autoimmunity) from patients with symptomatic DIL, because only the latter have IgG anti-[(H2A-H2B)-DNA] antibodies.[15]

4) Improvement and permanent resolution of symptoms generally occurs within days or weeks after discontinuation

of therapy. Serologic findings, especially autoantibody levels, often require months to resolve. Resolution of symptoms and laboratory abnormalities by withdrawing the offending drug is a defining feature of DIL. Although there is a strong temptation to treat patients suspected of DIL with anti-inflammatory agents, this maneuver may confound the diagnosis and should not be required for recovery from DIL.

Differential Diagnosis

It can be difficult to differentiate DIL from SLE, especially in the elderly, in whom clinical features have substantial overlap.[16,17] Because SLE is usually characterized by a much broader array of autoantibodies than is DIL (see "Laboratory Features of Drug-Induced Lupus" below), the serological profile can be very helpful in difficult cases. The differential diagnosis of DIL also includes viral syndromes and infectious diseases which may present with arthralgia, fever

and pleuropericarditis. Dressler's syndrome should be considered in a patient with a previous myocardial infarction. However, a recurrent ischemic myocardial event may also present with fever and pericarditis. The postpericardiotomy syndrome, which is similar to Dressler's syndrome and presents after cardiac surgery, can be confused with DIL because these patients are often treated with antiarrhythmics such as procainamide. Other diagnoses to be considered in the appropriate setting are rheumatoid arthritis, polymyalgia rheumatica, underlying malignancy, hypersensitive drug reactions (*vide infra*) and graft-versus-host disease.

Clinical Features of Drug-Induced Lupus

The range of clinical and laboratory features of lupus induced by procainamide and hydralazine can be described because of the numerous case reports involving these two drugs. The prevalence of symptoms and signs compared to idiopathic SLE are shown in Table 8-2. Musculoskeletal

Table 8-2 Prevalence of clinical and laboratory abnormalities in drug-induced lupus and SLE

Feature	Hydralazine-Induced Lupus*	Procainamide-Induced Lupus**	Systemic Lupus Erythematosus***
Symptoms			
Arthralgia	80%	85%	}80%
Arthritis	50%–100%	20%	
Pleuritis, pleural effusion	<5%	50%	44%
Fever, weight loss	40%–50%	45%	48%
Myalgia	<5%	35%	60%
Hepatosplenomegaly	15%	25%	5%–10%
Pericarditis	<5%	15%	20%
Rash	25%	<5%	71%
Glomerulonephritis	5%–10%	<5%	42%
CNS disease	<5%	<5%	32%
Signs			
ANA	>95%	>95%	97%
LE cell	>50%	80%	71%
Antihistone[†]	>95%	>95%	54%
Anti-[(H2A-H2B)-DNA][†]	43%	96%	70%
Anti-denatured DNA[†]	50%–90%	50%	82%
Anti-native DNA	<5%	<5%	28%–67%
Anticardiolipin	5%–15%	5%–20%	35%
Rheumatoid factor	20%	30%	25%–30%
Anemia	35%	20%	42%
Elevated ESR	60%	60%–80%	>50%
Leukopenia	5%–25%	15%	46%
+Coombs' test	<5%	25%	25%
Elevated gammaglobulins	10%–50%	25%	32%
Hypocomplementemia	<5%	<5%	51%

*Data compiled from Alarcón-Segovia, *et al,*[40] Hahn, *et al,*[41] Cameron and Ramsay[143] and Russell, *et al.*[126]
**Data compiled from Weinstein,[252] Harmon and Portanova,[253] Russell[254] and Hess and Mongey.[255]
***Data from Wallace.[235]
[†]From.[32,110,256]

Each prevalence represents consensus values ± 5 percentage points. Abnormalities occurring in fewer than 5% of patients may not be listed.

complaints, especially arthralgia, are commonly observed in DIL. There is some suggestion of a drug-specific symptomatology, with pleuritis and pericarditis common to procainamide-induced lupus, polyarthritis common to quinidine-induced lupus, and glomerulonephritis and rash in hydralazine-induced lupus. Lung involvement in procainamide-induced lupus occurs in approximately 50% of patients and consists of pleuritis, pleural effusions and/or pulmonary infiltrates; pericardial effusions are also common. Arthritis is less in lupus induced by procainamide (20%) than by hydralazine (50% to 100%). However, in any one patient, lupus induced by procainamide, hydralazine or other drugs cannot be distinguished by clinical features. Although a history of rheumatic disease independent of the suspected drug tends to negate a diagnosis of DIL, two diseases may develop concurrently. This situation is characteristic of patients with various forms of arthritis who also develop DIL during penicillamine or sulfasalazine therapy. In these difficult cases, serologic findings are especially informative.

The onset of symptoms in DIL can be insidious or acute, although an interval of one to two months typically passes before the diagnosis is made.[18–24] In most patients symptoms are mild and consist of fever, malaise, weight loss, polyarticular arthralgia and symmetrical myalgia. The symptoms of DIL usually resolve within days to weeks after discontinuing the offending drug. This removal of a suspected drug provides a key (although retrospective) diagnostic tool. The prevalence of musculoskeletal complaints in idiopathic SLE is very similar to that in procainamide-induced lupus. In contrast, skin, kidney and central nervous system involvement are much more common in SLE than in DIL. Although serious kidney disease is extremely rare for most lupus-inducing drugs, glomerulonephritis has been associated with hydralazine-induced lupus[25–29] and should not be a formal exclusion criterion for diagnosing DIL.

Laboratory Features of Drug-Induced Lupus

The prevalence of laboratory abnormalities in drug-induced lupus is shown in Table 8-2. The most commonly observed laboratory abnormality in DIL is a positive ANA, which is largely due to histone-reactive antibodies.[30,31] A systematic study of the antigenicity of histones, chromatin and nucleosome subunits revealed that the (H2A-H2B)-DNA complex contained the complete epitope for the bulk of the autoantibody activity in DIL, largely accounting for the capacity of DIL sera to bind to nucleosomes, chromatin and nuclei,[32] and to produce positive LE cells.[33] IgG anti-[(H2A-H2B)-DNA] antibodies occur in over 90% of patients prior to, or at the time of diagnosis of, procainamide-induced lupus.[32,34] These autoantibodies have also been detected in patients with lupus induced by penicillamine,[34,35] INH,[34,36] acebutalol,[34] methlydopa,[37] sulfasalazine[38] and opthalmic

timolol.[39] However, only approximately 50% of patients with quinidine- and 35% with hydralazine-induced lupus have detectable anti-[(H2A-H2B)-DNA] antibodies (Figure 8-1). IgG anti-[(H2A-H2B)-DNA] was found in 84% of patients with procainamide-induced lupus at the time of diagnosis, and low, but significantly elevated levels of this antibody activity were detected in 70% of patients up to one year before recognition of lupuslike symptoms.[16]

Autoantibodies to denatured (single-stranded) DNA (dDNA) are found in up to 50% of DIL sera.[34,40,41,42–48] These autoantibodies probably have multiple reactivities, and also bind to the nucleoside guanosine,[21,49] polyriboadenylic acid,[46,48] the phospholipid cardiolipin[50] and unusual conformations of DNA such as Z-DNA.[48,51] Anti-dDNA antibodies bearing the 16/6 and 32/15 idiotypes have been reported in one-third of patients with procainamide-induced lupus.[52] These idiotypes are also commonly expressed in idiopathic SLE. Anti-dDNA (but not anti-native DNA) antibodies are common in both DIL and SLE. However, the clinical significance of anti-dDNA is limited because these antibodies are commonly seen in asymptomatic patients and in those with a wide variety of rheumatic and inflammatory conditions.[53]

Less common laboratory features of DIL include circulating immune complexes,[54–56] positive Coombs' test (methyldopa,[57] chlorpromazine[58] and procainamide[59]), evidence of complement activation (procainamide),[13,60,61] hypocomplementemia (quinidine)[62] and a positive lupus band test.[63] However, unlike idiopathic SLE, low serum complement levels are not generally observed in DIL. Other laboratory features noted in a minority of DIL patients include mild anemia, leukopenia and thrombocytopenia,[13,42,59,64–66] hypergammaglobulinemia that is not as frequent as in SLE,[13,42,43,65–69] and an elevated erythrocyte sedimentation rate (ESR)[54,70,71] which commonly reverts toward normal as symptoms resolve.[62,65,71] Pancytopenia has been reported in association with procainamide therapy, but it is unlikely that these patients had DIL.[72,73] Agranulocytosis or severe neutropenia develops in about 1% of procainamide-treated patients,[74] but this condition is serologically and clinically distinct from DIL.[75] Hydralazine-induced lupus has been reported to be associated with acute neutrophilic dermatosis (Sweet's syndrome).[76,77] Rheumatoid factor (RF) has been reported in patients with procainamide-induced lupus.[42] Prospective studies suggest that RF is not drug-induced but rather reflects the increased prevalence of this autoantibody in the elderly population treated with the drug.[56,78] One study has reported the presence of antibodies in DIL sera directed against polyadenosine diphosphate-ribose.[79] Antinuclear ribonucleoprotein (RNP) antibodies were reported after short-term (prophylactic) procainamide treatment.[80] This observation has not been confirmed, and anti-RNP antibodies have not been observed in patients with DIL.[30,31,43,68] Cold-reactive lymphocytotoxic antibodies (LCTA) have been reported in procainamide-induced lupus,[81,82] but these

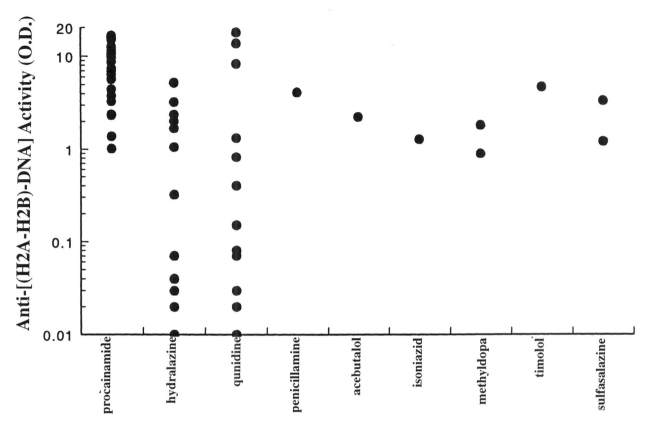

Fig. 8-1   IgG anti-[(H2A-H2B)-DNA] in lupus induced by various drugs. Each point represents the serum IgG anti-[(H2A-H2B)-DNA] activity in patients with lupus induced by the indicated drug.[32,34–39]

reactivities were also detected in procainamide-treated patients at the initiation of therapy and in asymptomatic procainamide-treated patients,[31,46,56] and therefore are unrelated to DIL. LCTA were also reported in four out of seven patients with hydralazine-induced lupus but also in 13 of 40 asymptomatic hydralazine-treated patients.[83,84] A recent study reported antibodies to high-mobility group proteins (HMG), especially HMG-14 and -17, in approximately half of the patients treated with procainamide, hydralazine and quinidine, whether or not they had symptomatic DIL.[85] This finding is of interest because HMG proteins bind to the core particle of the nucleosome, especially on transcriptionally active chromatin. This is consistent with the central role of chromatin in the autoantibody response observed in DIL.

Antibodies to the offending drugs have been detected in patients with lupus induced by procainamide[86] and hydralazine.[40] However, other studies have been unable to demonstrate drug-specific antibodies in patients treated with various lupus-inducing drugs.[31,43,68,87] In a prospective study of patients treated with hydralazine, only one of 27 sera showed binding to the drug.[46] The clinical significance of antibodies to drugs is unclear, because these antibodies have been reported in both asymptomatic and symptomatic indi-

viduals. In addition, it is unlikely that drug-binding antibodies represent cross-reactions with anti-dDNA or antichromatin autoantibodies.[87–89]

The presence of the lupus anticoagulant or of anticardiolipin antibodies has been described in patients using hydralazine,[90,91] procainamide[92–96] or chlorpromazine.[58,97–102] Up to 75% of patients treated with chlorpromazine for up to 2.5 years developed a lupus anticoagulant.[58,97] None of the patients developed features of SLE. In this setting, these antibodies are presumed to have no pathogenic significance because thrombosis is a rare (though it has been reported[92,95,103]) clinical event in lupus induced by procainamide, hydralazine or chlorpromazine.[104]

Neutrophil myeloperoxidase (MPO) and elastase antibodies were found in patients with hydralazine-induced lupus.[105,106] These specificities, as well as anti-proteinase-3 antibodies, were also reported in six patients treated with propylthiouracil,[107] and anti-MPO antibodies were observed in a patient with sulfasalazine-induced lupus.[108] These observations are of considerable interest because these antibodies contribute to the p- and c-ANCA neutrophil staining patterns that are associated with vasculitis of the capillaries and Wegener's granulomatosis, respectively.[109] The occurrence of glomerulonephritis in some patients with hydralazine-induced lupus may be related to anti-MPO antibodies.[28] Although anti-MPO antibodies occur in more than 50% of patients with hydralazine-induced lupus, they are not found in patients with lupus induced by procainamide (unpublished observations), consistent with the absence of kidney disease in procainamide-induced lupus.

It should be appreciated that many of these laboratory abnormalities are not linked to symptomatic DIL and can appear in asymptomatic drug-treated patients. Thus, appearance of antibodies to red blood cells (RBC), dDNA and total histones (but not the (H2A-H2B)-DNA complex) is independent of lupuslike symptoms. Nevertheless, like the clinical features, these autoantibodies are drug-induced and gradually subside after therapy with the offending agent is discontinued.

In summary, the serological abnormalities of lupus induced by procainamide and hydralazine are more restricted than those of idiopathic SLE. Although antihistone, anti-[(H2A-H2B)-DNA] and anti-dDNA antibodies are also common in SLE,[10] serum from these patients is rarely monospecific for these activities. Therefore, when a diagnosis cannot be clearly distinguished on clinical grounds, the presence of antibodies to native DNA, Sm, RNP, SS-A/Ro, SS-B/La or other nuclear antigens should be considered evidence against a diagnosis of DIL.

Kinetics of the Humoral Immune Response in Drug-Induced Lupus

Autoactivation of the humoral immune system is the overt expression of DIL. IgM, IgA and IgG autoantibodies reactive with native (H2A-H2B)-DNA, and denatured regions of chromatin (histones and dDNA) often develop simultaneously during procainamide treatment, although patients who remain asymptomatic fail to develop IgG anti-[(H2A-H2B)-DNA].[15] The high level of IgH autoantibody levels in procainamide-treated[15] and INH-treated[11] patients is remarkable, suggesting induction of autoantibody synthesis within the gastointestinal mucosal immune system where the drug concentration is presumably highest. The rather slow development of autoantibodies, the apparent concordance of IgG, IgA and IgM isotypes and the perpetuation of IgM autoantibodies for many years in asymptomatic, procainamide-treated patients suggest that the mechanism underlying drug induction of autoantibodies is unlike a classical immune phenomenon. Nevertheless, the restriction of the immune response to chromatin-derived antigens suggests that B cells with immunoglobulin receptors for various parts of chromatin become hyperactive in patients treated with diverse drugs. However, once induced, autoantibody secretion by these cells is not dependent upon the continuous presence of the drug because these autoantibodies have an apparent serum half-life of 2.5 to five months after withdrawal of procainamide,[15] approximately five times longer than the half-life of immunoglobulin in the circulation.[111]

Cellular Immune Abnormalities in Drug-Induced Lupus

Results of studies of cellular immune function in procainamide-treated patients have been somewhat conflicting. In one study, normal numbers and ratios of T helper and T suppressor cells were reported.[112] Procainamide enhanced immunoglobulin secretion *in vitro;* this was attributed to the inhibition of T suppressor cell activity.[113] Other investigators noted an increase of immunoglobulin secretion in the presence of pokeweed mitogen in patients treated with procainamide,[114,115] in agreement with the report of increased spontaneous IgM and especially IgG secretion by B cells from patients with procainamide-induced lupus.[116] Increased numbers of CD4+CD29+ activated T cells, interleukin-6 and soluble interleukin-2 receptors were observed in the pleural effusion of a patient with procainamide-induced lupus,[69] suggesting a role for local increased T-cell help in the pathogenesis of pleuritis.

Pathogenesis of Drug-Induced Lupus

Since symptoms and serologic features of DIL overlap with those of idiopathic SLE, it is presumed that similar pathogenic factors underlie both syndromes. However, immune complex formation and deposition in vital organs, one of the mechanisms shown to operate in SLE, have not been well documented in DIL. Immune complexes have been reported in patients with DIL,[54–56] but their composition, correlation with disease activity and pathogenic potential have not been evaluated. Evidence supporting the involvement of immune complexes in the pathogenesis of DIL includes the observations that complement breakdown products (for example, C3d and C4d) have been detected in individuals with DIL.[13,61] C4d/C4 ratios were significantly elevated in five of six procainamide-induced lupus patients,[13] and, in a prospective study, C4d levels gradually increased during the development of DIL and returned to normal 2.5 months after discontinuation of procainamide treatment.[60]

Immune complexes involving IgG anti-[(H2A-H2B)-DNA] and a chromatin-derived antigen are a candidate mediator of complement activation and subsequent inflammatory reactions. This possibility is consistent with the finding that anti-[(H2A-H2B)-DNA] activity is predominantly of IgG1 and IgG3[117] immunoglobulin subclasses, which are activators of the classical complement pathway when engaged by antigen. Detection of LE cells in patients with procainamide-induced lupus[33] also suggest the presence of complement-fixing autoantibodies. Although early studies of antihistone antibodies using indirect immunofluorescence failed to detect complement binding,[118,119] a subsequent study demonstrated deposition of C3, C4 and properdin mediated by anti-histone antibodies.[120] However, the lack of renal disease in DIL suggests that other factor(s), such as the form, amount or location of the target antigen, other autoantibodies such as anti-DNA or abnormalities in immune complex clearance, may account for the pathological features that are unique to SLE.

A small but significant reduction in the mean number of type 1 complement receptors for C3b on erythrocytes (CR1) was observed in patients with a prior history of hydralazine-induced lupus, and these individuals tended to have elevated circulating immune complexes.[55] However, based on restriction fragment polymorphism analysis, there was no difference between symptomatic and asymptomatic hydralazine-treated patients in the frequency of the allele encoding the low-expression CR1 phenotype,[121] indicating that patients with hydralazine-induced lupus may have an *acquired* deficiency (perhaps due to persisting immune complexes) in CR1 expression. Penicillamine[122] and procainamide-hydroxy-lamine,[123] a reactive metabolite of procainamide, inhibited C4—especially C4A—binding activity *in vitro*. It has been suggested, therefore, that these drugs may interfere with immune complex clearance by inhibiting classical complement pathway activation. However, measurements of Fc-receptor-mediated immune clearance in patients treated with chlorpromazine, procainamide, penicillamine or hydralazine with or without associated symptomatic disease has not demonstrated differences in clearance function.[54] These data suggest that, unlike in SLE, handling of circulating immune complexes by the reticuloendothelial system is not overloaded in DIL, possibly explaining the lack of kidney and CNS involvement.

Genetic Factors in Drug-Induced Lupus

HLA Phenotype

The immunogenetic factors that underlie DIL are of interest because only a small proportion of drug-treated patients develop symptomatic disease, and the immune response is restricted to a relatively narrow range of autoantigens. These observations implicate a role for major histocompatibility complex (MHC) encoded class II human leukocyte antigens (HLA), which are required for T-cell-dependent antibody responses. A study of 25 patients with hydralazine-induced lupus showed a 73% frequency of HLA-DR4 versus a frequency of 25% in asymptomatic patients, representing a relative risk of 8.1.[124–126] HLA-DR4 has been reported in individuals with penicillamine-induced lupus[127,128] and hydralazine-induced Sweet's syndrome.[76] However, a study of hydralazine-induced lupus from Australia[129] and a limited study of procainamide-induced lupus in Americans[21] failed to find a significant HLA association. Reexamination of

patients with hydralazine-induced lupus in the English study for complement protein phenotypes demonstrated that 76% of these patients had one or more C4 null alleles, compared to 43% of normal controls (p < 0.01).[130] The genes encoding the C4 complement proteins are situated between the HLA-B and HLA-DR loci, and the C4 null/DR4 haplotype displays linkage disequilibrium in Caucasians. Therefore the reported association of hydralazine-induced lupus with HLA-DR4 is probably a result of the C4 null trait,[131] and linkage disequilibrium between HLA-DR4 and C4 may not occur in the Australian study group.

HLA-Dw44 was suggested as a significant risk factor (relative risk equal to 3.6) for chlorpromazine-induced ANA.[131] Similarly, among procainamide-treated patients, there was a significant association between HLA-DQw7 and IgG antibodies to histones and H2A-H2B.[132] These results may suggest that these class II antigens have a propensity to present histone peptides to T cells. However, since most patients treated with hydralazine or procainamide develop ANA, it is unlikely that only one or a few HLA allotypes are necessary for autoantibody induction by these drugs. More controlled studies are required to determine whether MHC genes are important in the development of DIL.

Complement

The complement genes are part of the MHC class III region, and C4A and C4B are encoded by separate loci. Individuals with genetic deficiencies in one—and especially both—C4 genes have greatly increased susceptibility to SLE[134] presumably because insufficient classical pathway activation results in impaired immune complex clearance. As mentioned above, 76% of patients with hydralazine-induced lupus had one or more C4 null alleles, compared to 43% of normal subjects.[130] Therefore, a congenital defect in immune complex clearance may also predispose to DIL. It has not been determined, however, whether patients treated with hydralazine who remain asymptomatic have a low frequency of C4 null alleles. Similarly, it is not clear whether the occasional hypocomplementemia associated with procainamide-induced lupus[135] may be related to C4 deficiency. In most patients with DIL, serum complement levels are within the normal range.[55] There was no preferential association of C4A null versus C4B null with hydralazine-induced lupus.[130]

Acetylator Phenotype

Acetylator phenotype is the most well-characterized genetically determined predisposing factor in DIL, but its significance is often misunderstood. The studies of Perry and colleagues demonstrated that the activity of hepatic acetyl-transferase was inversely associated with the likelihood of development of DIL.[136] The acetyl group of acetyl-CoA can be transferred to the amino group of many small molecules by the action of acetyltransferases. Individuals who are slow acetylators are homozygous for a recessive gene that controls hepatic acetyltransferase activity and have an approximately twofold higher serum level of unacetylated drugs at equivalent therapeutic doses.

Compared to patients who are rapid acetylators, autoantibodies and clinical symptoms develop more quickly and in higher frequency during the treatment with hydralazine[124,136] and procainamide of patients who are slow acetylators.[24] Clinical symptoms also occur in up to 20% of patients who are rapid acetylators,[126] but both the dose and duration of drug administration are generally greater in these patients.[24] These studies support the hypothesis that the steady-state concentration of unacetylated procainamide and hydralazine and the duration of drug exposure are important determinants in the development of DIL. Such observations have led to the use of N-acetylprocainamide (NAPA) in the successful control of cardiac arrhythmias while bringing about the remission of procainamide-induced lupus.[137] NAPA has not been reported to reduce lupus or ANA or anti-dDNA.[138,139] Furthermore, if the procainamide dose is adjusted so that all patients have the same steady-state plasma concentration by increasing the dose for rapid acetylators, no difference has been observed between slow and rapid acetylators in the time for development of ANA or DIL.[20]

The importance of the free amino/hydrazino group of these drugs in the development of autoantibodies and DIL has been interpreted in two ways. A commonly held view is that these chemical moieties play a direct role in the induction of autoimmunity, and acetylation prevents this action. Alternatively, *in vivo* metabolism (other than acetylation) of the drug at this moiety may generate the active, autoimmunity-inducing compound, while N-acetylation blocks drug metabolism. In this view, the putative reactive metabolites, rather than the parent molecule, interact with a key immune target, leading to induction of autoimmunity ("Oxidative Metabolism of Lupus-Inducing Drugs" below). The association of the slow acetylator phenotype with symptomatic DIL can then be explained by a higher steady-state concentration of the metabolizable form of the drug. The lack of an association between acetylator phenotype and induction of ANA by INH[140] or by captopril[141] as well as idiopathic SLE[142] indicates that the slow acetylator phenotype is not a general predisposing factor for the autoimmune state, nor is it genetically linked to a putative autoimmunity-inducing or autoimmunity-accelerating gene.

Gender

The high female-to-male predominance characteristic of SLE (9:1 to 7:1) is not seen in DIL. This is largely because the majority of patients treated with the major lupus-inducing drugs are men. Nevertheless, procainamide-induced[18,21] and hydralazine-induced[19,124,126,143] lupus appear to be disproportionately more common in females. In the study by Totoritis and colleagues[18] the female-to-male ratio of procainamide-treated patients who developed lupuslike symptoms was 0.52, compared to a ratio of 0.19 for those who remained asymptomatic. A similar twofold-to-fourfold predominance of women over men for development of hydralazine-induced lupus has been reported.[124,126,143] In the study by Cameron and Ramsey,[143] the overall incidence of hydralazine-induced lupus during a four-year observation period was 11.6% in women and 2.8% in men. In this study, women treated with a daily dose of 200 milligrams of hydralazine had a 19.4% incidence of DIL during a three-year period. This contrasts with the rate of development of ANA in these patients, which demonstrated no gender differences.[19]

Race

Unlike SLE, the frequency of hydralazine-induced lupus in blacks was reported to be fourfold[22] to sixfold[14] lower than in whites. Whether this discordance between SLE and DIL reflects genetic factors or other demographic features is not know.

Oxidative Metabolism of Lupus-Inducing Drugs

The following features of drug-induced autoimmunity are difficult to explain by a direct action of the ingested, parent compound on some component of the immune system:

1) Lupus-inducing drugs are highly diverse in chemical structure and pharmacological action, yet the laboratory and clinical features of lupus induced by all the drugs are essentially the same.

2) Except for their pharmacological action, lupus-inducing drugs are largely inert at customary doses; nonspecific or generalized toxicity would preclude their use as therapeutic agents. Drug-induced lupus is therefore an idiosyncratic reaction not predicted by any known property of the implicated drugs.

3) Drugs reach a steady-state concentration within a few hours, but drug-induced autoimmunity and lupus require many months to develop.

Metabolic transformation of the ingested drug to a reactive compound may account for many features of DIL. *In vivo* metabolism of dissimilar drugs to a product with a common reactive property could explain how compounds with widely different pharmacological and chemical characteristics could produce the same adverse reaction. The low probability for a productive metabolic event could explain the long lag time for the development of autoimmunity.

Incubation of procainamide *in vitro* with human or rat liver microsomes which contain the "mixed function oxidases" results in the formation of an unstable product, procainamide-hydroxylamine (PAHA).[144,145] PAHA can be detected after the perfusion of rat liver with procainamide in a blood-free environment.[146] Hydralazine and INH are also susceptible to hepatic oxidative metabolism.[147,148] PAHA is cytotoxic under certain conditions,[149] and this biologic activity is enhanced by oxyhemoglobin in erythrocytes,[146,150] presumably by converting PAHA to nitroso-procainamide,[149–151] which has even greater cytotoxicity. Hepatic metabolism of drugs to reactive products demonstrates that the chemistry exists for generation of potentially toxic compounds, but these products typically bind to microsomes or macromolecules near their site of formation and fail to exit the liver in reactive forms. Although rats treated with procainamide showed increased liver lipid peroxide levels and antioxidant activity,[152] hepatotoxicity is not associated with drug-induced autoimmunity, making it unlikely that sufficient amounts of reactive metabolites of lupus-inducing drugs are generated in the liver to interact with lymphocytes or inflammatory cells *in situ*. The highly reactive nature of oxidative drug metabolites confers the capacity to interact with many kinds of self-molecules, but there appears to be no preferential binding to the chromatin-related structures that are the targets of the autoimmune response in DIL.

Rubin and colleagues[153] showed that activated peripheral blood neutrophils can metabolize procainamide to PAHA in the extracellular milieu; the role of the respiratory burst and degranulation associated with neutrophil and macrophage activation was confirmed[154] and analyzed in detail.[155] Metabolism of drugs by activated neutrophils provides a mechanism for generating highly reactive metabolites directly within lymphoid tissue, where autoimmunity presumably develops. Since neutrophils are present in high concentration in the circulation, local production of labile compounds can potentially occur in any lymphoid compartment, minimizing dilution effects.

Essentially all pharmacological classes of lupus-inducing drugs have been demonstrated to undergo oxidative metabolism by activated neutrophils.[154–169] The general mechanism responsible for neutrophil-mediated drug transformation is shown in Figure 8-2. Drug metabolism via this pathway requires the *enzymatic* action of MPO, as evidenced by the competitive inhibition of MPO activity by all lupus-inducing drugs tested and the correlation of this property with neutrophil-dependent drug cytotoxicity.[156]

Indirect evidence that neutrophil-mediated drug metabolism is required for induction of autoimmunity is suggested by the strong correlation between MPO-mediated oxidative drug transformation and propensity of the drug to induce lupus. Nitro-procainamide, a further oxidation product of PAHA,[149,151] has been detected in the urine of procainamide-treated patients.[133,170] Urinary metabolites of hydralazine have also been described.[78,171] Murine T cells sensitized to

oxidative metabolites of procainamide,[172] propylthiouracil or gold(I) thiomalate[173,174] displayed specific responses to lysates of phagocytic cells derived from mice subjected to long-term treatment with the respective parent compound, but did not respond to the parent compound itself. These data suggest that lupus-inducing drugs undergo oxidative metabolism *in vivo,* implicating these products in the induction of autoimmunity. N-acetylation of hydralazine and procainamide competes with N-oxidation of these drugs, accounting for the lower probability for development of autoimmunity in individuals with the rapid acetylation phenotype.

Animal Models of Autoimmunity Related to Lupus-Inducing Drugs

Attempts to induce ANA by oral administration of lupus-inducing drugs in mice have met with limited success.[175–181] These murine models are generally impractical because of the long treatment period required to develop even a partial response, the frequent spontaneous seroconversion of aging mice to ANA positivity, and the inability to achieve steady-state blood levels of the drug which are comparable to therapeutic levels in humans. More recently, a lupus-like chemopathological model, including autoantibodies and glomerulonephritis, has been produced in mice by injection of syngeneic splenocytes treated with procainamide *in vitro.*[182] For this effect to be manifested, splenocytes were first allogeneically activated and then treated *in vitro* with procainamide (50 μM) prior to their adoptive transfer monthly for six months into syngeneic mice.[182] A conalbumin-specific T-cell clone treated with procainamide or 5-azacytidine produced a similar *in vivo* pathology,[183] suggesting that this animal model did not require autoantigen-specific T cells exposed to procainamide. These phenomena appear similar to the autoimmune side effects accompanying the graft-versus-host reaction upon adoptive transfer of semiallogeneic T cells,[184] as has been proposed during T-cell sensitization to penicillamine,[185] diphenylhydantoin[186] and gold(III).[173,174]

Oral administration of propylthiouracil into mongrel cats for two months resulted in the development of ANA, direct anti-RBC antibodies and lupuslike symptoms in approximately half the animals.[187] Discontinuation of propylthiouracil or replacement with propyluracil caused resolution of symptoms and signs within one to four weeks,[187] indicating that this was a bona fide drug-induced lupuslike syndrome. Induction of autoimmunity was drug-dose-dependent, and cats which had previously developed propylthiouracil-induced lupus followed by a three-month washout period were not hyperresponsive to challenge with propylthiouracil (that is, they failed to redevelop disease at lower challenge doses).[188] Interestingly, the ANA was predominantly due to anti-native DNA antibodies; antihistone antibodies were not detected.[188] Therefore, this syndrome has

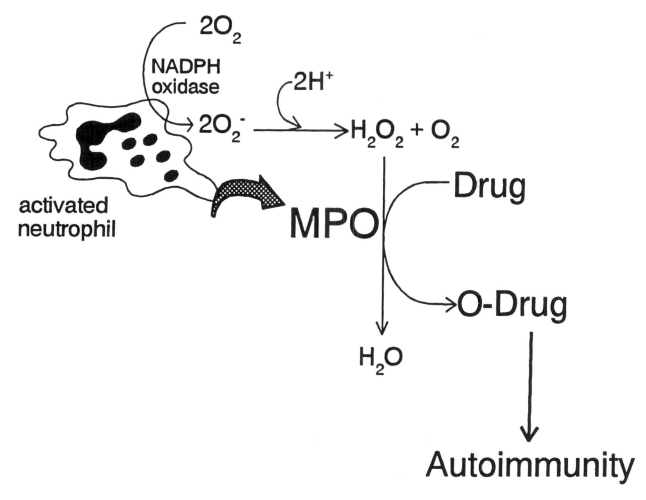

Fig. 8-2 Mechanism for transformation of drugs by activated neutrophils. Activation of neutrophils by opsonized particles or certain soluble factors triggers the ectoenzyme NADPH oxidase to produce superoxide anion (O_2^-) in the extracellular environment. O_2^- spontaneously dismutates to hydrogen peroxide (H_2O_2). Neutrophil granulation results in release of myeloperoxidase (MPO). Lupus-inducing drugs are MPO substrates and will participate in electron transfer with the H_2O_2-MPO intermediate. The functional group on the drug accepts an oxygen atom from H_2O_2, resulting in formation of a new compound. These unstable drug metabolites are candidates for initiating autoimmunity within an immune compartment. From.[155,156]

features of both drug-induced and idiopathic SLE, and may be a unique feline animal model.

A number of lupus-inducing drugs (hydralazine, chlorpromazine, carbamazepine, phenylbutazone and nitrofurantoin) will cause significant enlargement of the draining popliteal lymph node when injected subcutaneously into the hind foot pad of mice.[189] In this popliteal lymph node assay it is presumed that specific T_H cells respond to drug-altered self-proteins followed by B-cell expansion,[186,190,191] although nonspecific mitogenic or bystander effects have not been excluded. Procainamide, INH and propylthiouracil failed to induce lymphadenopathy in this assay[172,189,192] unless oxidatively metabolized by rat liver microsomes[192] or peritoneal macrophage,[172] or unless the metabolite itself, such as PAHA, was injected.[172] The requirement for a drug metabolite is in good agreement with the *in vitro* studies demonstrating neutrophil-mediated metabolism of the same drugs (see "Oxidative Metabolism of Lupus-Inducing Drugs" above). How-

ever, some drugs not reported to induce lupus were also positive in the popliteal lymph node assay,[173,174,189,193,194] indicating that this assay may be a general screening test for xenobiotics with immunostimulatory potential of various types. Appearance of antichromatin antibodies accompanying T-cell reactions to lupus-inducing drugs has not yet been reported.

DRUGS ASSOCIATED WITH EXACERBATION OF SLE OR INITIATION OF SLE FLARES

The report by Hoffman in 1945[1] and many similar subsequent studies helped to entrench the view that many cases of idiopathic SLE are "unmasked" during drug therapy in patients with a lupus diathesis.[195] This idea is difficult to discount or prove. Various drugs have been noted to have a temporal relationship with the exacerbation of SLE or with the onset of chronic SLE prior to diagnosis.[10] In the latter cases, SLE persists after withdrawal of the implicated agent. These drugs include antibiotics, anticonvulsants, hormones, nonsteroidal anti-inflammatory drugs (NSAIDs) and dermatologic agents. Sulfonamides,[196] tetracyclines,[197] griseofulvin,[198–200] piroxicam[201] and benoxaprofen[202] are reported to be photosensitizers of varying frequency. Drug-induced aseptic meningitis due to therapy with ibuprofen[203] and other NSAIDs (for example, sulindac,[204] tolmetin,[205] diclofenac[206]) is an important consideration for the physician involved in the care of SLE patients who present with signs of meningeal irritation. Hypersensitivity reactions that have been interpreted as initiating or aggravating factors in SLE are associated with hydralazine,[207] sulfonamides,[1,2,196,208] penicillin,[196] para-aminosalicylic acid,[209] hydrochlorothiazide,[210] cimetidine,[211] phenylbutazone,[212,213] mesantoin[8] and various NSAIDs.[10,214] Unknown or suspected environmental "chemicals" such as hair dyes and permanent wave preparations[215] are also occasionally implicated as causal agents in SLE and related diseases. Some reports have suggested that the incidence of SLE is increased following oral contraceptives, and that remissions follow cessation of their use.[217,218] These findings could not be substantiated.[10,219,220] An apparent immune-medicated syndrome develops in approximately 1% of gold-treated patients (see "Xenobiotics Related to Autoimmunity in Animals" below).

DRUGS OR ENVIRONMENTAL AGENTS ASSOCIATED WITH LUPUSLIKE SYMPTOMS OR SIGNS: DRUG-INDUCED IMMUNE HEMOLYTIC ANEMIA

Medications, certain foods, dietary supplements or contaminants in the diet have been associated with induction of autoimmunity displaying some lupuslike features. Non-drug-induced autoimmune syndromes are discussed in other chapters in this book (*vide supra*). Long-term therapy with certain drugs is associated with development of hemolytic anemia due to antibodies bound to red blood cells (RBC) *in vivo* (direct Coombs test positivity). In the penicillin-type reaction, antibody to the drug binds to RBC as a result of adsorption of the drug or its metabolite to the RBC membrane. In the methyldopa-type reaction, the drug is not required for (and does not affect) antibody binding, and anti-RBC antibodies typically have specificity for rhesus locus or other intrinsic RBC antigens. These antibodies rarely produce frank hemolytic anemia, possibly because their isotype or low avidity does not support complement fixation. Hemolytic anemia is commonly associated with the stibophen type of drug-induced antibodies (such as quinidine and quinine), in which immune complexes consisting of the drug metabolite bind to RBC presumably via Fc or complement receptors.

The mechanism underlying the penicillin type of anti-RBC response is frequently used as the basis for models for autoantibody elicitation in DIL. Interestingly, the autoantibodies associated with DIL behave more like the methyldopa type of immune response, in that the likelihood for autoantibody appearance is dose-dependent but the drug is not required for antibody binding to its target antigen. In fact, many of the drugs associated with Coombs' positivity of this drug-independent type (methyldopa, L-dopa, mefenamic acid (Ponstel), procainamide, chlorpromazine and streptomycin[221]) are also known to cause DIL or induce autoantibodies (Table 9-1), although there is generally no correlation between positive Coombs' test and ANA or DIL. However, patients with methyldopa-induced hemolytic anemia have been reported to have positive LE cells and ANA.[37,222–226] As with the autoantibodies associated with DIL, Coombs' positivity gradually disappears after cessation of therapy, and individuals with a history of methyldopa-induced anti-RBC autoantibodies do not display significantly increased propensity for induction of anti-RBC upon reinstitution of therapy with the same drug.[227] The mechanism for induction of this type of anti-RBC is unknown. However, despite the drug-independence of anti-RBC binding, a drug-altered RBC-antigen model is commonly invoked,[221] and this underlies most proposed mechanisms for induction of autoantibodies by drugs associated with induction of lupus (see "Mechanisms Underlying Xenobiotic-Induced Lupuslike Disease" below).

XENOBIOTICS RELATED TO AUTOIMMUNITY IN ANIMALS

Some xenobiotics are suspected of inducing autoimmunity based solely on studies in experimental animals. Parenteral, subcutaneous or intramuscular injection of mercuric chloride, gold(I) thiomalate or silver nitrate into mice possessing the H-2^S MHC class II phenotype results in an acute, self-limited autoimmune disease characterized by ANA and immune complex glomerulonephritis.[228,229] The major target of mercury-induced autoantibodies is the nucleolar protein fibrillarin,[230] a specific serologic marker for a subset of patients with scleroderma.[231] While this animal model is of considerable mechanistic interest, mercury has not been definitely implicated in autoimmune disease in humans, although it has been suggested that exposure to the heavy metals such as gold, silver and mercury in dental amalgam could underly autoimmunity in HLA-susceptible individuals.[232] Gold therapy for rheumatoid arthritis can result in leukopenia, thrombocytopenia or proteinuria in approximately 1% of treated patients.[233] These abnormalities are generally considered immune-mediated,[234] but they fall outside the usual presenting symptoms and clinical progression of SLE[235] or DIL. No report of gold-induced lupus has appeared, despite over six decades of treatment experience.

A prospective study of dietary intake of alfalfa seeds, alfalfa sprouts and L-canavanine, the suspected toxin in alfalfa, was undertaken in monkeys. Approximately half the animals developed ANA, anti-native DNA, hypocomplementemia and other symptoms and signs of SLE.[236,237] However, because this autoimmune effect required approximately a half-year of ingestion of a diet containing 40% to 45% (dried) alfalfa, it is unlikely that legumes are responsible for disease in most SLE patients. Nevertheless, several case reports of lupuslike disease associated with the ingestion of abnormally large amounts of alfalfa seeds or tablets[238,239] add another xenobiotic (presumably L-canavanine) to the list of compounds capable of inducing or exacerbating SLE.

MECHANISMS UNDERLYING XENOBIOTIC-INDUCED LUPUSLIKE DISEASE

Between 1954 and 1973, many examples appeared of the rapid recurrence of symptoms of DIL upon reintroduction of hydralazine,[5,14,22,240,241] procainamide,[242,243] INH,[244] penicillamine[245] and chlorpromazine.[246] Reports of DIL were often mixed with cases of drug-related lupus flares, drug-induced hemolytic anemia and drug allergies, leading to the notion that environmental agents operate in the same way to unmask incipient SLE. As a result, the view became ingrained in medical teachings that DIL behaves like a hypersensitivity reaction to the drug in individuals who are genetically predisposed to this side effect. The failure to recognize distinctions among various drug-associated illnesses was further confounded by the discovery of some drugs with capacity to bring about more than one syndrome. This confusion helped to promote the premise (modeled after penicillin-mediated allergic reactions) that stable drug-macromolecular complexes may initiate autoantibody and/or T-cell responses in drug-induced diseases. These concepts, variants of drug-hypersensitivity mechanisms involving an immune response to the drug or to a self-antigen altered directly or indirectly by the drug, were tested in numerous studies during the past 30 years (reviewed in[13,247,248]). Although positive immunological effects of drugs were reported, these studies invariably relied on nonpharmacologically relevant drug concentrations, artificial drug-macromolecular complexes, or addition of various types of adjuvants to elicit the observed effects. More recently, the capacity of drugs to enhance B- or T-cell function have been examined. Especially provocative are studies showing that inhibition of constitutive DNA methylation in lymphocytes by procainamide and hydralazine is associated with T-cell autoactivation *in vitro* and *in vivo* (*vide supra*).[249,250] Determining whether these phenomena are specific to lupus-inducing drugs and reflect the features characteristic of DIL (*vide supra*) will require further work.

The interpretation of the drug challenge studies in patients previously diagnosed with DIL is obscure. Reexamination of these reports reveals that in most cases, reintroduction of the implicated drug occurred within a few weeks after therapy was discontinued. Typically, these patients displayed symptom recurrence within one to two days after resuming therapy. It is now clear that although subjective symptoms of DIL may resolve in a few weeks, serological abnormalities, especially histone-reactive antibodies, persist for much longer. Thus, drug-induced immune abnormalities in most of these patients probably had not resolved when the rechallenge occurred, suggesting that a combination of autoantibody and another factor dependent on the drug is required for the pathology of DIL. Perhaps the most thorough study of this phenomenon was performed in 11 patients with hydralazine-induced lupus after a "long" (though unspecified) washout period.[15] In this study, three patients had symptom recurrence within one day, two within 14 days, two within two months and one after seven months, while three never developed symptom recurrence during the second treatment period of one to five years. It remains debatable whether variability in symptom recurrence reflects differences in putative predisposing factors for development of DIL, or differences in time for the autoimmune state to normalize. It is clear, however, that this process does not reflect a drug hypersensitivity reaction, which is characteristically drug dose-independent and recurs immediately after rechallenge with the inciting agent.[251]

Whether an environmental or pharmaceutical agent might aggravate or unmask incipient SLE should be considered a clinical problem distinct from DIL because, by definition, symptoms of DIL resolve after discontinuation of therapy. If drugs or environmental agents are truly causative in initiating or aggravating SLE, the mechanistic basis for this is probably different from that of DIL, because the steady-state blood levels of bona fide lupus-inducing drugs must generally be sustained for many months to years (that is, medications two to six times daily) for development of DIL. In contrast, for most cases of SLE believed to be xenobiotic-aggravated or -precipitated, chemical exposure is of very low level or infrequent when the suspected agent is environmental, or of relatively short duration when a drug is implicated. The association between drugs and the exacerbation or onset of SLE resembles the lupus flares following exposure to sunlight, exercise or pregnancy, and it is difficult to eliminate the possible occurrence of a spontaneous flare coincident with exposure to the xenobiotic.

CONCLUDING REMARKS

The similarities in duration of drug exposure, as well as laboratory and clinical features of SLE related to drugs in previously asymptomatic individuals, strongly suggest that the same mechanism underlies DIL regardless of the inciting agent. Oxidative metabolism of drugs transforms these heterogeneous parent compounds into products with similar, reactive properties, providing a starting point for investigating the underlying mechanism. In contrast, no single mechanism is likely to explain drug-related exacerbation of SLE, drug-induced hemolytic anemias, or the several well-documented examples of other environmental factors involved in initiating lupuslike disease. Nevertheless, DIL and other syndromes involving the associations between environmental factors and lupuslike symptoms indicate that autoimmunity can be acquired, and understanding these aberrations of immune tolerance may one day shed light on how the immune system discriminates self from foreign antigens.

REFERENCES

[1]Hoffman BJ. Sensitivity to sulfadiazine resembling acute disseminated lupus erythematosus. *Arch Dermatol Syphilol.* 1945;51:190–192.

[2]Honey M. Systemic lupus erythematosus presenting with sulphonamide hypersensitivity reaction. *Br Med J.* 1956;1:1272–1275.

[3]Morrow JD, Schroeder HA, Perry HM Jr. Studies on the control of hypertension by hyphex. II. Toxic reactions and side effects. *Circulation.* 1953;8:829–839.

[4]Dustan HP, Taylor RD, Corcoran AC, Page IH. Rheumatic and febrile syndrome during prolonged hydralazine treatment. *JAMA.* 1954;154:23–29.

[5]Perry HM, Schroeder HA. Syndrome simulating collagen disease caused by hydralazine (Apresoline). *JAMA.* 1954;154:670–673.

[6]Ladd AT: Procainamide-induced lupus erythematosus. *N Engl J Med.* 1962;267:1357–1358.

[7]Sanford HS, Michaelson AK, Halpern MM. Procainamide-induced lupus erythematosus syndrome. *Dis Chest.* 1967;51:172–176.

[8]Lindqvist T. Lupus erythematosus disseminatus after administration of mesantoin. Report of two cases. *Acta Med Scand.* 1957;158:131–138.

[9]Rothfield NF, Bierer WF, Garfield JW. Isoniazid induction of antinuclear antibodies. A prospective study. *Ann Intern Med.* 1978;88:650–652.

[10]Wallace DJ, Dubois EL. Drugs that exacerbate and induce systemic lupus erythematosus. In: Wallace DJ, Dubois EL, eds. *Dubois' Lupus Erythematosus.* 3rd edition. Philadelphia, PA: Lea and Febiger, 1987;450–469.

[11]Vázquez-Del Mercado M, Casiano CA, Rubin RL. IgA antihistone antibodies in isoniazid-treated tuberculosis patients. *Autoimmunity.* 1995;20:105–111.

[12]Tan EM, Cohen AS, Fries JF, *et al.* The 1982 revised criteria for the classification of systemic lupus erythematosus. *Arthritis Rheum.* 1982;25(11):1271–1277.

[13]Rubin RL. Autoimmune reactions induced by procainamide and hydralazine. In: Kammüller M, Bloksma M, Seimen W, eds. *Autoimmunity and Toxicology: Immune Disregulation Induced by Drugs and Chemicals.* Amsterdam: Elsevier, 1989;119–150.

[14]Perry HM Jr. Late toxicity of hydralazine resembling systemic lupus erythematosus or rheumatoid arthritis. *Am J Med.* 1973;54:58–72.

[15]Rubin RL, Burlingame RW, Arnott JE, Totoritis MC, McNally EM, Johnson AD. IgG but not other classes of anti-[(H2A-H2B)-DNA] is an early sign of procainamide-induced lupus. *J Immunol.* 1995;154:2483–2493.

[16]Cattogio LJ, Skinner RP, Smith G, Maddison PJ. Systemic lupus erythematosus in the elderly: Clinical and serological characteristics. *J Rheumatol.* 1984;11:175–181.

[17]Ward MM, Polisson RP: A meta-analysis of the clinical manifestations of older-onset systemic lupus erythematosus. *Arthritis Rheum.* 1989;32:1226–1232.

[18]Henningsen NC, Cederberg A, Hanson A, Johansson BW. Effects of long-term treatment with procainamide. *Acta Med Scand.* 1975;198:475–482.

[19]Mansilla-Tinoco R, Harland SJ, Ryan PJ, *et al.* Hydralazine, antinuclear antibodies, and the lupus syndrome. *Br Med J.* 1982;284:936–939.

[20]Sonnhag C, Karlsson E, Hed J. Procainamide-induced lupus erythematosus-like syndrome in relation to acetylator phenotype and plasma levels of procainamide. *Acta Med Scand.* 1979;206:245–251.

[21]Totoritis MC, Tan EM, McNally EM, Rubin RL. Association of antibody to histone complex H2A-H2B with symptomatic procainamide-induced lupus. *N Engl J Med.* 1988;318:1431–1436.

[22]Condemi JJ, Moore-Jones D, Vaughan JH, Perry HM. Antinuclear antibodies following hydralazine toxicity. *N Engl J Med.* 1967;276:486–490.

[23]Blomgren SE, Condemi JJ, Bignall MC, Vaughan JH. Antinuclear antibody induced by procainamide: A prospective study. *N Engl J Med.* 1969;281:64–66.

[24]Woosley RL, Drayer DE, Reidenberg MM, Nies AS, Carr K, Oates JA. Effect of acetylator phenotype on the rate at which procainamide induces antinuclear antibodies and the lupus syndrome. *N Engl J Med.* 1978;298:1157–1159.

[25]Ihle BU, Whitworth JA, Dowling JP, Kincaid-Smith P. Hydralazine and lupus nephritis. *Clin Nephrol.* 1984;22:230–238.

[26]Bjorck S, Svalander C, Westberg G. Hydralazine-associated glomerulonephritis. *Acta Med Scand.* 1985;218:261–269.

[27]Naparstek Y, Kopolovic J, Tur-Kaspa R, Rubinger D. Focal glomerulonephritis in the course of hydralazine-induced lupus syndrome. *Arthritis Rheum.* 1984;27:822–825.

[28]Torffvit O, Thysell H, Nassberger L. Occurrence of autoantibodies directed against myeloperoxidase and elastase in patients treated with hydralazine and presenting with glomerulonephritis. *Hum Exp Toxicol.* 1994;13:563–567.

[29]Shapiro KS, Pinn VW, Harrington JT, Levey AS. Immune complex glomerulonephritis in hydralazine-induced SLE. *Am J Kidney Dis.* 1984;3:270–274.

[30]Fritzler MJ, Tan EM. Antibodies to histones in drug-induced and idiopathic lupus erythematosus. *J Clin Invest.* 1978;62:560–567.

[31]Rubin RL, Reimer G, McNally EM, Nusinow SR, Searles RP, Tan EM. Procainamide elicits a selective autoantibody immune response. *Clin Exp Immunol.* 1986;63:58–67.

[32]Burlingame RW, Rubin RL. Drug-induced anti-histone autoantibodies display two patterns of reactivity with substructures of chromatin. *J Clin Invest.* 1991;88:680–690.

[33]Vivino FB, Schumacher HRJ. Synovial fluid characteristics and the lupus erythematosus cell phenomenon in drug-induced lupus. *Arthritis Rheum.* 1989;32:560–568.

[34]Rubin RL, Bell SA, Burlingame RW. Autoantibodies associated with lupus induced by diverse drugs target a similar epitope in the (H2A-H2B)-DNA complex. *J Clin Invest.* 1992;90:165–173.

[35]Enzenauer RJ, West SG, Rubin RL. D-penicillamine-induced systemic lupus erythematosus. *Arthritis Rheum.* 1990;33:1582–1585.

[36]Salazar-Paramo M, Rubin RL, Garcia-de la Torre I. Isoniazid-induced systemic lupus erythematosus. *Ann Rheum Dis.* 1992;51:1085–1087.

[37]Nordstrom DM, West SG, Rubin RL. Methyldopa-induced systemic lupus erythematosus. *Arthritis Rheum.* 1989;32:205–208.

[38]Bray VJ, West SG, Schultz KT, Boumpas DT, Rubin RL. Antihistone antibody profile in sulfasalazine induced lupus. *J Rheumatol.* 1994;21:2157–2158.

[39]Zamber R, Martens H, Rubin RL, Starkebaum G. Drug-induced lupus due to ophthalmic timolol. *J Rheumatol.* 1992;19:977–979.

[40]Alarcón-Segovia D, Wakin KG, Worthington JW, Wardd LE. Clinical and experimental studies on the hydralazine syndrome and its relationship to systemic lupus erythematosus. *Medicine.* 1967;46:1–33.

[41]Hahn BH, Sharp GC, Irvin WS, *et al.* Immune response to hydralazine and nuclear antigens in hydralazine-induced lupus erythematosus. *Ann Intern Med.* 1972;76:365–374.

[42]Blomgren SE, Condemi JJ, Vaughan JH. Procainamide-induced lupus erythematosus. *Am J Med.* 1972;52:338–348.

[43]Winfield JB, Davis JS. Anti-DNA antibody in procainamide-induced lupus erythematosus. *Arthritis Rheum.* 1974;17:97–110.

[44]Klajman A, Farkas R, Gold E, Ben-Efraim S. Procainamide-induced antibodies to nucleoprotein, denatured and native DNA in human subjects. *Clin Immunol Immunopathol.* 1975;3:525–530.

[45]Koffler D, Carr RI, Agnello V, Thoburn R, Kunkel HG. Antibodies to polynucleotides in human sera: Antigenic specificity and relation to disease. *J Exp Med.* 1971;134:294–312.

[46]Litwin A, Adams LE, Zimmer H, Foad B, Loggie JHM, Hess EV. Prospective study of immunologic effects of hydralazine in hypertensive patients. *Clin Pharmacol Ther.* 1981;29:447–456.

[47]Rubin RL, McNally EM, Nusinow SR, Robinson CA, Tan EM. IgG antibodies to the histone complex H2A-H2B characterize procainamide-induced lupus. *Clin Immunol Immunopathol.* 1985;36:49–59.

[48]Mongey A-B, Donovan-Brand R, Thomas TJ, Adams LE, Hess EV. Serologic evaluation of patients receiving procainamide. *Arthritis Rheum.* 1992;35:219–223.

[49]Weisbart RH, Yee WS, Colburn KK, Whang SH, Heng MK, Boucek RJ. Antiguanosine antibodies: A new marker for procainamide-induced systemic lupus erythematosus. *Ann Intern Med.* 1986;104:310–313.

[50]Lafer EM, Rauch J, Andrzejewski C Jr. *et al.* Polyspecific monoclonal lupus autoantibodies reactive with both polynucleotides and phospholipids. *J Exp Med.* 1981;153:897–909.

[51]Thomas TJ, Seibold JR, Adams LE, Hess EV. Hydralazine induces Z-DNA conformation in a polynucleotide and elicits anti(Z-DNA) antibodies in treated patients. *Biochem J.* 1993;294:419–425.

[52]Shoenfeld Y, Vilner Y, Reshef T, *et al.* Increased presence of common systemic lupus erythematosus (SLE) anti-DNA idiotypes (16/6 Id, 32/15 Id) is induced by procainamide. *J Clin Immunol.* 1987;7:410–419.

[53]Tan EM. Antinuclear antibodies: Diagnostic markers for autoimmune diseases and probes for cell biology. *Adv Immunol.* 1989;44:93–151.

[54]Fields TR, Zarrabi MH, Gerardi EN, Bennett RS, Zucker S, Hamburger MI. Reticuloendothelial system Fc receptor function in the drug-induced lupus erythematosus syndrome. *J Rheumatol.* 1986;13:726–731.

[55]Mitchell JA, Batchelor JR, Chapel H, Spiers CN, Sim E. Erythrocyte complement receptor type 1 (CR1) expression and circulating immune complex (CIC) levels in hydralazine-induced SLE. *Clin Exp Immunol.* 1987;68:446–456.

[56]Becker M, Klajman A, Moalem T, Yaretzky A, Ben-Efraim S. Circulating immune complexes in sera from patients receiving procainamide. *Clin Immunol Immunopathol.* 1979;12:220–227.

[57]Perry HM Jr, Chaplin H Jr, Carmody S, Haynes C, Frei C. Immunologic findings in patients receiving methyldopa: A prospective study. *J Lab Clin Med.* 1971;78:905–917.

[58]Zarrabi MH, Zucker S, Miller F, *et al.* Immunologic and coagulation disorders in chlorpromazine-treated patients. *Ann Intern Med.* 1979;91:194–199.

[59]Kleinman S, Nelson R, Smith L, Goldfinger D. Positive direct antiglobulin tests and immune hemolytic anemia in patients receiving procainamide. *N Engl J Med.* 1984;311:809–812.

[60]Rubin RL, Nusinow SR, Johnson AD, Rubenson DS, Curd JG, Tan EM. Serological changes during induction of lupus-like disease by procainamide. *Am J Med.* 1986;80:999–1002.

[61]Brandslund I, Ibsen HHW, Klitgaard NA, Svehag SE, Simonsen E, Diederichsen H. Plasma concentrations of complement split product C3d and immune complexes after procainamide-induced production of antinuclear antibodies. *Acta Med Scand.* 1986;220:431–435.

[62]Cohen MG, Kevat S, Prowse MV, Ahern MJ. Two distinct quinidine-induced rheumatic syndromes. *Ann Intern Med.* 1988;108:369–371.

[63]Kirby JD, Dieppe PA, Huskisson EC, Smith B. D-penicillamine and immune complex deposition. *Ann Rheum Dis.* 1979;38:344–346.

[64]Hess EV, Mongey A-B. Drug-related lupus: The same as or different from idiopathic disease? In: Lahita RG, ed. *Systemic Lupus Erythematosus.* 2nd edition. New York: Churchill Livingstone, 1993;893–904.

[65]Solinger AM. Drug-related lupus. Clinical and etiological considerations. *Rheumatic Dis Clinics N A.* 1988;14:187–202.

[66]Dubois EL. Procainamide induction of a systemic lupus erythematosus-like syndrome. Presentation of six cases, review of the literature, and analysis and follow-up of reported cases. *Medicine.* 1969;48:217–228.

[67]Davies P, Bailey PJ, Goldenberg MM. The role of arachidonic acid oxygenation products in pain and inflammation. *Annu Rev Immunol.* 1984;2:335–357.

[68]Klajman A, Camin-Belsky N, Kimchi A, Ben-Efraim S. Occurrence, immunoglobulin pattern and specificity of antinuclear antibodies in sera of procainamide-treated patients. *Clin Exp Immunol.* 1970;7:641–649.

[69]Klimas NG, Patarca R, Perez G, *et al.* Case report: Distinctive immune abnormalities in a patient with procainamide-induced lupus and serositis. *Am J Med.* 1992;303:99–104.

[70]Gorsulowsky DC, Bank PW, Golberg AD, Tennyson GL, Heinzerling RH, Burnham TK. Antinuclear antibodies as indicators for the procainamide-induced systemic lupus erythematosus-like syndrome and its clinical presentation. *J Am Acad Dermatol.* 1985; 12:245–253.

[71]Lavie CH, Biundo J, Quinet BJ, Waxman J. Systemic lupus erythematosus (SLE) induced by quinidine. *Arch Intern Med.* 1985; 145:700–702.

[72]Gill KS, Hayne OA, Zayed E. Another case of procainamide-induced pancytopenia (letter). *Am J Hematol.* 1989;31:298.

[73]Shields AF, Berenson JA. Procainamide-associated pancytopenia. *Am J Hematol.* 1988;27:299–301.

[74]Meyers DG, Gonzalez ER, Peters LL, *et al.* Severe neutropenia associated with procainamide: Comparison of sustained release and conventional preparations. *Am Heart J.* 1985;109:1393–1395.

[75]Starkebaum G, Kenyon CM, Simrell CG, Creamer JI, Rubin RL. Procainamide-induced agranulocytosis differs serologically and clinically from procainamide-induced lupus. *Clin Immunol Immunopathol.* 1996;78:112–119.

[76]Ramsey-Goldman R, Franz T, Solano FX, Medsger TAJ. Hyralazine-induced lupus and Sweet's syndrome. Report and review of the literature. *J Rheumatol.* 1990;17:682–684.

[77]Sequeira W, Polisky RB, Alrenga DP. Neutrophilic dermatosis (Sweet's syndrome). Association with a hydralazine-induced lupus syndrome. *Am J Med.* 1986;81:558–560.

[78]Litwin A, Adams LE, Hess EV, McManus J, Zimmer H. Hydralazine urinary metabolites in systemic lupus erythematosus. *Arthritis Rheum.* 1973;16:217–220.

[79]Hobbs RN, Clayton A-L, Bernstein RM. Antibodies to the five histones and poly(adenosine diphosphate-ribose) in drug induced lupus: Implications for pathogenesis. *Ann Rheum Dis.* 1987;46:408–416.

[80]Winfield JB, Koffler D, Kunkel HG. Development of antibodies to ribonucleoprotein following short-term therapy with procainamide. *Arthritis Rheum.* 1975;18:531–534.

[81]Bluestein HG, Zvaifler NJ, Weisman MH, Shapiro RF. Lymphocyte alteration by procainamide: Relation to drug-induced lupus erythematosus syndrome. *Lancet.* 1979;2:816–819.

[82]Bluestein HG, Redelman D, Zvaifler NJ. Procainamide lymphocyte reactions: A possible explanation for drug-induced autoimmunity. *Arthritis Rheum.* 1981;24:1019–1023.

[83]Hughes GRV, Rynes RI, Gharavi A, Ryan PFJ, Sewell J, Mansilla R. The heterogeneity of serologic findings and predisposing host factors in drug-induced lupus erythematosus. *Arthritis Rheum.* 1981;24:1070–1073.

[84]Ryan PFJ, Hughes GRV, Bernstein R, Mansilla R, Dollery CT. Lymphocytotoxic antibodies in hydralazine-induced lupus erythematosus. *Lancet.* 1979;ii:1248–1249.

[85]Ayer LM, Rubin RL, Dixon GH, Fritzler MJ. Antibodies from patients with drug-induced autoimmunity react with high mobility group (HMG) proteins. *Arthritis Rheum.* 1994;37:98–103.

[86]Russell AS, Ziff M. Natural antibodies to procainamide. *Clin Exp Immunol.* 1968;3:901–909.

[87]Adams LE, Roberts SM, Donovan-Brand R, Zimmer H, Hess EV. Study of procainamide hapten-specific antibodies in rabbits and humans. *Int J Immunopharmacol.* 1993;15:887–897.

[88]Carpenter JR, McDuffie FC, Sheps SG, Spiekerman RE, Brumfield H, King R. Prospective study of immune response to hydralazine and development of antideoxyribonucleoprotein in patients receiving hydralazine. *Am J Med.* 1980;69:395–400.

[89]McDuffie FC. Relationship between immune response to hydralazine and to deoxyribonucleoprotein in patients receiving hydralazine. *Arthritis Rheum.* 1981;24:1079–1081.

[90]Mongey AB, Hess EV. Drug-related lupus. *Curr Opinion Rheumatol.* 1989;1:353–359.

[91]Anderson B, Stillman MT. False-positive FTA-ABS in hydralazine-induced lupus. *JAMA.* 1978;239:1392–1393.

[92]Asherson RA, Zulman J, Hughes GRV. Pulmonary thromboembolism associated with procainamide-induced lupus syndrome and anticardiolipin antibodies. *Ann Rheum Dis.* 1989;48:232–235.

[93]Chokron R, Robert A, Rozensztajn L. Procainamide-induced lupus with circulating anticoagulant (letter). *Nouv Presse Med.* 1982;11:2568.

[94]Davis S, Furie BC, Griffin JH, Furie B. Circulating inhibitors of blood coagulation associated with procainamide-induced lupus erythematosus. *Am J Hematol.* 1978;4:401–407.

[95]Edwards RL, Rick ME, Wakem CJ. Studies on a circulating anticoagulant in procainamide-induced lupus erythematosus. *Arch Intern Med.* 1981;141:1688–1690.

[96]Triplett DA, Brandt JT, Musgrave KA, Orr CA. The relationship between lupus anticoagulants and antibodies to phospholipid. *J Am Med Assoc.* 1988;259:550–554.

[97]Canoso RT, deOliveira RM. Chlorpromazine-induced anti-cardiolipin antibodies and lupus anticoagulant: absence of thrombosis. *Am J Hematol.* 1988;27:272–275.

[98]Canoso RT, Sise HS. Chlorpromazine-induced lupus anticoagulant and associated immunologic abnormalities. *Am J Hematol.* 1982;13:121–129.

[99]Derksen RHMW, Kater L. Lupus anticoagulant: Revival of an old phenomenon. *Clin Exp Rheumatol.* 1991;3:349–357.

[100]Tollefson G, Rodysill K, Cusulos M. A circulating lupus-like coagulation inhibitor induced by chlorpromazine. *J Clin Psych Pharmacol.* 1984;4:49–51.

[101]Zucker S, Zarrabi MH, Romano GS, Miller F. IgM inhibitors of the contact phase of coagulation in chlorpromazine-treated patients. *Br J Hematol.* 1978;40:447–457.

[102]McNeil HP, Chesterman CN, Krilis SA. Immunology and clinical importance of antiphospholipid antibodies. *Adv Immunol.* 1991;49:193–280.

[103]Steen VD, Ramsey-Goldman R. Phenothiazine-induced systemic lupus erythematosus with superior vena cava syndrome: Case report and review of the literature. *Arthritis Rheum.* 1988;31:923–926.

[104]Gastineau DA, Holcomb GR. Lupus anticoagulant in drug-induced systemic lupus erythematosus (SLE). *Arch Intern Med.* 1985;145:1926–1927.

[105]Nässberger L, Sjöholm AG, Jonsson H, Sturfelt G, Åkesson A. Autoantibodies against neutrophil cytoplasm components in systemic lupus erythematous and in hydralazine-induced lupus. *Clin Exp Immunol.* 1990;81:380–383.

[106]Nässberger L, Johansson AC, Björck S, Sjöholm AG. Antibodies to neutrophil granulocyte myeloperoxidase and elastase: Autoim-

mune responses in glomerulonephritis and due to hydralazine treatment. *J Intern Med.* 1991;229:261–265.

[107]Dolman KM, Gans RO, Vervaat TJ, *et al.* Vasculitis and antineutrophil cytoplasmic autoantibodies associated with propylthiouracil therapy. *Lancet.* 1993;342:651–652.

[108]Caulier M, Dromer C, Andrieu V, Le Guennec P, Fournie B. Sulphasalazine-induced lupus in rheumatoid arthritis. *J Rheumatol.* 1994;21:750–751.

[109]Jennette JC, Wilkman AS, Falk RJ. Anti-neutrophil cytoplasmic autoantibody-associated glomerulonephritis and vasculitis. *Am J Pathol.* 1989;135:921–930.

[110]Burlingame RW, Boey ML, Starkebaum G, Rubin RL. The central role of chromatin in autoimmune responses to histones and DNA in systemic lupus erythematosus. *J Clin Invest.* 1994;94:184–192.

[111]Waldmann TA, Strober W. Metabolism of immunoglobulins. *Prog Allergy.* 1969;13:1–110.

[112]Yu CL, Ziff M. Effects of long-term procainamide therapy on immunoglobulin synthesis. *Arthritis Rheum.* 1985;28:276–284.

[113]Ochi T, Goldings EA, Lipsky PE, Ziff M. Immunomodulatory effect of procainamide in man. *J Clin Invest.* 1983;71:36–45.

[114]Green BJ, Wyse DG, Duff HJ, Mitchell LB, Matheson DS. Procainamide in vivo modulates suppressor T cell activity. *Clin Invest Med.* 1988;11:425–429.

[115]Miller KB, Salem D. Immune regulatory abnormalities produced by procainamide. *Am J Med.* 1982;73:487–492.

[116]Forrester J, Golbus J, Brede D, Hudson J, Richardson B. B cell activation in patients with active procainamide-induced lupus. *J Rheumatol.* 1988;15:1384–1388.

[117]Rubin RL, Tang F, Chan EKL, Pollard KM, Tsay G, Tan EM. IgG subclasses of autoantibodies in systemic lupus erythematosus, Sjögren's syndrome, and drug-induced autoimmunity. *J Immunol.* 1986;137:2528–2534.

[118]Fritzler M, Ryan P, Kinsella TD. Clinical features of systemic lupus erythematosus patients with antihistone antibodies. *J Rheumatol.* 1982;9(1):46–51.

[119]Klajman A, Farkas R, Ben-Efraim S. Complement-fixing activity of antinuclear antibodies induced by procainamide treatment. *Isr J Med Sci.* 1973;9:627–630.

[120]Kanayama Y, Peebles C, Tan EM, Curd JG. Complement-activating abilities of defined antinuclear antibodies. *Arthritis Rheum.* 1986;29:748–754.

[121]Mitchell JA, Sim RB, Sim E. CR1 polymorphism in hydralazine-induced systemic lupus erythematosus: DNA restriction fragment length polymorphism. *Clin Exp Immunol.* 1989;78:354–358.

[122]Sim E. Drug-induced immune complex disease. *Biochem Soc Trans.* 1991;19:164–170.

[123]Sim E, Stanley L, Gill EW, Jones A. Metabolites of procainamide and practolol inhibit complement components C3 and C4. *Biochem J.* 1988;251:323–326.

[124]Batchelor JR, Welsh KL, Tinoco RM, *et al.* Hydralazine-induced systemic lupus erythematosus: Influence of HLA-DR and sex on susceptibility. *Lancet.* 1980;1:1107–1109.

[125]Spears CJ, Batchelor JR. Drug-induced autoimmune disease. *Adv Nephrol.* 1987;16:219–230.

[126]Russell GI, Bing RF, Jones JAG, Thurston H, Swales JD. Hydralazine sensitivity: Clinical features, autoantibody changes and HLA-DR phenotype. *Q J Med.* 1987;65:845–852.

[127]Chin GL, Kong NCT, Lee BC, Rose IM. Penicillamine-induced lupus-like syndrome in a patient with classical rheumatoid arthritis. *J Rheumatol.* 1991;947–948.

[128]Chalmers A, Thompson D, Stein HE. Systemic lupus erythematosus during penicillamine therapy for rheumatoid arthritis. *Ann Intern Med.* 1982;97:659–663.

[129]Brand C, Davidson A, Littlejohn G, Ryan P. Hydralazine-induced lupus: No association with HLA-DR4. *Lancet.* 1984;i:462.

[130]Speirs C, Chapel H, Fielder AHL, Davey NJ, Batchelor JR. Complement system protein C4 and susceptibility to hydralazine-induced systemic lupus erythematosus. *Lancet.* 1989;i:922–924.

[131]Batchelor JR. Autoantibodies and HLA-DR phenotype in hydralazine induced lupus. In: *Proceedings of the Second International Conference on Systemic Lupus Erythematosus, 26th–30th November, Singapore.* Professional Postgraduate Services, International, 1989;166–168.

[132]Canoso RT, Lewis ME, Yunis EJ. Association of HLA-Bw44 with chlorpromazine-induced autoantibodies. *Clin Immunol Immunopathol.* 1982;25:278–282.

[133]Adams LE, Balakrishnan K, Roberts SM, *et al.* Genetic, immunologic and biotransformation studies of patients on procainamide. *Lupus.* 1993;2:89–98.

[134]Howard PF, Hochberg MC, Bias WB, Arnett FC, McLean RH. Relationship between C4 null genes, HLA-D region antigens, and genetic susceptibility in systemic lupus erythematous in Caucasian and Black Americans. *Am J Med.* 1986;81:187–193.

[135]Utsinger PD, Zvaifler NJ, Bluestein HG. Hypocomplementemia in procainamide-associated systemic lupus erythematosus. *Ann Intern Med.* 1976;84:293.

[136]Perry HMJ, Tan EM, Carmody S, Sakomoto A. Relationship of acetyl transferase activity to antinuclear antibodies and toxic symptoms in hypertensive patients treated with hydralazine. *J Lab Clin Med.* 1970;76:114–125.

[137]Stec GP, Lertora JJL, Atkinson AJ Jr *et al.* Remission of procainamide-induced lupus erythematosus with N-acetylprocainamide therapy. *Ann Intern Med.* 1979;90:799–801.

[138]Lahita R, Kluger J, Drayer DE, Koffler D, Reidenberg MM. Antibodies to nuclear antigens in patients treated with procainamide or acetylprocainamide. *N Engl J Med.* 1979;301:1382–1385.

[139]Roden DM, Reele SB. Higgins SB, *et al.* Antiarrhythmic efficacy, pharmacokinetics and safety of N-acetylprocainamide in human subjects: Comparison with procainamide. *Amer J Cardiol.* 1980;46:463–468.

[140]Alarcón-Segovia D, Fishbein E, Alcala H. Isoniazid acetylation rate and development of antinuclear antibodies upon isoniazid treatment. *Arthritis Rheum.* 1971;14:748–752.

[141]Reidenberg MM, Chase DB, Drayer DE, Reis S, Lorenzo B. Development of antinuclear antibody in patients treated with high doses of captopril. *Arthritis Rheum.* 1984;27:579–581.

[142]Baer AN, Woosley RL, Pincus T. Further evidence for the lack of association between acetylator phenotype and systemic lupus erythematosus. *Arthritis Rheum.* 1986;29:508–514.

[143]Cameron HA, Ramsay LE: The lupus syndrome induced by hydralazine: A common complication with low-dose treatment. *Br Med J.* 1984;289:410–412.

[144]Uetrecht JP, Sweetman BJ, Woosley RL, Oates JA. Metabolism of procainamide to a hydroxylamine by rat and human hepatic microsomes. *Drug Metab Dispos.* 1984;12:77–81.

[145]Budinsky RA, Roberts SM, Coates EA, Adams L, Hess EV. The formation of hydroxylamine by rat and human liver microsomes. *Drug Metab Dispos.* 1987;15:37–43.

[146]Roberts SM, Adams LE, Donovan-Brand R, *et al.* Procainamide hydroxylamine lymphocyte toxicity. 1. Evidence for participation by hemoglobin. *Int J Immunopharmacol.* 1989;11:419–427.

[147]Streeter AJ, Timbrell JA. Enzyme-mediated covalent binding of hydralazine to rat liver microsomes. *Drug Metab Dispos.* 1983; 11:179–183.

[148]Hein DW, Weber WW. Metabolism of procainamide, hydralazine, and isoniazid in relation to autoimmune(-like) reactions. In: Kammueller ME, Bloksma N, Seinen W, eds. *Autoimmunity and Toxicology: Immune Disregulation Induced by Drugs and Chemicals.* Amsterdam: Elsevier Science, 1989;239–265.

[149]Rubin RL, Uetrecht JP, Jones JE. Cytotoxicity of oxidative metabolites of procainamide. *J Pharmacol Exp Ther.* 1987;242: 833–841.

[150]Adams LE, Sanders CE Jr, Budinsky RA, Donovan-Brand R, Roberts SM, Hess EV. Immunomodulatory effects of procainamide metabolites. Their implications in drug-related lupus. *J Lab Clin Med.* 1989;113:482–492.

[151]Uetrecht JP. Reactivity and possible significance of hydroxylamine and nitroso metabolites of procainamide. *J Pharmacol Exp Ther.* 1985;232:420–425.

[152]Magner-Wróbel K, Toborek M, Drózdz M, Danch A. Increase in antioxidant activity in procainamide-treated rats. *Pharmacol Toxicol.* 1993;72:94–97.

[153]Rubin RL, Jones JE, Uetrecht JP. Metabolism of procainamide to the reactive hydroxylamine by leukocytes. *Fed Proc.* 1987;46: 1380(Abstract).

[154]Uetrecht J, Zahid N, Rubin R. Metabolism of procainamide to a hydroxylamine by human neutrophils and mononuclear leukocytes. *Chem Res Toxicol.* 1988;1:74–78.

[155]Rubin RL, Curnutte JT. Metabolism of procainamide to the cytotoxic hydroxylamine by neutrophils activated *in vitro*. *J Clin Invest.* 1989;83:1336–1343.

[156]Jiang X, Khursigara G, Rubin RL: Transformation of lupus-inducing drugs to cytotoxic products by activated neutrophils. *Science.* 1994;266:810–813.

[157]Waldhauser L, Uetrecht J. Oxidation of propylthiouracil to reactive metabolites by activated neutrophils. Implications for agranulocytosis. *Drug Metab Dispos.* 1991;19:354–359.

[158]Hofstra AH, Matassa LC, Uetrecht JP. Metabolism of hydralazine by activated leukocytes: Implications for hydralazine-induced lupus. *J Rheumatol.* 1991;18:1673–1680.

[159]Hofstra AH, Li-Muller SMA, Uetrecht JP. Metabolism of isoniazid by activated leukocytes. Possible role in drug-induced lupus. *Drug Metab Dispos.* 1992;20:205–210.

[160]Kelder PP, De Moal NJ, 't Hart BA, Janssen LHM. Metabolic activation of chlorpromazine by stimulated human polymorphonuclear leukocytes. Induction of covalent binding of chlorpromazine to nucleic acids and proteins. *Chem Biol Interact.* 1991;79:15–30.

[161]Uetrecht J, Zahid N. N-chlorination of phenytoin by myeloperoxidase to a reactive metabolite. *Chem Res Toxicol.* 1988;1:148–151.

[162]Uetrecht J, Zahid N, Shear NH, Biggar WD. Metabolism of dapsone to a hydroxylamine by human neutrophils and mononuclear cells. *J Pharmacol Exp Ther.* 1988;245:274–279.

[163]Van Zyl JM, Basson K, Uebel RA, Van Der Walt BJ. Isoniazid-mediated irreversible inhibition of the myeloperoxidase antimicrobial system of the human neutrophil and the effect of thyronines. *Biochem Pharmacol.* 1989;38:2363–2373.

[164]Mahlis E, Christophidis N. Modulation of the iodination reaction in normal human neutrophils and in whole blood by penicillamine, congeners and intracellular enzyme catalase and superoxide dismutase. *Clin Exp Rheumatol.* 1989;7:365–371.

[165]Van Zyl JM, Basson K, Kriegler A, Van Der Walt BJ. Activation of chlorpromazine by the myeloperoxidase system of the human neutrophil. *Biochem Pharmacol.* 1990;40:947–954.

[166]Lee E, Miki Y, Katsura H, Kariya K. Mechanism of inactivation of myeloperoxidase by propylthiouracil. *Biochem Pharmacol.* 1990;39:1467–1471.

[167]Uetrecht J, Sokoluk B. Comparative metabolism and covalent binding of procainamide by human leukocytes. *Drug Metab Dispos.* 1992;20:120–123.

[168]Hill CM, Lunec J, Griffiths HR, Herbert KE. Characterization of tumour necrosis factor a release by human granulocytes in response to procainamide challenge. *Biochem Pharmacol.* 1995;49:1837–1849.

[169]Schopf RE, Hanauske-Abel HM, Tschank G, Schulte-Wissermann H, Günzler V. Effects of hydrazyl group containing drugs on leucocyte functions: An immunoregulatory model for the hydralazine-induced lupus-like syndrome. *J Immunopharmacol.* 1985;7:385–401.

[170]Wheeler JF, Adams LE, Mongey A-B, Roberts SM, Heineman WR, Hess EV. Determination of metabolically derived nitroprocainamide in the urine of procainamide-dosed humans and rats by liquid chromatography with electrochemical detection. *Drug Metab Dispos.* 1991;19:691–695.

[171]Timbrell JA, Facchini V, Harland SJ, Mansilla-Tinoco R. Hydralazine-induced lupus: Is there a toxic metabolic pathway? *Eur J Clin Pharmacol.* 1984;27:555–559.

[172]Kubicka-Muranyi M, Goebels R, Goebel C, Uetrecht J, Gleichmann E. T lymphocytes ignore procainamide, but respond to its reactive metabolites in peritoneal cells: Demonstration by the adoptive transfer popliteal lymph node assay. *Toxicol Appl Pharmacol.* 1993;122(1):88–94.

[173]Schuhmann D, Kubicka-Muranyi M, Mirtschewa J, Kind P, Gleichmann E. Adverse immune reactions to gold. I. Chronic treatment with an Au(I) drug sensitizes mouse spleen cells not to Au(I), but to Au(III) and induces autoantibody formation. *J Immunol.* 1990;145:2132–2139.

[174]Goebel C, Kubicka-Muranyi M, Tonn T, Gonzalez J, Gleichmann E. Phagocytes render chemicals immunogenic: Oxidation of gold(I) to the T cell-sensitizing gold(III) metabolite generated by mononuclear phagocytes. *Arch Toxicol.* 1995;69:450–459.

[175]Tannen RH, Weber WW. Antinuclear antibodies related to acetylator phenotype in mice. *J Pharmacol Exp Ther.* 1980;213:485–490.

[176]Weber WW, Tannen RH. Pharmacogenetic studies on the drug-related lupus syndrome. Differences in antinuclear antibody development and drug-induced DNA damage in rapid and slow acetylator animal models. *Arthritis Rheum.* 1981;24:979–986.

[177]Whittingham S, Mackay IR, Whitworth JA, Sloman G. Antinuclear antibody response to procainamide in man and laboratory animals. *Am Heart J.* 1972;84:228–234.

[178]Ten Veen JH, Feltkamp TEW. Studies on drug-induced lupus erythematosus in mice. I. Drug-induced antinuclear antibodies (ANA). *Clin Exp Immunol.* 1972;11:265–276.

[179]Ten Veen JH. Studies on drug-induced lupus erythematosus in mice. II. Drug-induced smooth muscle and skeletal muscle antibodies. *Clin Exp Immunol.* 1973;15:375–384.

[180]Cannat A, Seligmann M. Possible induction of antinuclear antibodies by isoniazid. *Lancet.* 1966;1:185–187.

[181]Cannat A, Seligmann M. Induction of isoniazid and hydralazine of antinuclear factors in mice. *Clin Exp Immunol.* 1968;3:99–105.

[182]Quddus J, Johnson KJ, Gavalchin J, et al. Treating activated CD4+ T cells with either of two distinct DNA methyltransferase inhibitors, 5-azacytidine or procainamide, is sufficient to induce a lupus-like disease in syngeneic mice. *J Clin Invest.* 1993;92:38–52.

[183]Yung RL, Quddus J, Chrisp CE, Johnson KJ, Richardson BC. Mechanisms of drug-induced lupus. I. Cloned Th2 cells modified with DNA methylation inhibitors *in vitro* cause autoimmunity *in vivo. J Immunol.* 1995;154:3025–3035.

[184]Gleichmann E, Pals ST, Rolink AG, Radaskiewicz T, Gleichmann H. Graft-versus-host reactions: Clues to the etiopathology of a spectrum of immunological diseases. *Immunol Today.* 1984;5:324–332.

[185]Nagata N, Hurtenbach U, Gleichmann E. Specific sensitization of Lyt-1+2- T cells to spleen cells modified by the drug D-penicillamine or a stereoisomer. *J Immunol.* 1986;136:136–1820.

[186]Gleichmann H. Studies on the mechanism of drug sensitization: T-cell-dependent popliteal lymph node reaction to diphenylhydantoin. *Clin Immunol Immunopathol.* 1981;18:203–211.

[187]Aucoin DP, Peterson ME, Hurvitz AI, et al. Propylthiouracil-induced immune-mediated disease in the cat. *J Pharmacol Exp Ther.* 1985;234:13–18.

[188]Aucoin DP, Rubin RL, Peterson ME, et al. Dose-dependent induction of anti-native DNA antibodies by propylthiouracil in cats. *Arthritis Rheum.* 1988;31:688–692.

[189]Kammüller ME, Thomas C, De Bakker JM, Bloksma N, Seinen W. The popliteal lymph node assay in mice to screen for the immune disregulation potential of chemicals—A preliminary study. *Int J Immunopharmacol.* 1989;11:293–300.

[190]Gleichmann E, Vohr H-W, Stringer C, Nuyens J, Gleichmann H. Testing the sensitization of T cells to chemicals. From murine graft-versus-host (GVH) reactions to chemical-induced GVH-like immunological diseases. In: Kammüller ME, Bloksma N, Seinen W, eds. *Autoimmunity and Toxicology.* Amsterdam: Elsevier Science Publishers B.V., 1989;363–390.

[191]Gleichmann HIK, Pals ST, Radaszkiewicz T. T cell-dependent B-cell proliferation and activation induced by administration of the drug diphenylhydantoin to mice. *Hematol Oncol.* 1983;1:165–176.

[192]Katsutani N, Shionoya H. Popliteal lymph node enlargement induced by procainamide. *Int J Immunopharmacol.* 1992;14:681–686.

[193]Thomas C, Punt P, Warringa R, Högberg T, Seinen W, Bloksma N. Popliteal lymph node enlargement and antibody production in the mouse induced by zimeldine and related compounds with varying side chains. *Int J Immunopharmacol.* 1990;12:561–568.

[194]Thomas C, Lippe W, Seinen W, Bloksma N. Popliteal lymph node enlargement and antibody production in the mouse induced by drugs affecting monoamine levels in the brain. *Int J Immunopharmacol.* 1991;13:621–629.

[195]Alarcón-Segovia D. Drug-induced lupus syndrome. *Mayo Clin Proc.* 1967;44:664–681.

[196]Gold S. Role of sulphonamides and penicillin in the pathogenesis of systemic lupus erythematosus. *Lancet.* 1951;1(260):268–272.

[197]Domz CA, McNamara DH, Holzapfel HF. Tetracycline provocation in lupus erythematosus. *Ann Intern Med.* 1959;50:1217–1226.

[198]Alexander S. Lupus erythematosus in two patients after griseofulvin treatment of *Trichophyton rubrum* infection. *Br J Dermatol.* 1962;74:72–74.

[199]Anderson WA, Torre D. Griseofulvin and lupus erythematosus. *J Med Soc NJ.* 1982;63:161–162.

[200]Watsky MS, Lynfield YL. Lupus erythematosus exacerbated by griseofulvin. *Cutis.* 1976;17:361–363.

[201]Bigby M, Stern R. Cutaneous reactions to nonsteroidal anti-inflammatory drugs. A review. *J Am Acad Dermatol.* 1985;5:866–876.

[202]Smythe HA, ed. Prostaglandins and benoxaprofen (editorial). Proceedings of the International Symposium on Benoxaprofen. *J Rheumatol.* 1980;6(Suppl. 1):1–3.

[203]Widener HL, Littman BH. Ibuprofen-induced meningitis in systemic lupus erythematosus. *JAMA.* 1978;239:1062–1064.

[204]Ballas ZK, Donta ST. Sulindac-induced aseptic meningitis. *Arch Intern Med.* 1982;142:165–166.

[205]Ruppert GB, Barth WF. Tolmetin-induced aseptic meningitis. *JAMA.* 1981;245:67–68.

[206]Codding C, Targoff IN, McCarty GA. Aseptic meningitis in association with diclofenac treatment in a patient with systemic lupus erythematosus. *Arthritis Rheum.* 1991;34:1340–1341.

[207]Alarcón-Segovia D, Worthington JW, Ward LE, Wakim KG. Lupus diathesis and the hydralazine syndrome. *N Engl J Med.* 1965;272:462–466.

[208]Rallison ML, O'Brien J, Good RA. Severe reactions to long-acting sulfonamides. Erythema multiforme exudativum and lupus erythematosus following administration of sulfamethoxypyridazine and sulfadimethoxine. *Pediatr.* 1961;28:908–917.

[209]Simpson DG, Walker JH. Hypersensitivity to para-aminosalicylic acid. *Am J Med.* 1960;29:297–306.

[210]Reed BR, Huff JC, Jones SK, Orton DW, Lee LA, Norris DA. Subacute cutaneous lupus erythematosus associated with hydrochlorothiazide therapy. *Ann Intern Med.* 1985;103:49–51.

[211]Davidson BL, Gilliam JN, Lipsky PE. Cimetidine-associated exacerbation of cutaneous lupus erythematosus. *Arch Intern Med.* 1982;142:166–167.

[212]Handley AJ. Thrombocytopenia and L.E. cells after oxyphenbutazone. *Lancet.* 1971;1:245–246.

213Farid N, Anderson J. SLE-like reaction after phenylbutazone (letter). *Lancet.* 1971;1:1022–1023.

214Sonnenblick M, Abraham AS. Ibuprofen hypersensitivity in systemic lupus erythematosus. *Br Med J.* 1978;1:619–620.

215Pereyo-Torrellas N. p-Aminobenzoic acid-related compounds and systemic lupus. *Arch Dermatol.* 1978;114:1097.

216Removed in proofs.

217Kay DR, Bole GG Jr, Ledger WJ. Antinuclear antibodies, rheumatoid factor and C-reactive protein in serum of normal women using oral contraceptives. *Arthritis Rheum.* 1971;14:239–248.

218Bole GG Jr, Friedlaender MH, Smith CK. Rheumatic symptoms and serological abnormalities induced by oral contraceptives. *Lancet.* 1969;1:323–326.

219Tarzy BJ, Wallach EE, Garcia C-R, Zweiman B, Myers AR. Rheumatic disease, abnormal serology, and oral contraceptives. *Lancet.* 1972;ii:501–503.

220Travers RL, Hughes GR. Oral contraceptive therapy and systemic lupus erythematosus. *J Rheumatol.* 1978;5:448–451.

221Petz LD. Autoimmune and drug-induced immune hemolytic anemia. In: Rose NR, de Macario EC, Fahey JL, Friedman H, Penn GM, eds. *Manual of Clinical Laboratory Immunology.* 4th edition. Washington, DC: American Society for Microbiology, 1992; 325–343.

222Hodge JV, Casey TP. Methyldopa and the direct antiglobulin (Coombs') test. *N Z Med J.* 1968;68:240–246.

223Sherman JD, Love DE, Harrington JF. Anemia, positive lupus and rheumatoid factors with methyldopa. Report of 3 cases. *Arch Intern Med.* 1967;120:321–326.

224Harth M. LE cells and positive direct Coombs' test induced by methyldopa. *Can Med Assoc J.* 1968;99:277–280.

225Mackay IR, Cowling DC, Hurley TH. Drug-induced autoimmune disease: Hemolytic anemia and lupus cells after treatment with methyldopa. *Med J Aust.* 1968;2:1047–1050.

226Booth RJ, Wilson J, Bullock J. Beta-adrenergic-receptor blockers and anti nuclear antibodies in hypertension. *Clin Pharmacol Ther.* 1982;31:555–558.

227Breckenridge A, Dollery CT, Worlledge SM, Holborow EJ, Johnson GD. Positive direct Coombs tests and antinuclear factor in patients treated with methyldopa. *Lancet.* 1967;2:1265–1267.

228Robinson CJG, Abraham AA, Balazs T. Induction of anti-nuclear antibodies by mercuric chloride in mice. *Clin Exp Immunol.* 1984;58:300–306.

229Robinson CJG, Balazs T, Egorov IK. Mercuric chloride-, gold sodium thiomalate-, and D-penicillamine-induced antinuclear antibodies in mice. *Toxicol Appl Pharmacol.* 1986;86:159–169.

230Hultman P, Enestrom S, Pollard KM, Tan EM. Anti-fibrillarin autoantibodies in mercury-treated mice. *Clin Exp Immunol.* 1989; 78:470–472.

231Reimer G, Steen VD, Penninger CA, Medsger TA, Tan EM. Correlates between autoantibodies to nucleolar antigens and clinical features in patients with systemic sclerosis (scleroderma). *Arthritis Rheum.* 1996;31:525–532.

232Hultman P, Johansson U, Turley SJ, Lindh U, Enestrom S, Pollard KM. Adverse immunological effects and autoimmunity induced by dental amalgam and alloy in mice. *FASEB J.* 1996;8: 1183–1190.

233Lockie LM, Smith DM. Forty-seven years experience with gold therapy in 1,019 rheumatoid arthritis patients. *Semin Arthritis Rheum.* 1985;14:238–246.

234Romagnoli P, Spinas GA, Sinigaglia F. Gold-specific T cells in rheumatoid arthritis patients treated with gold. *J Clin Invest.* 1992;89:254–258.

235Wallace DJ. The clinical presentation of systemic lupus erythematosus. In: Wallace DJ, Hahn BH, eds. *Dubois' Lupus Erythematosus.* 4th edition. Philadelphia: Lea and Febiger, 1993;317–321.

236Malinow MR, Bardana EJ, Pirofsky B, Craig S. Systemic lupus erythematosus-like syndrome in monkeys fed alfalfa sprouts: Role of a non-protein animo acid. *Science.* 1982;216:415–417.

237Bardana EJ, Malinow MR, Houghton DC, *et al.* Diet-induced systemic lupus erythematosus (SLE) in primates. *Am J Kidney Dis.* 1982;1:345–352.

238Malinow MR, Bardana EJ, Goodnight SH. Pancytopenia during ingestion of alfalfa seeds. *Lancet.* 1981;1:615–617.

239Roberts JL, Hayashi JA. Exacerbation of SLE associated with alfalfa ingestion. *N Engl J Med.* 1983;308:1361.

240Slonim NB. Arthralgia, headache, prostration, and fever during hydralazine therapy. *JAMA.* 1954;154:1419.

241Reinhardt DJ, Waldron JM. Lupus erythematosus-like syndrome complicating hydralazine (apresoline) therapy. *JAMA.* 1954;155: 1491–1492.

242Mehta BR. Lupus-like syndrome after procainamide. *Hawaii Med J.* 1968;28:120–121.

243Prockop LD. Myotonia, procaine, amide, and lupus-like syndrome. *Arch Neurol.* 1966;14:326–330.

244Masel MA. A lupus-like reaction to antituberculosis drugs. *Med J Aust.* 1967;2:738–740.

245Elsas LJ, Hayslett JP, Spargo BH, Durant JL, Rosenberg LE. Wilson's disease with reversible renal tubular dysfunction. Correlation with proximal tubular ultrastructure. *Ann Intern Med.* 1971; 75:427–433.

246Dubois EL, Tallman E, Wonka RA. Chlorpromazine-induced systemic lupus erythematosus. *JAMA.* 1972;221:595–596.

247Rubin RL: Drug-induced lupus. In: Wallace DJ, Hahn BH, eds. *Dubois' Lupus Erythematosus.* 5th edition. Baltimore, MD: Williams and Wilkens, 1997;871–901.

248Yung RL, Richardson BC. Drug-induced lupus. *Rheum Dis Clin North Am.* 1994;20:61–86.

249Cornacchia E, Golbus J, Maybaum J, Strahler J, Hanash S, Richardson B. Hydralazine and procainamide inhibit T cell DNA methylation and induce autoreactivity. *J Immunol.* 1988;140:2197–2200.

250Richardson B, Cornacchia E, Golbus J, Maybaum J, Strahler J, Hanash S. N-acetylprocainamide is a less potent inducer of T cell autoreactivity than procainamide. *Arthritis Rheum.* 1988;31:995–999.

251Pohl LR, Satoh H, Christ DD, Kenna JG. The immunologic and metabolic basis of drug hypersensitivities. *Ann Rev Pharmacol.* 1988;28:367–387.

252Weinstein A. Drug-induced lupus erythematosus. *Prog Clin Immunol.* 1980;4:1–21.

253Harmon CE, Portanova JP. Drug-induced lupus: Clinical and serological studies. *Clin Rheum Dis.* 1982;8:121–135.

[254]Russell AS. Drug-induced autoimmune disease. *Clin Immunol Allergy.* 1981;1:57–76.

[255]Hess EV, Mongey A. Drug-related lupus. *Bull Rheum Dis.* 1991;40:1–8.

[256]Suzuki T, Burlingame RW, Casiano CA, Boey ML, Rubin RL. Antihistone antibodies in systemic lupus erythematosus: Assay dependency and effects of ubiquitination and serum DNA. *J Rheumatol.* 1994;21:1081–1091.

9

Pulmonary Hypertension Associated with Drugs and the Environment

Lewis J. Rubin

INTRODUCTION

The normal pulmonary circulation is a low-resistance circuit capable of accommodating increases in cardiac output, which can rise fourfold during physical activity, without altering its perfusion pressure. In pulmonary hypertensive states, however, afterload to the right ventricle increases as pulmonary artery pressure rises, eventually leading to right ventricular failure and death. Pulmonary hypertension, defined as a mean pulmonary artery pressure greater than 25 mm Hg at rest or 30 mm Hg with exercise, can occur as a distinct entity—primary pulmonary hypertension (PPH)—or as a complication of a variety of respiratory, cardiac or systemic diseases.[1] This chapter will focus on pulmonary vascular disease which occurs as the result of identifiable exogenous factors—an increasingly frequent cause of severe pulmonary vascular disease.

PPH is an uncommon disease (approximate incidence of two per million in the general population). The presenting symptoms and physical signs of PPH are often nonspecific and subtle. Furthermore, sensitive and specific noninvasive diagnostic tests are lacking. These factors may result in a delay in diagnosis, frequently of a year or more, from the onset of symptoms.[2]

There is no cure for PPH, although spontaneous remissions have been reported. Medical management includes therapy with anticoagulants, oral vasodilators (which are effective in 20% to 25% of cases), continuous intravenous infusion of prostacyclin, diuretics and supplemental oxygen.[3–6] Thoracic transplantation, either lung or combined heart-lung, is performed for severe pulmonary vascular disease which is refractory to medical therapy.[7,8]

Although most cases of PPH are spontaneous, several factors have been associated with its development. These include portal hypertension, infection with the human immunodeficiency virus (HIV), inhaled cocaine use and the use of diet-suppressant (anorexic) agents (Table 9-1).[1,9–11]

Additionally, 7% to 10% of cases of PPH are familial, with an autosomal pattern of transmission and incomplete penetrance.[3,12] These observations have led to the speculation that a predisposition, possibly genetically determined, must be present for the development of PPH in response to potential triggers.

ANOREXIGEN-ASSOCIATED PULMONARY HYPERTENSION

The first suggestion that anorexigen use may be associated with the development of PPH originated from the observation of a sharp increase in the incidence of PPH in the western European countries where aminorex fumarate was marketed in the late 1960s.[13] Less than 1% of aminorex users developed PPH—supporting the notion of individual susceptibility—and approximately one-third of the affected patients improved after drug discontinuation. The incidence of PPH returned to its baseline level with the withdrawal of aminorex from the market. Subsequently, several centers reported cases of PPH in individuals using anorexigens. Both amphetamine-like drugs and serotonin uptake inhibitor agents (SSRIs) have been associated with PPH.[11,14,15] While a few cases were reversible upon discontinuation of the putative offending agents, most were not.[16,17]

The widespread use of fenfluramine and dexfenfluramine in Europe, coupled with the impending approval of dexfenfluramine for long-term use in the United States by the Food and Drug Administration (FDA) prompted a multinational, prospective case-control study of risk factors in PPH—the International Primary Pulmonary Hypertension Study (IPPHS).[18] Ninety-five PPH cases were collected from 35 centers in four European countries (France, Belgium, England and Holland) and 355 controls matched for gender and age were obtained from the general population. The use of any anorexigen within the previous year was associated

Table 9-1 Exogenous agents reported to be associated with
pulmonary hypertension

- Anorexigens
- Cocaine
- Intravenous substance abuse
- HIV infection
- Contaminated rapeseed cooking oil (toxic oil syndrome)
- Contaminated L-tryptophan (eosinophilia myalgia syndrome)
- Chemotherapeutic drugs
  - Mitomycin C
  - Carmustine (BCNU)
  - Etoposide
  - Cyclophosphamide
- Pyrrolizidine alkaloids (herbal extracts)

---

with a tenfold increase in risk of developing PPH, and the risk increased to over twentyfold with anorexigen use of over three months. Although long-term use (more than one year) was uncommon in this study, the risk of PPH appears to be even greater in long-term users, and may be as high as fiftyfold. Dexfenfluramine and fenfluramine were the most commonly used agents in this study, constituting 90% of all anorexigen use. As in the NIH Registry, a database established to gather information on the natural history and risk factors for PPH, a delay in establishing a diagnosis was common, averaging one year from the onset of symptoms.

The IPPHS report provides the first definitive evidence for an association between anorexic agent use and PPH based on a prospective, case-control epidemiologic study design. Recent studies suggest that fenfluramine, dexfenfluramine and aminorex inhibit potassium channels in isolated rat pulmonary artery smooth muscle cells, leading to vasoconstriction[19]; preliminary evidence also suggests that potassium channel activity is altered in pulmonary artery smooth muscle cells obtained from PPH patients.[20] Thus, anorexigens may trigger the pulmonary vasculopathic cascade in individuals with a predisposition at the pulmonary smooth muscle cell membrane level, initially by promoting vasoconstriction, followed by progressive vascular growth and remodelling. Alternatively, drug-mediated alterations in local serotonin and/or catecholamine metabolism could be responsible for vascular changes via other pathways. Furthermore, serotonin is a pulmonary vasoconstrictor, and its levels have been reported to be increased in patients with PPH.[21]

The IPPHS found no significant association between the risk of PPH and other variables such as obesity, smoking, recent pregnancy or the use of thyroid preparations. Future studies on the pathogenesis of PPH may, however, provide further insight into potential predispositions for developing PPH. Additionally, it is unclear whether the risk of developing PPH increases with long-term use, or whether the risk plateaus or even decreases with time. This question is cru-

cial, since dexfenfluramine has now been approved by the FDA for long-term use.

The reversibility of anorexigen-induced pulmonary vascular disease is also unknown. In one study, no case was found of anorexigen-associated PPH which was reversible upon drug discontinuation.[11] However, the referral center in this study is likely to see the most serious cases in need of complex management. Reversibility of PPH has been observed with several agents, including aminorex. The factors responsible for determining reversibility (that is, duration of anorexigen use, time from symptom onset to diagnosis, age and so on) remain unknown.

Extrapolation from recent studies suggests that the widespread and long-term use of anorexigen drugs may result in a sharp increase in the incidence of PPH. The practicing physician must therefore carefully assess the available information regarding risks and benefits of anorexigen therapy, and should be particularly attentive for any signs or symptoms suggestive of the development of pulmonary vascular disease in patients taking these drugs.

PULMONARY VASCULAR DISEASE ASSOCIATED WITH OTHER DRUGS

Cocaine is a potent vasoconstrictor of pulmonary and systemic vessels. Both inhaled and intravenous use of cocaine have been associated with the development of pulmonary hypertension.[22,23] Pathologically, the medium-sized and small pulmonary arteries demonstrate medial thickening and intimal proliferation similar to the changes seen in PPH. Intravenous drug use may also be associated with a granulomatous pulmonary arteritis, most likely due to an inflammatory response to talc, starch and cotton fibers, which are common constituents of illicit drugs.[24]

Pulmonary veno-occlusive disease, a rare form of pulmonary hypertension in which the small and medium-sized pulmonary veins are the predominant site of vascular involvement, has been reported with the use of chemotherapeutic agents,[25] and after bone marrow transplantation.[26]

HIV-ASSOCIATED PULMONARY HYPERTENSION

The first case of HIV infection associated with pulmonary hypertension was reported in 1987.[27] Since that time, nearly 100 patients with HIV-associated pulmonary hypertension have been described.[28] The incidence of pulmonary hypertension in HIV-positive individuals appears to be approximately 0.5%, and is unrelated to the mode of transmission of HIV or the severity of immune deficiency. Pulmonary hypertension tends to be severe and contributes significantly to morbidity and mortality.[28,29] A recent report suggests that aggressive antiretroviral therapy may slow the progression of pulmonary vascular disease, but long-term studies are lacking.[28]

PULMONARY HYPERTENSION IN TOXIC OIL SYNDROME (TOS)

In 1981, an epidemic of a systemic illness characterized by eosinophilia, rash, neuromuscular abnormalities, and hepatic and cardiopulmonary disease was recognized in Spain.[30] The syndrome, which affected more than 20,000 people, was subsequently attributed to the use of adulterated rapeseed cooking oil. Although the mechanism responsible for the syndrome remains obscure, the evidence suggests that aniline derivatives, which were added to the oil to denature it, may have induced the disease process either by a direct toxic effect or through an immune mechanism. The acute phase of the syndrome, characterized by eosinophilia, pulmonary edema and rash, was associated with substantial morbidity and mortality. Of those who survived the acute phase, approximately 10% developed pulmonary hypertension. Pathologically, the pulmonary vessels demonstrated intimal vacuolization and thickening, medial hypertrophy and, in some cases, arteritis. Progressive pulmonary vascular disease was a common cause of late mortality in patients with TOS.[31,32]

PULMONARY HYPERTENSION IN THE EOSINOPHILIA MYALGIA SYNDROME

A syndrome characterized by severe muscle pain and marked peripheral eosinophilia was first recognized in the United States in late 1989 and was subsequently attributed to the ingestion of manufactured L-tryptophan (LTP).[33] This syndrome, termed the eosinophilia myalgia syndrome (EMS), reached epidemic proportions prior to the removal of LTP from the market, with over 1500 cases reported to the Center for Disease Control (CDC).[34] The spectrum of illness associated with EMS was broad, with some patients having a brief and self-limiting illness while others developed a multiorgan system disease which was debilitating or even fatal. Cardiopulmonary disease was among the most serious complications of EMS and, after neuromuscular disease, was the most commonly occurring complication of EMS in fatal cases.[35]

As with other forms of pulmonary disease, the true incidence of pulmonary involvement in EMS is unknown. This is most likely due in large part to the nonspecific mode of presentation and the lack of specific screening and sensitive noninvasive diagnostic tests to establish its presence. Additionally, transient and reversible lung disease has been observed in this condition and could have been obscured in some patients whose extrathoracic symptoms dominated the clinical picture. However, when pulmonary hypertension

was present and persistent, this serious complication resulted in death in at least two patients[35] and had probably contributed to the demise of several others by 1991.

The pathologic features of pulmonary disease seen with EMS range from potentially reversible inflammation to alveolar fibrosis.[36–38] Chronic pneumonitis or bronchiolitis has been observed in several EMS patients who presented with shortness of breath,[39] some of whom undoubtedly had secondary pulmonary hypertension due to the effects of chronic hypoxemia. Blood vessel involvement can produce narrowing of the vessel due to growth of smooth muscle, inflammation around the vessel wall or endothelial proliferation.

The respiratory system can also be involved indirectly by EMS as a result of nerve or muscle disease, leading to respiratory muscle weakness. In this setting, the lung parenchyma and vasculature are normal, but the weakness leads to an inability to ventilate adequately.

Most patients with EMS presented with complaints within several months of using LTP, although the range of time from the onset of LTP use to the development of symptoms ranged from one month to over a year.[34] As is typical of patients with pulmonary disease regardless of the etiology, shortness of breath was the most common presenting complaint. Physical examination and laboratory studies were remarkable only for the characteristic systemic features of this syndrome, which in some patients were less marked than the cardiopulmonary findings. Chest radiographs often show changes of fibrosis, particularly in the lower zones of the lung, but may be normal even in the presence of significant disease. Sophisticated tests of respiratory muscle function, which are not usually available in many pulmonary function laboratories, are required to demonstrate neuromuscular disease causing impaired lung function. It should also be noted that many patients who ingested LTP developed some features of EMS but did not meet the CDC definition of EMS; indeed, it has been estimated that as many as 3000 individuals developed some form of this syndrome without having significant peripheral eosinophilia.

Twelve patients with EMS and chronic respiratory disease were referred to the University of Maryland Medical System for evaluation between 1990 and 1993. The female to male ratio was 5:1 and the mean age was 38 years. All subjects had ingested LTP prior to the onset of their illness, which ranged from fairly isolated pulmonary vascular disease to a severe systemic illness which also involved skin, muscle and the central nervous system. All presented with dyspnea, and five had evidence of right heart dysfunction. Six patients had isolated pulmonary hypertension, four had interstitial lung disease, and two had neuromuscular disease. Cardiac catheterization demonstrated moderately severe pulmonary hypertension in the six patients with isolated pulmonary vascular disease, with hemodynamic abnormalities similar to those typical of PPH.

The natural history of the six patients with pulmonary vascular disease was consistent with PPH, with one exception:

while three of the six died within two years, one patient experienced a complete regression within one year of the diagnosis. Spontaneous remission has been reported with PPH but it is exceedingly rare, with the exception of anorexic-agent-induced pulmonary hypertension. One of the fatalities was a patient with progressive disease who underwent single lung transplantation but died from postoperative complications one month after the procedure. Pathological examination of the explanted lung demonstrated changes of severe pulmonary hypertension. Two remaining patients have severe but stable pulmonary vascular disease. The remaining six patients have experienced persistent symptoms of shortness of breath, with four of the six demonstrating stable but impaired lung function. Two patients have demonstrated a slow decline in lung function over time.

There are limited data regarding the treatment of pulmonary vascular disease in EMS. Patients with pulmonary interstitial disease or neuromuscular-cutaneous manifestations have been reported to be responsive to corticosteroids,[39,40] and it is possible that those patients with occult pulmonary vascular inflammation may have responded to this therapeutic approach. Oral vasodilator therapy with calcium channel blockers has proved disappointing with this disease, and transplantation may prove unfeasible due to the systemic nature of this illness.

As with other forms of "spontaneous" or exogenous pulmonary vascular disease, a predisposition to its development may be necessary, providing an explanation for the low incidence of pulmonary hypertension in the populations exposed to toxic oil and contaminated LTP. Management of pulmonary hypertension has been largely supportive. Transplantation should be considered for patients with severe, isolated lung involvement. Although these epidemics were limited in scope (due to the withdrawal of LTP from the market and removal of implicated cooking oil from the affected communities by the Spanish government), efforts should continue to elucidate the mechanisms responsible, since this may lead to a clearer understanding of the pathogenesis of other forms of pulmonary disease. Furthermore, other exogenous substances may result in a similar process in the future.

PYRROLIZIDINE ALKALOIDS

The pyrrolizidine alkaloids are extracts from the plant species *Crotalaria,* which is widely used in the Caribbean and parts of Africa for making herbal teas. Fulvine, the extract from crotalaria fulva, is known to produce hepatic veno-occlusive disease and cirrhosis in individuals ingesting Jamaican bush tea, which is prepared from this plant. An African patient with fatal primary pulmonary hypertension attributed to the heavy ingestion of tea made from crotalaria laburnoides has also been reported.[41] Monocrotaline derivatives administered to laboratory animals produces pulmonary arteritis and progressive pulmonary hypertension.[42]

SUMMARY

A variety of exogenous substances have been shown to be associated with, and presumably causative of, pulmonary hypertension in humans. Some of these exposures are associated with systemic illnesses which resemble systemic sclerosis (LTP, toxic oil), while others appear exclusively to injure the pulmonary circulation (anorexigens). Although the mechanisms responsible for the development of pulmonary vascular disease after these exposures remain unclear, only a minority of exposed individuals develop this complication. A predisposition, possibly genetically determined, may be necessary for the development of pulmonary hypertension in response to a "trigger." Clarification of the cellular and molecular responses to known triggers may shed light on the mechanisms responsible for "spontaneous" PPH and may be useful in preventing future epidemics due to exogenous inducers.

REFERENCES

[1]Rubin LJ, Barst RJ, Kaiser LR, *et al.* ACCP consensus statement: Primary pulmonary hypertension. *Chest.* 1993;104:236–250.

[2]D'Alonzo GE, Barst RJ, Ayres SM, *et al.* Survival in primary pulmonary hypertension. Results from a national prospective registry. *Ann Intern Med.* 1991;115:343–349.

[3]Rich S, Dantzker DR, Ayres SM, *et al.* Primary pulmonary hypertension: A national prospective study. *Ann Intern Med.* 1987;107:216–223.

[4]Rich S, Kaufmann E, Levy PS. The effect of high doses of calcium-channel blockers on survival in primary pulmonary hypertension. *N Eng J Med.* 1992;327:76–81.

[5]Fuster V, Steele PM, Edwards WD, *et al.* Primary pulmonary hypertension: Natural history and the importance of thrombosis. *Circulation.* 1984;70:580–587.

[6]Barst RJ, Rubin LJ, Long WA, *et al.* A comparison of continuous intravenous epoprostenol (prostacyclin) with conventional therapy for primary pulmonary hypertension. *N Eng J Med.* 1996;334:296–301.

[7]Pasque MK, Trulock EP, Kaiser LR, Cooper JD. Single-lung transplantation for pulmonary hypertension. *Circulation.* 1991;84:2275–2279.

[8]Higenbottam TW, Spiegelhalter D, Scott JP, *et al.* Prostacyclin (epoprostenol) and heart-lung transplantation as treatments for severe pulmonary hypertension. *Br Heart J.* 1993;70:366–370.

[9]Petitprez P, Brenot F, Azarian R, *et al.* Pulmonary hypertension in patients with human immunodeficiency virus infection: A comparison with primary pulmonary hypertension. *Circulation.* 1994;89:2722–2727.

[10]McDonnell PJ, Toye PA, Hutchins GM. Primary pulmonary hypertension and cirrhosis: Are they related? *Am Rev Respir Dis.* 1983;127:437–441.

[11]Brenot F, Herve P, Petitprez P, *et al.* Primary pulmonary hypertension and fenfluramine use. *Br Heart J.* 1993;70:537–541.

[12]Loyd JE, Butler MG, Foroud TM, *et al.* Genetic anticipation and abnormal gender ratio at birth in familial primary pulmonary hypertension. *Am J Resp Crit Care Med.* 1995;152:93–97.

[13]Gurtner HP. Aminorex and pulmonary hypertension. *Cor Vasa.* 1985;27:160–171.

[14]McMurray J, Bloomfield P, Miller HC. Irreversible pulmonary hypertension after treatment with fenfluramine. *Br Med J.* 1986; 293:51–52.

[15]Pouwels HM, Smeets JL, Cheriex EC, Wouters EF. Pulmonary hypertension and fenfluramine. *Eur Respir J.* 1990;3:606–607.

[16]Loogen F, Worth H, Schwan G, *et al.* Long-term follow-up of pulmonary hypertension in patients with and without anorectic drug intake. *Cor Vasa.* 1985;27:111–124.

[17]Nall KC, Rubin LJ, Lipskind S, Sennesh JD. Reversible pulmonary hypertension associated with anoexigen use. *Am J Med.* 1991;91:97–99.

[18]Abenhaim L, Moride Y, Brenot F, *et al.* Appetite-suppressant drugs and the risk of primary pulmonary hypertension. *N Eng J Med.* 1996;335:609–616.

[19]Michelakis ED, Archer SL, Huang JMC, Nelson DP, Weir EK. Anorexic agents inhibit potassium current in pulmonary artery smooth muscle cells. *Am J Resp Crit Care Med.* 1995;151:A725 (abstract).

[20]Yuan XJ, Aldinger AM, Orens JB, Conte JV, Rubin LJ. Dysfunctional voltage-gated potassium channels in the pulmonary artery smooth muscle cells of patients with primary pulmonary hypertension. *Circulation.* 1997;94:I–48 (abstract).

[21]Herve P, Launey JM, Scrobohaci ML, *et al.* Increased plasma serotonin in primary pulmonary hypertension. *Am J Med.* 1995;99:249–254.

[22]Schaiberger PH, Kennedy TC, Miller FC, Gal J, Petty TL. Pulmonary hypertension associated with long-term inhalation of "crank" methamphetamine. *Chest.* 1993;104:614–616.

[23]Tomashefski JF, Hirsch CS. The pulmonary vascular lesions of intravenous drug abuse. *Hum Pathol.* 1980;11:133–145.

[24]Robertson CH, Reynolds RC, Wilson JE. Pulmonary hypertension and foreign body granulomas in intravenous drug abusers: Documentation by cardiac catheterization and lung biopsy. *Am J Med.* 1976;61:657–664.

[25]Joselson R, Warnock M. Pulmonary veno-occlusive disease after chemotherapy. *Hum Pathol.* 1983;13:88–91.

[26]Troussard X, Bernaudin JF, Cordonnier C. *et al.* Pulmonary veno-occlusive disease after bone marrow transplantation. *Thorax.* 1984;39:956–957.

[27]Goldsmith GH, Baily RG, Brettler DB, *et al.* Primary pulmonary hypertension in patients with classic hemophilia. *Ann Intern Med.* 1988;108:797–799

[28]Opravil M, Pechere M, Speich R, *et al.* HIV-associated primary pulmonary hypertension. *Am J Resp Crit Care Med.* 1997;155: 990–995.

[29]Petitprez P, Brenot F, Azarian R, *et al.* Pulmonary hypertension in patients with human immunodeficiency virus infection: Comparison with primary pulmonary hypertension. *Circulation.* 1994;89: 2722–2727.

[30]Kilbourne EM, *et al.* Clinical epidemiology of toxic-oil syndrome. *N Eng J Med.* 1983;309:1408–1414.

[31]Garcia-Dorado D, Miller DD, Garcia EJ, *et al.* An epidemic of pulmonary hypertension after toxic rapeseed oil ingestion in Spain. *J Am Coll Cardiol.* 1991;18:1539–1545.

[32]Gomez-Sanchez MA, Saenz De La Calzada C, Gomez-Pajuelo C, *et al.* Clinical and pathologic manifestations of pulmonary vascular disease in the toxic oil syndrome. *J Am Coll Cardiol.* 1991;18: 1539–1545.

[33]Hertzman PA, Blevins WL, Mayer J, *et al.* Association of the eosinophilia-myalgia syndrome with the ingestion of tryptophan. *N Eng J Med.* 1990;322:869–873.

[34]Centers for Disease Control. Eosinophilia-myalgia syndrome associated with ingestion of L-tryptophan: United States as of January 9, 1990. *MMWR.* 1990;39:14–15.

[35]Swygert LA, Back EE, Auerbach SB, *et al.* Eosinophilia-myalgia syndrome: Mortality data from the US national surveillance system. *J Rheumatol.* 1993;20:1711–1717.

[36]Tazelaar HD, Myers JL, Drage CW, *et al.* Pulmonary disease associated with L-tryptophan-induced eosinophilic-myalgia syndrome. *Chest.* 1990;97:1032–1036.

[37]Banner AS, Borochovitz D. Acute respiratory failure caused by pulmonary vasculitis after L-tryptophan ingestion. *Am Rev Respir Dis.* 1991;143:881–884.

[38]Yakovlevitch M, Siegel M, Hoch DH, *et al.* Pulmonary hypertension in a patient with tryptophan-induced eosinophilia-myalgia syndrome. *Am J Med.* 1991;90:272–273.

[39]Strumpf IJ, Drucker RD, Anders KH, *et al.* Acute eosinophilic pulmonary disease associated with the ingestion of L-tryptophan-containing products. *Chest.* 1991;99:8–13.

[40]Catton CK, Elmer JC, Whitehouse AC, *et al.* Pulmonary involvement in the eosinophilia-myalgia syndrome. *Chest.* 1991;99:327–329.

[41]Harris P, Heath D, eds. *The Human Pulmonary Circulation.* Edinburgh: Churchill Livingstone, 1977;409.

[42]Rabinovitch M. Insights into the pathogenesis of primary pulmonary hypertension from animal models. In: Rubin LJ, Rich S, eds. *Primary Pulmonary Hypertension,* New York: Marcel Dekker, 1997;63–82.

10

Cigarette Smoking and Other Acquired Risk Factors for Rheumatoid Arthritis

Alfonse T. Masi and Huan J. Chang

INTRODUCTION

Rheumatoid arthritis (RA) is a multifactorial disease of unknown etiology that is believed to be influenced by both genetically related[1] and environmentally associated[2] determinants. These factors interact with each other in complex fashion and exert their influences upon RA in complicated ways that have been difficult to study. Monozygotic (MZ) twin studies show only 15% to 30% concordance for disease,[3–6] but interpretation of heritability from such simple twin data should be treated with caution. Monozygotic twins are not entirely identical, and can differ in terms of somatic rearrangement/mutation of immunoglobulin and T cell receptor genes, X chromosome inactivation in females, genomic imprinting and *in utero* immune relationships.[7] Calculations of heritability by more specific methods put the genetic component in RA higher than those derived from MZ twin concordance studies.[7]

Environmental or lifestyle behavioral contributions to the development of RA in susceptible populations are issues of long-standing interest.[8,9] These have been difficult to identify and to differentiate from ethnic and genetic factors. Environmental causality has not been proven in RA, despite its biological plausibility. Notwithstanding the heterogeneity of disease[10] and diverse, long-term pathophysiology,[1,2] the prevailing assumption is that RA has an underlying etiology resulting from particular inherited major histocompatibility complex (MHC) class II alleles.[11] Unlike other organ failures, for example of the circulatory system, little is known about precursor events in RA that eventually lead to joint and other tissue inflammation or necrosis during the active disease phases. Recent studies attempting to examine these issues illustrate the complex and often controversial relationships between proposed risk factors.[1,10]

Prevalence studies of RA were performed in an Inuit population during the 1960s.[12] The results suggested that either ethnic factors or possibly a high dietary intake of polyunsaturated fish oils associated with that culture may protect against the disease. Such fatty acids have since been found to decrease inflammatory activity in RA.[13] Studies of Bantu tribespeople living their original village lifestyle reported a low incidence of RA.[14] RA incidence increased after Bantu migration to an urban environment.[15] Behavioral and dietary changes and psychological stresses in the new environment were suspected to increase the risk of RA in these people.[14,15] Early studies of socioeconomic status reported an increased prevalence of RA among males in the United States of lower socioeconomic status.[16] A recent prospective population-based study from Britain, however, failed to confirm a relationship between the incidence of RA and indicators of socioeconomic deprivation.[17]

The relationship between current cigarette smoking and RA is also unsettled. Although current cigarette smoking has been implicated as a risk factor or marker for RA in men and women in many epidemiological studies,[18–24] these results have not been unanimous.[18,25] One prospective study failed to show consistent results between the sexes,[18] and a retrospective case-control study found that history of any cigarette smoking protected against RA in younger women.[25] The relationship between cigarette smoking and RA is further complicated by their conjoint association with serum rheumatoid factor (RF). Smoking was associated with the presence of RF in two population surveys.[26,27] RF is a strong predictive marker for development of clinical RA.[28–32] The complex interaction of smoking, RF and familial predisposition in RA is discussed in a later section (*vide infra*).

The objective of this chapter is to present a broad overview of possible environmentally related factors which may contribute to the risk of developing RA, and to review in greater detail the reported associations with cigarette smoking, which is currently the most likely behavioral or nocuous contributor to this disease. Its potential impact on the risk of RA may rival that of genetic mechanisms.

THE "ENVIRONMENT" AND "NATURE VERSUS NURTURE" DILEMMAS

Complicated chronic diseases like RA cannot be interpreted within a simple dichotomy of environmental versus genetic determinants, because the respective factors are imperceptibly intertwined. This complex interrelationship is illustrated in Figure 10-1. The host and its innate predisposition to health or illness is a by-product of dynamic evolution, which is determined by behavioral, developmental and environmental factors interacting with each other and with genetic controls.[2] The complex biological process of "normal" human growth, development, maturation, physiological decline and death result from continuous interactions of

Behavioral, Developmental and Environmental Factors Interacting with Host Biology in Predisposing to Development of Rheumatoid Arthritis

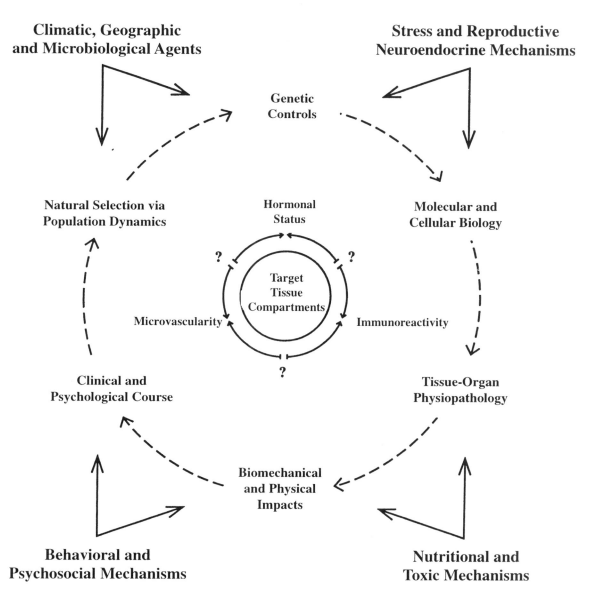

Fig. 10-1 Interactions among a complex set of behavioral, developmental and environmental factors with the host biology in predisposing to development of rheumatoid arthritis. A simplified wholistic model of rheumatoid arthritis indicating hormonal-immunological-vascular interactions at target tissue sites within a larger framework of environmental-genetic-biological-host processes.

the constellations of endowed genetic and nongenetic ("acquired") somatic factors, all operating upon the individual within his or her "personal" environment.

Somatic or "intrinsic" factors may be viewed as the individual's total biological status at a particular time, including but not restricted to the component genetic control processes. Genetic mechanisms interact with other somatic and environmental influences via intrinsic biological processes.[33] A particular gene interacts with a virus following a complex sequence of host-viral exposures and intrinsic biological processing of signals and stimuli from the agent.[33] Nonhereditary somatic and environmental mechanisms can influence the degree to which a particular genotype or a potentially pathogenic agent may interact or cause disease.[33]

The environment or "extrinsic" factors may be conceptualized as all influences external to the host, but only in the broadest context. Environs or environment may be a physical area, a behavioral interaction or the totality of living circumstances. In contradistinction to heredity ("nature"), environment ("nurture") includes extrinsic physical conditions that can affect and influence growth and development as well as social and cultural conditions which may otherwise affect the individual's personal behaviors or community interactions. Still, one must differentiate extrinsic factors that are objectively evident in the "public" physical and social domain from "private" dynamics of the individual. The latter may include behaviors, habits and reactions, nutritional variation and other personal aspects of lifestyle, all of which may influence the degree of environmental adaptation but may not be easily documented. Even in MZ twins, with presumably identical genetic endowment and similar biological development, disease predisposition may differ considerably within the same public environment, perhaps influenced by private behaviors and personalized life patterns.

The degree to which acquired somatic and developmental factors (for example, "personal healthfulness"), distinct from either genetic endowment or objective extrinsic factors, may influence the risk of RA is unknown. Objective methods can be employed to study risk factors related to heredity and the physical or objective social environment; however, investigations of personal behaviors and lifestyle rely upon historical reports and subjective interpretations. Nevertheless, each component in the spectrum of risk factors for RA needs to be investigated for a more comprehensive understanding of the dynamic evolution of this disease in a particular person or population. Major determinants of disease likely manifest objectively across various populations and are not unique to particular individuals, restricted families or socioeconomic clusters.

MAJOR HOST RISK FACTORS IN RA: AGING, GENDER AND HEREDITY

The major recognized host determinants of increased risk in RA are advancing age, female gender and a positive family history of erosive, seropositive disease in a first-degree relative.[1–9,28–32,34–36] Familial factors will not be reviewed here in detail, but are described for purposes of indicating their comparative strength and influences upon other recognized determinants.

The incidence of RA increases with age in the adult years, more so in women than in men (Figure 10-2).[36] From ages 20 to 50, men have significant relative sparing compared to women. The female to male (F:M) ratio of incidence is approximately 5:1 in these age groups, whereas it approaches equality in juvenile and older age groups.[36] Over all ages, the F:M ratio is about 2:1 or 3:1 in diverse populations that have been studied.[2,8,9,14–17] The characteristic incidence risk pattern of RA,[36] when combined with the marked improvement of disease during pregnancy,[34,35] suggest that hormonally related factors are important in the pathophysiology of this disease.

Familial predisposition to RA is complex.[7,37–41] It varies with the individual's onset age and gender, disease severity and genotype specificity. Heritability of RA is believed to be stronger when the individual has disease onset under the age of 45 years,[37–39] is male[39] or demonstrates severe disease,[40] rather than minor disease, as may occur in a population-based sample of cases.[41] In fact, under the latter circumstances,[41] a genetic effect is weak (risk ratio 1.6) and may not be evident in first-degree relatives. Such complex interactions of genetic and acquired somatic determinants of RA suggest that multiple factors are operating in different degrees at various life stages of each gender.[1,2,10,35] These data are consistent with a multifactorial "threshold" model of RA, in which an accumulation of genetic and environmental influences is needed for the disease to manifest in a particular individual.[42]

Environmental exposures or lifestyle behaviors may contribute to RA in varying degrees, depending upon the host's onset age, gender or disease severity.[1,2,34–42] The relative contributions of aging, female gender and heritability are seen in Table 10-1.[34] In each category, the baseline risk is the favorable population incidence (that is, without the accentuating risk factor). Aging in males increases the incidence of RA by about twentyfold, from a baseline at the age of 20 years to the highest risk at the age of 70 or older (Table 10-1). Acquired somatic factors or lifestyle determinants may be presumed to contribute to such marked age differentials in onset risk.[34]

ORAL CONTRACEPTIVES AND THE RISK OF DEVELOPING RA

Studies of oral contraceptive (OC) and other female sex hormone usage are inconclusive and conflicting with respect to the risk of developing RA or treating active disease.[43–51] Observational studies of this type have many inherent self-selection and ascertainment biases which compromise the reliability of conclusions drawn about cause-effect relationships.[40,52–56]

A protective effect of OCs against RA might be suggested

Composite, Age-Specific Incidence of Rheumatoid Arthritis Per 100,000 Person-Years in Females and Males

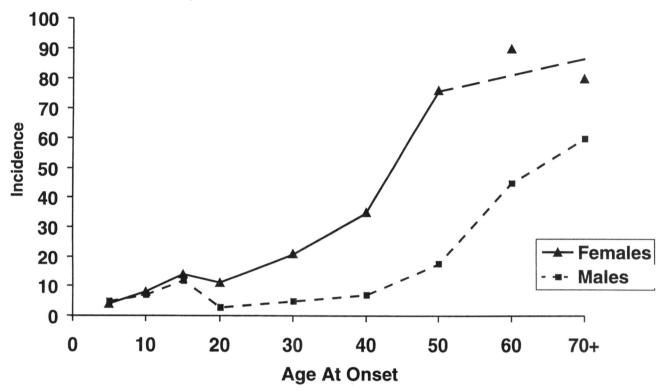

Fig. 10-2 Composite, age-specific incidence of RA per 100,000 person-years in females and males.[36] Figure reproduced with permission of Oxford University Press.

Table 10-1 Estimated relative risks of the aging (70+ years), female gender and heritability accentuating factors compared with baseline frequencies of RA

Accentuating Risk Factors	Accentuated Frequencies	Baseline Frequencies	Accentuating RRs
Age (70+ yr)	Incidence (70+ yr)*	Incidence (20 yr)*	
F	80	10	8
M	60	≈ 3	≈ 20
Female gender	Incidence (female)†	Incidence (male)†	
Adult ages (20+ yr)	45	15	3
Reproductive ages	20	4	5
Heritability	Co-twin RR‡	Population Prevalence§	
DZ twin pairs	3.4	1%	3.4
MZ twin pairs	8.6	1%	8.6

Abbreviations: RR, relative risks; RA, rheumatoid arthritis; DZ, dizygotic; MZ, monozygotic.
*Female and male age-specific incidence rates per 100,000 person-years.[36]
†Female and male incidence rates estimated from Figure 10–2 composite data.[36]
‡Observed/expected RR of RA among those DZ and monozygotic MZ co-twin pairs having an affected member with RA, adjusted by age and gender.[4]
§Prevalence of RA in the total twin sample studied.[4]
Reproduced from Masi *et al.*[34] with permission.

if normal comparison women used OCs more frequently than patients. However, self-selection factors that influence OC usage or nonusage must be critically considered before drawing conclusions.[55,56] For example, women predisposed to RA may be less likely to use OCs than comparison women not so predisposed, for as yet unproven reasons. In such a circumstance, "nonuse of OCs" would be a marker for the development of RA. Two separate meta-analyses of available data had differing conclusions regarding a protective effect of OCs on the development of RA.[48,50]

Differences concerning OC use and development of RA exist mainly between hospital-based and population-based groups.[43] In meta-analyses, the pooled data from hospital-based studies showed a protective effect of OCs (OR = 0.49; 95% CI: 0.39, 0.63), but population-based samples did not (OR = 0.95; 95% CI: 0.78, 1.16).[43,47,48,50] Hospital-based data have suggested that OC usage protects against progression of RA to severe disease.[50,57] Recently, a population-based case-control study found that although cases and controls reported a similar level of "ever use" of oral contraceptives (OR = 0.88; 95% CI: 0.47, 1.64), cases were less likely to report oral contraceptive use at the time of disease onset (OR = 0.22; 95% CI: 0.6, 0.88).[43] Unknown selection and comorbidity factors may be operating, however, which could bias those results.[52,55,56]

A recent report found that women with severe RA (mean age of 61 years) had a significantly lower history of past OC usage for more than 5 years than women with mild RA (mean age of 55.6 years), after adjustment for age of first childbirth, parity and breast-feeding (odds ratio 0.1, 95% CI: 0.01–0.06).[58] Importantly, the women with mild RA had a higher rate of OC usage (25.8) than controls (19.3) of comparable age. No data were available in this study on educational level or social class of the women,[58] which could bias past OC usage and course of RA (*vide infra*). Biological mechanisms that would explain a distant-past OC usage markedly predisposing to severe RA but not affecting the risk of mild RA are not defined.[58]

Associations observed with either use or nonuse of OCs and the development of RA seem to be due to self-selection or indexing by the type of women using these products, rather than reflecting a protective effect of these hormones.[54–56] Such assessment also seems to apply to women who develop more severe RA.[50,58] Similar conclusions have been drawn about peri- or postmenopausal women using noncontraceptive replacement hormones.[51,59] In summary, the available data on the use of OC and RA indicate that the relationship is complex precluding definitive conclusions at this time.[34,42,56]

ETHNIC AND GEOGRAPHIC DISTRIBUTIONS OF RA

People of all races may develop RA. Although differences in case definition and criteria for RA[60,61] make comparisons of prevalence from various sources difficult, estimates for definite disease in adult white populations are relatively constant, at about 1.0% or greater.[2,62,63] The prevalence of RA was similar for Caucasians and African-Americans in the United States,[16] but has been shown to vary among other ethnic groups.[2,62–65] A high prevalence of RA-like disease was observed in young adult Yakima females, but was not associated with either HLA-Dw4 or HLA-DR4,[66,67] in contrast to

most other populations.[2,7,10,11] A Chippewa band was reported with a prevalence of RA of at least 5.3%. A significant correlation of HLA-DR4 and RA was found in this population, paralleling the high prevalence (68%) of HLA-DR4.[68] When American Rheumatism Association (ARA) criteria[60] for definite disease were used, the prevalence of RA in major reported surveys for adults (age 15 and older) has ranged from as low as 0.1% in a rural South African black community[14] to 3.0% among Finnish whites.[64] Reported differences in RA prevalence rates among various ethnic and racial populations seem to be genuine and not accounted for entirely by genetic factors, as shown in the low frequency of disease among the Chinese.[63,65] Climate does not seem to be an important factor in determining the prevalence of RA.

Most population studies of RA do not permit estimation of its incidence; however, average annual incidence varies from 0.5 to 3 per 1000 persons at risk.[62,63] Several reports have suggested a secular decline in the incidence of RA since 1950, but the results could be due to differences in methodology among the studies.[44,46,69,70] A more recent report found no secular change in RA incidence compared with similarly ascertained historical data.[71]

Analyses of mortality in RA are even more difficult to interpret than incidence or prevalence studies.[72] Besides differences in criteria, which apply to all population surveys, selection factors for mortality and death certification must be considered in comparing results.[72] Age and gender influences upon disease susceptibility and incidence[36] may not be translated into mortality risks from RA.[72]

Emphasis in future field studies of RA in populations should be directed at critically evaluating criteria, incidence, and disease course among groups that offer particular logistical advantages or suggest unusually high or low frequencies. Further emphasis should also be placed on controlled analyses of historical, personal, and environmental factors with which the disease may be associated, in order to gain clues to etiology or pathogenesis.

SOCIOECONOMIC FACTORS AND RA

The relationship between socioeconomic factors, such as educational level or marital (coupling) status, and RA has evoked much interest but is difficult to analyze and is controversial. The marked increase in the rate of definite RA in a South African black urban population compared with a genetically similar rural population implicates both sociological and physical environmental factors in disease occurrence.[14,15]

Studies pertaining to education in patients with established RA are more difficult to interpret. Worse outcomes were reported among those with lower education levels,[73–75] particularly among men.[73,74] These retrospective or cross-sectional studies, however, have not demonstrated that the prospective risk of developing RA correlates with years of formal education completed. Furthermore, most studies have been performed on data of patients with more than 10 years of disease duration before entry into study.[76] A consistent association between education level and disease outcome has not been found in other studies.[76-79] Various factors may confound the association of RA outcome with education level, for example, age, severity of disease at medical presentation, disease duration and type of work or number of hours worked.[76] In a study of 138 women with RA of recent onset (mean 1.5 years) who were followed for 5.8 years,[76] findings suggested that differences in severity of RA between patients with different educational levels may be attributed to variations in the initial disease presentation between patient groups.

Preliminary published results suggested higher RA prevalence in men with lower income levels.[16,80] However, recent incidence data do not support this relationship.[17] Marital status is another sociodemographic variable associated with RA in some studies. An increased prevalence of RA has been noted in single and divorced women.[81] Being divorced, separated or widowed, or never having been married may be a predictor of functional disability in RA.[74,75,82,83]

Suggestions that RA is a communicable disease have not been substantiated. No significant association of RA has been found in marital partners,[84] and evidence of an infectious agent has not been demonstrated.[42] Failure to find disease similarity in sibling pairs with RA suggests that various environmental factors contribute to heterogeneity in RA.[85]

PSYCHOLOGICAL AND STRESS FACTORS RELATED TO RA

Over the past half-century, many investigators have addressed the issue of psychological and life stress factors influencing the onset or course of RA.[86-88] Increased stress does not necessarily associate with progression to an advanced disease state,[89] while improved mood may have a positive effect on outcome.[90] However, measurement and methodological complexities on both sides of the observational relationships have yielded indefinite data and contradictory conclusions.[86-90] In a recent study, data suggested that RA patients were more reactive to interpersonal stressors than persons with osteoarthritis.[86] In a second report, patients with definite RA reported more stress at disease onset than a comparison group with osteoarthritis.[87] In a third study, no excess of stressful life events during the 12 months before onset of RA was found.[88]

One report describes the influence of a 6.7-magnitude earthquake on the clinical status of 13 RA patients who had been evaluated within 45 days before and after this experience. None of the patients experienced a clinical flare, and all prednisone doses remained stable.[91] Another report of 26 RA patients found that mirthful laughter improved mood and was associated with decreased pain and decreased mean serum levels of cortisol, interleukin-6, and interferon-β 30 minutes after exposure compared to one hour before exposure.[92] In a prospective study of 238 patients with early RA, the experience of positive life events during the past year was significantly related to a reduction in disability.[93] Patient interaction in the setting of a support group has also been shown to improve RA patients' global assessment over a short term.[94]

The biological basis of psychological and stress mechanisms operating in RA is not defined (Figure 10-1), but numerous theories have been postulated.[91] Gender dimorphism in stress response was postulated, whereby stressful life events might initiate or exacerbate RA in men but ameliorate the disease in women.[95] Hypothalamic-pituitary-adrenal axis function is believed to play an important role in RA.[1,35,95-97] One case report in support of this theory describes a patient with severe destructive RA who went into spontaneous remission after the onset of Cushing's disease but experienced subsequent disease recurrence when the hypercortisolemia was normalized.[96] Also, elevated plasma ACTH levels without hypercortisolemia were reported in untreated RA, as might occur in adrenal cortical dysfunction.[1,35,97] Androgenic-anabolic hormone function is also believed to play a role in RA.[1,35,55,56,95] These steroids can be altered under stress or in circumstances that elevate circulating ACTH levels.[1,35,95] Psychoneuroendocrine physiology could theoretically influence susceptibility to RA, but specific mechanisms and pathways have not been documented in humans.[1,35,95-97]

JUVENILE-TYPE RHEUMATOID ARTHRITIS OF CHILDHOOD OR ADULT ONSET

Epidemiological patterns of RA are less well-defined in juveniles than in adults due to fewer studies and greater diversity of classification criteria.[2,62,98] Space does not permit review of the complex issues of juvenile rheumatoid arthritis (JRA) classification,[98] nor of data that might reflect environmental contributions to disease. However, a recent Canadian cooperative study of the seasonal onset of juvenile Still's disease (that is, systemic-onset JRA) may be mentioned.[99] Across Canada the onset of Still's disease was constant throughout the seasons, without evidence that viral infections correlated with the disease incidence. A matched case-control study of 60 patients with adult Still's disease indicated that stressful life events in the year preceding onset were significantly associated with risk of disease.[100] A considerable number of other factors were found not to be significantly associated with disease risk, including OC usage in the preceding year.[100]

PROSPECTIVE STUDIES OF CIGARETTE SMOKING AND RA IN WOMEN

A significant association was first reported between cigarette smoking and RA in 1987, as shown in Table 10-2.[20]

Table 10-2   Rates per 100,000 person-years (P-Ys) and relative risks (RRs) of developing rheumatoid arthritis (RA) after entry to study by categories of current cigarette smoking histories in published prospective studies

| First Author (yr) | Study Characteristics | | | Rates (per 100,000 P-Ys) of RA and RRs by Current Cigarette Smoking Categories | | | | |
| | Enrollment Period | Number of Subjects | Outcomes | | Rheumatoid Arthritis | | | p values or Confidence Intervals (CIs) |
				Cigs/d	Nos.	Rates	RRs	
Vessey (1987)[20]	1968–1974	17,032F[1]	RA Onset[2]	Never	34	27[3]	1.0[4]	X[2]trend,
				Ex	10	38	1.41	8.1, 1d.f.
				1–14	15	38	1.41	p<0.01.
				15+	19	64	2.37	
				1+	34	51	1.89	N.A.
Hernández-Avila (1990)[21]	1976	116,779F[5]	RA Onset	Never	40	10.5[6]	1.0[7]	—
				Ex	36	15.8	1.5	(0.9–2.3)
				1–14	5	6.6	0.6	(0.3–1.5)
				15–24	21	18.3	1.5	(0.9–2.6)
				25+	11	14.1	1.4	(0.7–2.7)
				1+	37	13.8	1.3	(0.9–2.1)
				15+	32	16.6	1.5	(1.0–2.1)
Heliövaara (1993)[18]	1966–1972	24,445F[8]	RA Onset (seropositive)	Never	180	49.7[9]	1.0	—
				Ex	8	38.2	0.8	(0.4–1.7)
				1–14	36	49.7	1.1	(0.8–1.6)
				15+	5	49.7	1.1	(0.4–2.6)
				1+	41	49.7	1.1[9]	(0.7–1.3)[9]
		28,364M[8]	RA Onset (seropositive)	Never	12	7.5[9]	1.0	—
				Ex	23	24.1	2.8	(1.4–5.6)
				1–14	37	33.0	4.4	(2.3–8.5)
				15+	39	30.0	4.0	(2.1–7.7)
				1+	76	31.5	4.2[9]	(3.2–5.1)[9]

[1]White, married women aged 25–39 yrs recruited at 17 family planning clinics in England and Scotland.

[2]First ever visit to hospital (outpatient or inpatient) for RA.

[3]Rate per 100,000 women-years, standardized for age.

[4]Relative risk, using never smokers as the reference category, i.e., 1.0.

[5]Female nurses aged 30–55 followed at least once in the Nurses' Health Study.

[6]Nonadjusted rates derived from Table 5 of article.

[7]Age-adjusted relative risk of RA among US nurses aged 30–55 in 1976.

[8]Adult (16+ years) Finns examined by the Social Insurance Institution's Mobile Clinic Health Examination Survey, followed until the end of 1989.

[9]Estimated from data in the original article, not age-adjusted nor corrected for deaths.

Analyses were performed on 17,032 married premenopausal women aged 25 to 39 who were recruited between 1968 and 1974 at 17 family planning clinics in England and Scotland. Information on cigarette smoking was obtained as the women entered the study. The estimated average follow-up was 12.9 years per enrolled woman, yielding a total crude observation of 219,404 person-years at risk. The outcome variable was the onset of RA after entry to the study of sufficient severity to be referred to hospital (outpatient or inpatient), which was discovered in 78 women (crude incidence of 35.6 cases per 100,000 person-years). The cases had a young median RA onset age of 37.6 years.

Among women who smoked 15 or more cigarettes daily at entry, the rate of developing RA was 64 per 100,000 person-years compared with women who never smoked (27 per 100,000 person-years) (p < 0.01) all standardized for age, yielding a risk ratio (RR) of 2.37 (Table 11-2). The risks for ex-smokers and those who smoked less than 15 cigarettes daily were intermediate (38 per 100,000 person-years; RR = 1.41), which is not significantly higher than the rate for women who never smoked. Linear association of gradients of cigarette smoking and RA is also significant by chi-square test (p < 0.01).

A second prospective study analyzed female nurses aged 30 to 55 years who were recruited in 1976 and were followed at least once in the U.S. Nurses' Health Study.[21] Table 10-2 shows results from information on cigarette smoking obtained from completed mailed questionnaires on entry to the study. The estimated average follow-up of the 116,779 enrolled women who provided information on smoking habits was 7.3 years, yielding a total crude observation of 883,187 person-years at risk. A total of 113 women were identified who developed definite RA after entry to study (a crude incidence of 12.8 cases per 100,000 person-years). Compared to women who had never smoked, those who reported smoking 15 to 24 cigarettes daily at entry had an age-adjusted RR of developing RA of 1.5 (95% CI: 0.9, 2.6) (Table 10-2). However, when this level of cigarette smoking was analyzed in a multivariate model, adjusting for additional factors, the RR for RA was statistically significant at 1.6 (1.1, 2.3). Most (53.1%) of the women in this study were postmenopausal on entry.[21]

A third prospective study included 24,445 Finnish women older than 16 who were enrolled between 1966 and 1972 in the Social Insurance Institution's Mobile Clinic Health Examination Survey and were followed until the end of 1989.[18] Information on smoking history was obtained as part of the entry examination (Table 10-2). The estimated average duration of follow-up per study subject was 19.1 years, yielding a total crude observation of 467,037 person-years at risk. A total of 229 women were detected who developed seropositive RA after entry to the study (crude incidence: 49.0 cases/100,000 person-years). No significant difference in risk of developing RA by any category of smoking history was found in these women.[18] However, only five (2.2%) of the 229 seropositive women with RA smoked 15 or more cigarettes daily on entry, a markedly lower proportion than was found in the other prospective studies.[20,21,24]

There was also no association between smoking and seronegative RA among women in this study. However, only 524 (2.1%) of the total 24,445 female participants smoked 15 or more cigarettes daily on entry to the study, yielding a crude observation of 10,008 person-years at risk in this exposed subgroup. A total of five seropositive RA cases were found in this subgroup cohort, whereas 11.6 and 7.8 cases would have been expected based on RRs of 2.37 and 1.6 found in the previous studies.[20,21] The beta error of failing to detect an association between smoking 15 or more cigarettes daily and RA, assuming these magnitudes of RRs[20,21] exceeds a probability level of 0.05. Insufficient exposure risk to 15 or more cigarettes daily in this female population[18] may have been responsible, at least in part, for not detecting an association with RA. In a population where smoking is rare, it is difficult to show an association with disease in a prospective study, even if a causal relationship exists.[101,102]

The most recent prospective study evaluated an inception cohort of 21,061 adult residents of Washington County, Maryland who were enrolled in 1974 and followed for 20 years.[24] A history of cigarette smoking was obtained from all participants at entry. The cases were defined as members of the cohort who developed definite RA after entry to the study and who were referred to the sole rheumatologist in the community. Similarly, the controls were defined as members of the cohort who did not develop RA after entry into the study, as determined by not having been referred to this rheumatologist. Four controls were individually matched to each case on age and sex; all case-control study participants were Caucasian.

A significantly (p < 0.01) increased frequency of current cigarette smoking in 1974 was found among 54 identified cases compared to their matched controls (50.9% versus 31.1% percent; cross-products odds ratio [OR] 2.3; 95% CI: 1.07, 4.31). Results were significant in the 36 female sets (p < 0.025), but not among the 18 males, due to their smaller number.[24]

RETROSPECTIVE STUDIES OF CIGARETTE SMOKING AND RA IN WOMEN

The first retrospective clinical study of cigarette smoking and RA in women was performed at the University Hospital in Leiden between 1982 and 1986.[25] The study recruited 135 women from 20 to 50 years old with definite or classical RA and onset of symptoms within five years before their first clinic visit. Information on cigarette smoking was obtained with reference to the time of the first clinic visit and not with respect to onset of first symptoms or the initial diagnosis of RA. The median age at onset of symptoms of RA was 37.1 years; 89% of the women were premenopausal.[25] Reported cigarette smoking histories were compared to those of 378 women with soft tissue rheumatism or osteoarthritis of similar demographic characteristics.

Employing a baseline of nonsmokers, a negative association was found between any amount of cigarette smoking at first clinic visit and RA (OR = 0.61; 95% CI: 0.42, 0.89), as shown in Table 10-3. A proposed explanation for the negative association observed among current smokers of at least one cigarette a day and RA was that these patients may have been more inclined to stop smoking after disease onset and before referral to clinic than the controls.[25] Alternatively, the authors suggested that cigarette smoking may have been a protective factor (or marker) for developing RA. Higher concentrations of adrenal androgens such as dehydroepiandrosterone sulfate and androstenedione were reported in postmenopausal female cigarette smokers than in nonsmokers[103] and were cited as possible support for a "protective" smoking hypothesis.[25] In the Leiden study, the OR of 21 or more cigarettes daily was 0.82 (95% CI: 0.44, 1.50), which is not a significant negative association at that level.

The second retrospective study recruited 349 women between the ages of 18 and 64 with incident RA (92% definite or classical disease) from November 1986 to February 1991 from residents of King County, WA, or from persons enrolled in the Group Health Cooperative of Puget Sound.[22] Subjects' reported data on cigarette smoking histories were compared to those of 1457 women without arthritis from the same population base. Information on cigarette smoking was

Table 10-3 Odds Ratios of Having Rheumatoid Arthritis vs Control Status in Women by Categories of Current Cigarette Smoking Histories at First Clinic Visit or Symptomatic Onset of RA in Published Retrospective Studies.

First Author (Year)	Enrollment Period	Cases	Controls	Cigs/d	Nos.	ORs	Confidence Intervals (CIs)
		Study Characteristics			Odds Ratios (ORs) of Developing RA by Current Cigarette Smoking Categories		
					Rheumatoid Arthritis		
Hazes (1990)[25]	1982–86	135 female RA[1] (definite or classical)	378 female[1] STR or OA	None[2]	91	1.0[3]	—
				1–10	N.S.	0.60	(0.33–1.08)
				11–20	N.S.	0.53	(0.32–0.89)
				21+	N.S.	0.82	(0.44–1.50)
				1+[4]	44	0.61	(0.42–0.89)
Voigt (1994)[22]	1986–1991	349 female RA[5] (92% diagnosed definite or classical)	1457 female nonarthritis population residents[6]	Premenopausal:			
				Never	N.S.	1.0	—
				Ex	N.S.	1.2	(0.8–1.7)
				Current	N.S.	1.3	(0.9–1.8)
				P–Ys[7]			
				<5	N.S.	1.0	(0.7–1.6)
				5–10	N.S.	1.5	(0.9–2.5)
				10–20	N.S.	1.0	(0.6–1.7)
				21+[8]	N.S.	1.6	(1.0–2.7)
				Postmenopausal:			
				Never	N.S.	1.0	—
				Ex	N.S.	1.4	(0.9–2.2)
				Current	N.S.	1.4	(0.8–2.2)
				P–Ys[7]			
				<5	N.S.	1.2	(0.6–2.3)
				5–10	N.S.	0.9	(0.4–2.2)
				10–20	N.S.	1.8	(0.9–3.6)
				21+[8]	N.S.	1.4	(0.9–2.3)

[1]Age at first visit between ages 20 to 50 years and onset of symptoms within 5 years: RA = rheumatoid arthritis; STR = soft tissue rheumatism; OA = osteoarthritis.

[2]Cigarette smoking status at the time of first outpatient clinic visit, not at onset of RA.

[3]Odds ratios adjusted for age and other variables in a logistic regression model.

[4]Current smoking in RA (33%) was less than controls (48%) or the general population (44%).

[5]Women aged 18–64 years diagnosed with RA in the King County, WA, USA area.

[6]Women identified using random digit dialing of households in King County (N = 1289) and random sampling of enrolled non-arthritis patients in Group Health Cooperative (N = 168).

[7]Pack-years of cigarette smoking.

[8]Combined pre- and post-menopausal OR for 21+ P-Ys ever smoked = 1.5 (95% CI = 1.0–2.0).

obtained in person by trained interviewers with respect to the time of the first physician visit for symptoms ultimately diagnosed as RA. Controls were assigned a comparable reference date for purposes of determining their smoking history. At entry to the study, the median age of RA patients was 42.8 years and 65.3% were pre- or perimenopausal.

The ORs of current cigarette smoking for premenopausal and postmenopausal onset of RA were 1.3 and 1.4, respectively (95% CIs: 0.9, 1.8 and 0.8, 2.2).[22] An OR for any cigarette smoking and RA was not reported for all the women, but was significant (OR = 1.3; 95% CI: 1.0, 1.7) (personal communication, Dr. LF Voight). For all women who had a history of ever having smoked 21 or more pack-years of cigarettes (one pack-year is the equivalent of one pack a day for a year), the OR is 1.5 (95% CI: 1.0, 2.0). Among the premenopausal women alone, this cumulative level of smoking experience also associates significantly with RA (OR = 1.6; 95% CI: 1.0, 2.7), as shown in Table 10-3.

The third and most recent retrospective study includes data from the Women's Health Cohort Study of female health professionals.[23] Mailed questionnaires were completed by 386,564 subjects and included information on RA diagnosis, date of diagnosis and cigarette smoking history. RA was self-reported by 8376 women, with 3648 being seropositive (0.94%).

Compared to women who never smoked, the age-adjusted RR of RA among current smokers of more than 25 cigarettes daily was 1.40 (95% CI: 1.28, 1.53). The linear trend of cigarette smoking gradients and ORs of RA was highly significant (p < 0.0001). The corresponding RR for developing seropositive RA was 1.44 (95% CI: 1.27, 1.65), with a similarly significant linear trend (p < 0.001). Adjustments for other factors (menopausal status, age at menarche, pregnancy history, hormone use, body-mass index, race, income and educational level) did not significantly alter the findings. The authors concluded that cigarette smoking is associated with an increased risk of RA in women and that a dose-response relationship exists.

One recent retrospective study of primary-care-based incident RA cases and controls also found that a history of having ever smoked cigarettes was associated with an increased OR for developing RA (OR = 1.66; 95% CI: 0.95, 3.06).[104]

DISCORDANT TWIN STUDY OF CIGARETTE SMOKING AND RA IN WOMEN

A twin study from Britain[19] recruited 71 pairs of monozygotic twins and 79 pairs of dizygotic like-sexed twins nationwide. Analyses were restricted to disease- and smoking-discordant twin pairs from this sample. History of cigarette smoking at the time of disease onset was obtained by interview. No information was provided on the age distribution of the twins analyzed or the degree of smoking experience.

Among the total 24 discordant female twin pairs, the RA member alone smoked in 19 pairs, whereas the unaffected twin alone smoked in five pairs (OR 3.8; 95% CI: 1.37, 13.0). The relationship was also significant among the subset of 15 discordant dizygotic pairs, but not the nine monozygotic pairs, possibly due to their smaller number (Table 10-4).

SUMMARY OF PREVIOUS STUDIES OF CIGARETTE SMOKING AND RA IN WOMEN

The preceding studies of cigarette smoking and RA in women[18–25] support an overall positive association, either at a level of more than 15 cigarettes currently smoked daily or a cumulative exposure of 21 or more pack-years. The studies that do not support this hypothesis are likely explained by their particular characteristics.[18,25] In the Finnish prospective study that found no association,[18] a small proportion (2.1%) of women in the population reported moderate or heavier (15 or more cigarettes daily) smoking behaviors. In the retrospective study that found a negative association with any degree of cigarette smoking,[25] some RA patients may have discontinued smoking after the onset of disease but before their first clinic visit. Also, this cohort was young at onset of RA (median age 37.1 years) and may not have had sufficient duration of cigarette smoking exposure to detect a risk relationship.[25]

PREVIOUS STUDIES OF CIGARETTE SMOKING AND RA IN MEN

Among men, the prospective study from Finland shows an association only between any past or current smoking experience and seropositive RA, but not seronegative disease.[18]

Table 10-4 Odds ratios (ORs) of rheumatoid arthritis (RA) by retrospective history of current cigarette smoking at symptomatic onset of RA in disease- and smoking-discordant, like-sexed twin pairs recruited nationwide in UK.

First Author (Year)	Recruitment Period	Total Twin Pairs		Type of Twins	Discordant Pairs			95% Confidence Intervals
		Cases: RA Twins	Controls (CN) non-RA Twins		RA Only Smoker	CN Only Smoker	ORs	
Silman (1996)[19]		71 MZ	71 MZ	F,MZ	7	2	3.5	(0.67–34.5)
		79 DZ	79 DZ	F,DZ	12	3	4.0	(1.08–22.1)
				F, Total	19	5	3.8	(1.37–13.0)
				M,MZ	4	0	∞	—
				M,DZ	3	2	1.5	(0.17–18.0)
				M, Total	7	2	3.5	(0.67–34.5)
				All MZ	11	2	5.5	(1.20–51.1)
				All DZ	15	5	3.0	(1.04–10.6)
				Total	26	7	3.7	(1.57–10.1)

MZ = monozygotic
DZ = dizygotic

However, this positive association with seropositive RA in men is complicated. Among the control men who had never smoked, a significantly decreasing incidence of RA was observed over time during the extended course of observation (from entry between 1966 and 1972 until follow-up in late 1989). In contrast, a significantly increasing incidence trend was observed over time among smokers,[18] as would be expected due to their increasing age during follow-up.[36] The significantly elevated relative risks of seropositive RA among male smokers in this study may have to some extent been contributed to by the decreasing incidence of RA over time among men who had never smoked.[18]

In the twin study,[19] only nine male discordant pairs were analyzed. This sample showed a positive association between smoking and RA (seven versus two pairs; OR = 3.5), but the numbers are small and the difference is not significant (95% CI: 0.67, 34.5). A similar OR of 2.3 was found in male cigarette smokers from the prospective case-control study,[24] but this result was also nonsignificant due to the small number of male study subjects.

LIMITATIONS OF A SINGLE TIME-POINT HISTORY OF SMOKING EXPOSURE

Precise, quantitative, cumulative, lifetime histories of cigarette smoking prior to onset of disease among cases and controls would be the ideal data for determining risk relationships.[101,102] However, most data about smoking have been obtained at only one time-point on entry to studies.[18-21,23-25] The limited data on smoking behaviors from most but not all studies[22] necessarily qualify conclusions that may be drawn with respect to risk of developing RA. One must assume that the amount of cigarette smoking reported at the single time-point is correlated with cumulative exposure to cigarettes. Tracking of lifestyle risk factors over a period of 14 years covering adolescence and young adulthood revealed moderately high stability coefficients only for smoking, indicating good longitudinal predictability for this factor.[105]

LIMITATIONS OF OBSERVATIONAL STUDY DESIGNS

Alternative explanations for the observed associations of current cigarette smoking and RA might be chance circumstances or distorting effects of other variables causing undetected, systematic methodological biases, particularly in retrospective studies which suffer from recall bias.[101,102] Any one observational study allows less potential to draw definitive conclusions than an experimental trial, because of its random allocation design and control of exposures. However, such trials are not ethically feasible in this issue. Therefore, the goal of nonexperimental research is to simulate the results of an experiment, had one been possible.[102]

RA AND LUNG CANCER

Excess respiratory or lung cancer frequencies have been reported following onset of RA, although no information on smoking habits was available.[106-109] Standardized incidence ratios, which are the ratios of observed to expected frequencies, ranged from 1.2 to 1.4 for lung cancers developing after a diagnosis of RA. However, two further studies did not confirm such excess cancer risks, with standardized incidence ratios of 1.1 and 0.7.[110,111] Such data are difficult to interpret with respect to a shared comorbidity of respiratory cancers and RA resulting from cigarette smoking, since interstitial lung disease in RA may also predispose to lung cancer.[112]

POTENTIAL CONFOUNDING OF ANDROGENICITY, CIGARETTE SMOKING AND RA

Increased serum androgen levels have been reported in female[103] and male[113] smokers. Serum androgenic-anabolic hormone levels are also genetically influenced.[114,115] Low serum testosterone levels are associated with increased risk of RA in women[114] and men,[115] as well as with immunogenetic markers that associate with RA, including HLA-DR4 in younger women[114,116] and HLA-B15 in men.[38,115] If increased androgenicity associates positively with smoking behaviors[103,113] but negatively with risk of developing RA, particularly in premenopausal females[1,35,55] and males,[1,35,115] then confounding could occur in analyzing the relationship of current cigarette smoking to risk of RA.[25]

BIOLOGICAL PLAUSIBILITY OF AN ASSOCIATION BETWEEN CURRENT CIGARETTE SMOKING AND RA

Cigarette smoking induces endothelial injury, which may act as a precursor to macro- and microvascular diseases,[117-122] including RA.[1,42] Cigarette smoking also facilitates platelet formation of proaggregatory thromboxane A_2 and increases fibrinogen levels, which could enhance endothelial dysfunction and microcirculatory insufficiency.[118] Smoking results in decreased nitric oxide synthase activities of placental vessels.[123] The nitric oxide molecule is believed to play a central role in protecting against vascular disease.[120,124] Nitric oxide is produced in many tissues and cells of the body by either the constitutive or inducible form of nitric oxide synthase,[125] and thereby subsumes multiple homeostatic and pathological roles.[126] In RA, nitric oxide is believed to modulate both microvascular and inflammatory processes.[127]

The primary mechanisms whereby cigarette smoking could predispose to RA are not known. However, microvascular and inflammatory pathways deserve further investigation.[1,42,127] Because aging is also a strong determinant of RA, prodegenerative actions of cigarette smoking should also be investigated as a possible risk mechanism.[36,118] To this end, data from studies on smoking and knee osteoarthritis are relevant. In one report, smoking, or some unidentified factor associated with smoking, appears to protect modestly against the development of knee osteoarthritis[128]; another report found no protection from smoking.[20]

ESTIMATED POPULATION ATTRIBUTABLE FRACTION OF CURRENT CIGARETTE SMOKING AND RA

Given the emphatic qualification that observed associations between cigarette smoking and RA may not yet be judged as causal, the importance of findings from previous studies are underscored by estimates of the population attributable fraction (PAF) of RA which could be associated with current cigarette smoking. Hypothetically, if the OR of current cigarette smoking and RA were estimated to be 2.0 among the combined genders, and the proportion of current cigarette smokers in a base population (Pe) were 0.30,[129] the PAF would be estimated to be 0.23, using the following equation[101,102]:

$$PAF = \frac{Pe \; (0.30) \; (OR = 2.0 - 1)}{Pe \; (0.30) \; (OR = 2.0 - 1) + 1} = \frac{0.30}{1.30} = 0.23$$

If the exposure-associated relationship of current cigarette smoking and RA is judged as causal, and if such magnitude of PAF (2.0 or higher) is supported, the overall morbidity and economic costs from such exposure would be considerable. An estimated 2.1 million adults in the United States have classical or definite RA,[130] at a cost of $8.7 billion annually.[131]

The PAF estimates the proportion of cases in the target population related to the exposure of interest and does not differentiate between causal and marker relationships.[132,133] Caution should be expressed in the interpretation of PAF estimates in diseases that demonstrate biological interactions. The exposure of interest may accelerate onset of illness in persons destined to develop the disease later, rather than be an etiological factor among those not so predisposed.[132,133] Severity of outcome is a further conceptual problem in interpreting attributable fractions of disease following exposures of interest. Different degrees of severity outcomes may manifest in the presence or absence of exposures.[133] Estimates of PAF cannot be considered as biological constants, but must be judged within the context of each study as well as in terms of the overall empirical evidence and biomedical plausibility.[102,103]

GENETIC AND ENVIRONMENTAL INFLUENCES ON RHEUMATOID FACTOR

In simple terms, rheumatoid factor (RF) is a circulating antibody (for example, agglutinin) to antigenic determinants on the crystallizable fraction (Fc) of altered immunoglobulin G (IgG).[42] Characteristically, such reactivity results from the IgM isotype molecules of human whole serum, but may also be found in other Ig isotypes, that is, IgA and IgG.[134] Historically, the antigen for RF reactivity has been human IgG, but goat or rabbit protein may be substituted[134] in an attempt to increase the utility of this test for diagnosing RA.[134–137] Thus, serum RF reactivity may result from IgM, IgG or IgA isotype molecules, and RF may be measured in aggregate, or its specific isotype antibodies may be separately assayed against human, goat or rabbit IgG antigens. The conventional latex test measures whole serum RF reactivity, using altered human IgG as the antigen, and is assayed by either aggregation or nephelometry techniques.[134] Also, enzyme-linked immunosorbent assay (ELISA) techniques may be used to detect either whole serum or isotype-specific RF reactivity against human, goat or rabbit IgG.[134–137]

Assay results of the several whole serum RF methods are attributable mainly to the IgM antibody reactivity and tend to correlate closely with each other. Various studies have compared the clinical utility of Ig isotype RF reactivity, as measured by ELISA, to the results of whole serum methods, for example, nephelometric.[134–137] The ELISA method of assaying IgM RF is more sensitive than the latex agglutination or nephelometry techniques and has only recently been incorporated in routine clinical laboratory use as a standardized test system.[134]

Studies of RF in populations have revealed an association with smoking,[26,27] and RF also predicts the subsequent development of RA in longitudinal studies.[28–31] Cigarette smoking of sufficient degree and duration[18–24] and RF[28–31] can each significantly predict the onset risk of RA; an important issue is whether or not these factors may be operating conjointly or independently in the development of RA.[138] If RF is an important contributor to the pathogenesis of RA, a corollary issue is whether its formation may be influenced mainly by environmental or genetic mechanisms.

Regarding the latter question, RF reactivity clusters in disease-free members of multiplex RA families,[139,140] suggesting either shared environmental or genetic mechanisms, or their combination. In order to analyze this issue more critically, the occurrence of IgM, IgG and IgA RFs were determined in disease-unaffected monozygotic versus dizygotic twins of seropositive RA co-twins from a nationwide British study.[141] A genetic influence would be supported by a higher proportion of RF occurrence among the unaffected monozygotic co-twins than among the unaffected dizygotic co-twins, whereas no genetic influence would be expected to result in equal proportions among the two types of co-twins. A monozygotic:dizygotic seropositivity odds ratio was further adjusted for potential confounding effects of age, sex and either HLA-DRB1*04 or DRB1*01 status of the unaffected twin.[141]

After accounting for the confounding variables, the monozygotic unaffected twins had roughly twofold to threefold increased seropositivity for IgM and IgG RF but an equivalent odds ratio for IgA RF.[141] Thus, genetic-related factors may be assumed to be important in determining IgM and IgG RF levels, which were found to be independent of HLA-DR in this study.[141] In healthy persons, HLA-DR4 also did not predispose to higher amounts of rheumatoid factor.[142]

Since RF frequency was not measured in a population control group adjusted for age, sex and HLA-DR status,[141] the possible influences of environmental factors on RF reactivity of the monozygotic and dizygotic twins could not be determined. IgM RF was detected in 11 of 69 (15.9%) unaffected dizygotic twins, which is higher than expected and could have resulted from either environmental or genetic factors. IgM RF was detected in 18 of 57 (31.6%) unaffected monozygotic twins. The excess seropositivity of the monozygotic above the dizygotic twins probably reflects a major genetic component, independent of HLA-DR4. However, early shared environmental effects cannot be excluded as influencing these findings.[141]

The greater occurrence of RF in the unaffected monozygotic than dizygotic twins may also reflect their fourfold increased risk of developing RA. Further longitudinal and prospective studies are needed to identify environmental and genetic effects on RF production and to analyze their relationships to the onset risks of RA.

The presence of RF may be either a determinant or simply a long-term predictive marker. The fact that rheumatoid factors long precede clinical onset of RA[28-31] does not necessarily indicate that they play a direct pathogenetic role in the onset of RA. RF production may be one of the first consequences of a disturbed immune system, eventually leading to clinical RA, or it may be an indicator of other pathogenetic mechanisms. The immune system might be imbalanced or perturbed by many endogenous and exogenous factors (Figure 10-1). RFs that are highly specific and highly avid for human IgG are important in the course of RA, possibly by RF immune complex formation.[143] If smoking interacts with RF to modulate RA, it may add to vascular damage during the course of disease. Smoking is associated with vasculitis in RA,[144,145] which may be augmented by RF. The relative contributions of environmental,[26,27] familial[140] and nongenetic somatic[144] influences on RF production in RA are presently not well defined, nor is the relationship of RF to current cigarette smoking in predisposing to RA onset[141,146] or to vasculitis.[144,145]

SUMMARY

Until the present, no lifestyle or environmental risk factor or marker for RA has been documented, with the exception of cigarette smoking. Among community-derived cases, familial factors have not been demonstrated to be significant risks for RA, implying that acquired or environmental determinants predominate among those individuals.[41]

The nine reported studies on the association of cigarette smoking and RA are heterogeneous, including prospective, retrospective and disease-discordant twin pair designs.[18-25,104] Each report includes data from females. Males were specifically investigated only in three studies, two of which employed national samples, that is, a prospective analysis from Finland[18] and a disease-discordant twin study from Britain.[19] The third report was a community-based, nested, case-control study.[24]

Among men, results from the Finnish prospective study show a significant association only between history of any smoking (past or current of any degree) and seropositive RA.[18] In the discordant twin study, the RA-affected members reported currently smoking cigarettes more frequently than the unaffected co-twins, but the numbers are small and the difference is not significant (Table 10-4).[19] The prospective case-control study showed a similarly increased odds ratio of RA among male cigarette smokers, as did the twin analysis,[18] but was also not significant due to a small sample size.[24]

Among women, results favor an association between history of cigarette smoking and RA, particularly at a level of 15 or more cigarettes daily or a cumulative exposure of 21 or more pack-years.[19-24] However, the large-scale prospective analysis from Finland found no increased relative risk in women (OR = 1.1; 95% CI: 0.4, 2.6).[18] Also, the retrospective clinic-based study from Leiden found a negative association between any degree of reported cigarette smoking (one or more daily) and RA (OR = 0.61; 95% CI: 0.42, 0.89).[25] The study of disease-discordant twins[19] did not quantitate the degree of current smoking (one cigarette or more daily), but found a significant association with RA (OR = 3.8, 1.4–13.0). Similar results were found in the nested, case-control study.[24]

RF positivity is a strong predictor of RA[28-31] and is significantly associated with smoking in the population at large.[26,27] Data are few, but RF and current cigarette smoking seem to predict RA independently of each other and of a positive family history in first-degree relatives.[146,147]

Investigation of pathogenetic mechanisms operating during the onset of RA should include the host factors of increasing age, gender, obesity[104], a positive family history (or comparable immunogenetic predictors), smoking behavior, blood transfusion[104], and other influences on acquiring RF positive status. The interactions of these various factors upon the host's hormonal, immunological and vascular systems likely determine susceptibility to RA and the course of disease. The roles of psychological, stress and sociodemographic factors upon RA risk are more difficult to interpret and have not yet been well established.

In conclusion, among the behavioral and environmental influences, significant associations have been found between current cigarette smoking and the development of RA among males and females. Further investigation of this and other lifestyle influences may provide new research avenues into the complex pathogenesis of this disease and possible behavioral or other host interventions.

Supported in part by grants from the HealthCORE Fund, Methodist Medical Center Foundation, and The Proctor Foundation.

We express sincere appreciation to Mrs. Kay Paul for her dedicated and effective assistance in preparing this manuscript.

REFERENCES

[1]Masi AT, Feigenbaum SL, Chatterton RT, Cutolo M. Integrated hormonal-immunological-vascular (H-I-V triad) systems interactions in rheumatic diseases. *Clin Exp Rheumatol.* 1995;13:203–216.

[2]Masi AT, Medsger TA Jr. Epidemiology of the rheumatic diseases. In: McCarty DJ, ed. *Arthritis and Allied Conditions.* 11th edition. Philadelphia: Lea & Febiger, 1989;16–54.

[3]Lawrence JS. Rheumatoid arthritis—nature or nurture? *Ann Rheum Dis.* 1970;29:357–359.

[4]Aho K, Koskenvuo M, Tuominen J, Kaprio J. Occurrence of rheumatoid arthritis in a nationwide series of twins. *J Rheumatol.* 1986;3:899–902.

[5]Silman AJ, MacGregor AJ, Thomson W, *et al.* Twin concordance rates for rheumatoid arthritis: Results from a nationwide study. *Br J Rheumatol.* 1993;32:903–907.

[6]Järvinen P, Aho K. Twin studies in rheumatic diseases. *Semin Arthritis Rheum.* 1994;24:19–28.

[7]Ollier ER, MacGregor A. Genetic epidemiology of rheumatoid disease. *Br Med Bull.* 1995;51:267–285.

[8]Masi AT. Population studies in rheumatic disease. *Annu Rev Med.* 1967;18:185–206.

[9]Lawrence JS. *Rheumatism in Populations.* London: William Heinemann Medical Books, Ltd, 1977; chap. 6, "Rheumatoid arthritis," 156–271.

[10]Weyand CM, Goronzy JJ. Inherited and noninherited risk factors in rheumatoid arthritis. *Curr Opin Rheum.* 1995;7:206–213.

[11]Winchester R. The molecular basis of susceptibility to rheumatoid arthritis. *Adv Immunol.* 1994;56:389–466.

[12]Blumberg BS, Bloch KJ, Black RL, Dotter C. A study of the prevalence of arthritis in Alaska Eskimos. *Arthritis Rheum.* 1961; 4:325–341.

[13]Levinthal LJ, Boyce EG, Zurier JB. Treatment of rheumatoid arthritis with gammalinolenic acid. *Ann Intern Med.* 1993;119: 867–873.

[14]Beighton P, Solomon L, Valkenburg HA. Rheumatoid arthritis in a rural South African Negro population. *Ann Rheum Dis.* 1975;34:136–141.

[15]Solomon L, Robin G, Valkenburg HA. Rheumatoid arthritis in an urban South African Negro population. *Ann Rheum Dis.* 1975;34: 128–135.

[16]National Center for Health Statistics. *Rheumatoid Arthritis in Adults, United States, 1960–1962.* Public Health Service Publication No. 1000, Series 11, No. 17. Washington DC: United States Government Printing Office, Sept. 1966.

[17]Bankhead C, Silman A, Barrett B, Scott D, Symmons D. The incidence of rheumatoid arthritis is not related to indicators of socio-economic deprivation. *J Rheumatol.* 1996;23:2039–2042.

[18]Heliövaara M, Aho K, Aromaa A, Knekt P, Reunanen A. Smoking and risk of rheumatoid arthritis. *J Rheumatol.* 1993;20:1830–1835.

[19]Silman AJ, Newman J, MacGregor AJ. Cigarette smoking increases the risk of rheumatoid arthritis: Results from a nationwide study of disease-discordant twins. *Arthritis Rheum.* 1996;39: 732–735.

[20]Vessey MP, Villard-Mackintosh L, Yeates D. Oral contraceptives, cigarette smoking and other factors in relation to arthritis. *Contraception.* 1987;35:457–465.

[21]Hernández-Avila M, Liang MH, Willett WC, *et al.* Reproductive factors, smoking, and the risk for rheumatoid arthritis. *Epidemiology.* 1990;1:285–291.

[22]Voigt LF, Koepsell TD, Nelson JL, Dugowson CE, Daling JR. Smoking, obesity, alcohol consumption, and the risk of rheumatoid arthritis. *Epidemiology.* 1994;5:525–532.

[23]Karlson EW, Lee IM, Cook NR, *et al.* Cigarette smoking and risk of rheumatoid arthritis in the Women's Health Cohort Study. *Arthritis Rheum.* 1996;39:S310.

[24]Masi AT, Fecht T, Aldag JC, Comstock GW, Hoffman S, Malamet RL. History of currently smoking cigarettes, but not years of education, correlated with the subsequent development of rheumatoid arthritis: Preliminary findings from a community-wide, prospective, nested, case-control study. *Arthritis Rheum.* 1996;39:S301.

[25]Hazes JMW, Dijkmans BAC, Vandenbroucke JP, de Vries RRP, Cats A. Lifestyle and the risk of rheumatoid arthritis: Cigarette smoking and alcohol consumption. *Ann Rheum Dis.* 1990;49:980–982.

[26]Mathews JD, Whittingham S, Hooper BM, Mackay JR. Association of autoantibodies with smoking, cardiovascular morbidity, and death in the Busselton population. *Lancet.* 1973;2:754–758.

[27]Tuomi T, Heliövaara M, Palosuo T, Aho K. Smoking, lung function, and rheumatoid factors. *Ann Rheum Dis.* 1990;49:753–756.

[28]Aho K, Palosuo T, Raunio V, Puska P, Aromaa A, Salonen JT. When does rheumatoid arthritis disease start? *Arthritis Rheum.* 1985;28:485–489.

[29]del Puente A, Knowler WC, Pettit DJ, Bennett PH. The incidence of rheumatoid arthritis is predicted by rheumatoid factor titer in a longitudinal population study. *Arthritis Rheum.* 1988;31:1239–1244.

[30]Aho K, Heliövaara M, Maatela J, Tuomi T, Palosuo T. Rheumatoid factors antedating clinical rheumatoid arthritis. *J Rheumatol.* 1991;18:1282–1284.

[31]Masi AT, Chatterton RT, Lu YC, *et al.* Low serum dehydroepiandrosterone sulfate (DHAS) levels, rheumatoid factor (RF) and elevated serum tumor necrosis factor (TNF) *without* cytokine receptor (CR) elevations predict long-term onset of RA in women: A controlled, prospective study. *Arthritis Rheum.* 1995;38:S214.

[32]Aho K, Palosuo T, Kurki P. Marker antibodies of rheumatoid arthritis: diagnostic and pathogenic implications. *Semin Arthritis Rheum.* 1994;23:379–387.

[33]Barnes P, Karin M. Nuclear factor—*kB*—a pivotal transcription factor in chronic inflammatory diseases. *N Engl J Med.* 1997;336: 1066–1071.

[34]Masi AT, Feigenbaum SL, Chatterton RT. Hormonal and pregnancy relationships to rheumatoid arthritis: Convergent effects with immunologic and microvascular systems. *Semin Arthritis Rheum.* 1995;25:1–27.

[35]Masi AT, Da Silva JAP, Cutolo M. Perturbations of hypothalamic-pituitary-gonadal (HPG) axis and adrenal androgen (AA) functions in rheumatoid arthritis. *Bailliere's Clin Rheum.* 1996;10:295–332.

[36]Masi AT. Incidence of rheumatoid arthritis: Do the observed age-sex interaction patterns support a role of androgenic-anabolic (AA) steroid deficiency in its pathogenesis? *Br J Rheumatol.* 1994;33: 697–699.

[37]Del Junco DJ, Luthra HS, Annegers JF, *et al.* The familial aggregation of rheumatoid arthritis and its relationship to the HLA-DR4 association. *Am J Epidemiol.* 1984;119:813–829.

[38]Hasstedt SJ, Clegg DO, Ingles L, Ward RH. HLA-linked rheumatoid arthritis. *Am J Human Genet.* 1994;55:738–746.

[39]Kwoh CK, Venglish C, Lynn AH, Whitley DM, Young E, Chakravarti A. Age, sex, and the familial risk of rheumatoid arthritis. *Am J Epidemiol.* 1996;144:15–24.

[40]Deighton CM, Roberts DF, Walker DJ. Effect of disease severity on rheumatoid arthritis concordance in same sexed siblings. *Ann Rheum Dis.* 1992;51:943–945.

[41]Jones MA, Silman AJ, Whiting S, Barrett EM, Symmons DPM. Occurrence of rheumatoid arthritis is not increased in the first-degree relatives of a population-based inception cohort of inflammatory polyarthritis. *Ann Rheum Dis.* 1996;55:89–93.

[42]Harris ED Jr. *Rheumatoid Arthritis.* Philadelphia: W.B. Saunders Company, 1997.

[43]Brennan P, Bankhead C, Silman A, *et al.* Oral contraceptives and rheumatoid arthritis: Results from a primary care-based incident case-control study. *Semin Arthritis Rheum.* 1997;26:817–823.

[44]Wingrave SJ, Kay CR. Reduction in incidence of rheumatoid arthritis associated with oral contraceptives. *Lancet.* 1978;1:569–571.

[45]Linos A, Worthington JW, O'Fallon MW, Kurland LT. The epidemiology of rheumatoid arthritis in Rochester, Minnesota: A study of incidence, prevalence and mortality. *Am J Epidemiol.* 1980;1:87–98.

[46]Silman AJ. Has the incidence of RA declined in the United Kingdom? *Br J Rheumatol.* 1988;27:77–79.

[47]Silman AJ, Vandenbroucke JP, eds. Female sex hormones and rheumatoid arthritis. Proceedings of an International Workshop. Leiden, The Netherlands, 20–21 March, 1989. *Br J Rheumatol.* 1989;28(suppl):1–73.

[48]Hernández-Avila M, Liang MH, Willett WC, *et al.* Exogenous sex hormones and the risk of rheumatoid arthritis. *Arthritis Rheum.* 1990;33:947–953.

[49]Dugowson CE, Koepsell TD, Voigt LF, *et al.* Rheumatoid arthritis in women. Incidence rates in Group Health Cooperative, Seattle, Washington, 1987–1989. *Arthritis Rheum.* 1991;34:1502–1507.

[50]Spector TD, Hochberg MC. The protective effect of the oral contraceptive pill on rheumatoid arthritis: An overview of the analytical epidemiological studies using meta-analysis. *J Clin Epidemiol.* 1990;43:1221–1230.

[51]Spector TD, Brennan P, Harris P, *et al.* Does estrogen replacement therapy protect against rheumatoid arthritis? *J Rheumatol.* 1991;18: 1473–1476.

[52]Esdaile JM, Horwitz RI. Observational studies of cause-effect relationships: An analysis of methodological problems as illustrated by the conflicting data for the role of oral contraceptives in the etiology of rheumatoid arthritis. *J Chron Dis.* 1986;39:841–852.

[53]Silman AJ. The role for epidemiology in rheumatology. *Clin Exper Rheumatol.* 1992;10:105–108.

[54]Silman AJ. The genetic epidemiology of rheumatoid arthritis. *Clin Exper Rheumatol.* 1992;10:309–312.

[55]James WH. Rheumatoid arthritis, the contraceptive pill, and androgens. *Ann Rheum Dis.* 1993;52:470–474.

[56]Masi AT. Sex hormones and rheumatoid arthritis: Cause or effect relationships in a complex pathophysiology? *Clin Exper Rheumatol.* 1995;13:227–240.

[57]van Zeben D, Hazes JMW, Vandenbrouke JP, Dijksman BAC, Cats A. Diminished incidence of severe rheumatoid arthritis associated with oral contraceptive use. *Arthritis Rheum.* 1990;33:1462–1465.

[58]Jorgensen C, Picot MC, Bologna C, Sany J. Oral contraception, parity, breast feeding, and severity of rheumatoid arthritis. *Ann Rheum Dis.* 1996;55:94–98.

[59]Carette S, Marcoux S, Gingras S. Postmenopausal hormones and the incidence of rheumatoid arthritis. *J Rheumatol.* 1989;16:911–913.

[60]Ropes MW, Bennett CA, Cobb S, Jacox R, Jessar R. A revision of diagnostic criteria for rheumatoid arthritis. *Bull Rheum Dis.* 1958;9:175–176.

[61]Arnett FC, Edworthy SM, Bloch DA, *et al.* The American Rheumatism Association 1987 revised criteria for the classification of rheumatoid arthritis. *Arthritis Rheum.* 1988;31:315–324.

[62]Hochberg MC. Adult and juvenile rheumatoid arthritis: Current epidemiologic concepts. *Epidemiol Rev.* 1981;3:27–44.

[63]Peacock DJ, Cooper C. Epidemiology of the rheumatic diseases. *Curr Opin Rheumatol.* 1995;7:82–86.

[64]Laine VAI. Rheumatic complaints in an urban population in Finland. *Acta Rheum Scand.* 1962;8:81–88.

[65]Lau EMC, Symmons DPM, Croft P. The epidemiology of hip osteoarthritis and rheumatoid arthritis in the orient. *Clin Orthop.* 1996;323:81–90.

[66]Willkens RF, Blandau RL, Aoyama DT, Beasley RP. Studies of rheumatoid arthritis among a tribe of Northwest Indians. *J Rheumatol.* 1976;3:9–14.

[67]Willkens RF, Hansen JA, Malmgren JA, *et al.* HLA antigens in Yakima Indians with rheumatoid arthritis: lack of association with HLA-Dw4 and HLA-DR4. *Arthritis Rheum.* 1982;25:1435–1439.

[68]Harvey J, Lotze M, Arnett FC, Bias WB, *et al.* Rheumatoid arthritis in a Chippewa band. II. Field study with clinical serologic and HLA-D correlations. *J Rheumatol.* 1983;10:28–32.

[69]Hochberg MC. Changes in the incidence and prevalence of rheumatoid arthritis in England and Wales, 1970–1982. *Semin Arthritis Rheum.* 1990;19:294–302.

[70]Hazes JMW, Silman AJ. Review of UK data on the rheumatic diseases. II. Rheumatoid arthritis. *Br J Rheumatol.* 1990;29:310–312.

[71]Chan K-WA, Felson DY, Yood RA, Walker AM. Incidence of rheumatoid arthritis in Central Massachusetts. *Arthritis Rheum.* 1993;36:1691–1696.

[72]Anderson ST. Mortality in rheumatoid arthritis: Do age and gender make a difference? *Semin Arthritis Rheum.* 1996;25:291–296.

[73]Callahan LF, Pincus T. Formal educational level as a significant marker of clinical status in rheumatoid arthritis. *Arthritis Rheum.* 1988;31:1346–1357.

[74]Leigh JP, Fries JF. Education level and rheumatoid arthritis: Evidence from five data centers. *J Rheumatol.* 1991;18:24–34.

[75]Verbrugge LM, Gates DM, Ike RW. Risk factors for disability among U.S. adults with arthritis. *J Clin Epidemiol.* 1991;44: 167–182.

[76]Vlieland TPMV, Buitenhuis NA, van Zeben D, Vandenbrouke JP, Breedveld FC, Hazes JMW. Sociodemographic factors and the outcome of rheumatoid arthritis in young women. *Ann Rheum Dis.* 1994;53:803–806.

[77]Meenan RF, Kazis LE, Anderson JJ. The stability of health status in rheumatoid arthritis: A five-year study of patients with established disease. *Am J Public Health.* 1988;78:1484–1487.

[78]Lorish CD, Abraham N, Austin J, Bradley LA, Alarcon GS. Disease and psychosocial factors related to physical functioning in rheumatoid arthritis. *J Rheumatol.* 1991;18:1150–1157.

[79]Wolfe F, Cathey MA. The assessment and prediction of functional disability in rheumatoid arthritis. *J Rheumatol.* 1991;18:1298–1306.

[80]Engel A. Rheumatoid arthritis in US adults 1960–62. In: Bennett PH, Wood PHN, eds. *Population Studies of the Rheumatic Diseases.* Amsterdam: Excerpta Medica, 1968;83–89.

[81]Medsger AR, Robinson H. Comparative study of divorce in rheumatoid arthritis and other rheumatic diseases. *J Chronic Dis.* 1972;25:269–275.

[82]Leigh JP, Fries JF. Predictors of disability in a longitudinal sample of patients with rheumatoid arthritis. *Ann Rheum Dis.* 1992;51:581–587.

[83]Ward MM, Leigh JP. Marital status and the progression of functional disability in patients with rheumatoid arthritis. *Arthritis Rheum.* 1993;36:581–588.

[84]Hellgren L. Rheumatoid arthritis in both marital partners. *Acta Rheum Scand.* 1969;15:135–138.

[85]Silman AJ, Ollier WER, Currey HLF. Failure to find disease similarity in sibling pairs with rheumatoid arthritis. *Ann Rheum Dis.* 1987;46:135–138.

[86]Zautra AJ, Burleson MH, Matt KS, Roth S, Burrows L. Interpersonal stress, depression, and disease activity in rheumatoid arthritis and osteoarthritis patients. *Health Psychol.* 1994;13:139–148.

[87]Latman NS, Walls R. Personality and stress: An exploratory comparison of rheumatoid arthritis and osteoarthritis. *Arch Phys Med Rehab.* 1996;77:796–800.

[88]Conway SC, Creed FH, Symmons DPM. Life events and the onset of rheumatoid arthritis. *J Psychosom Res.* 1994;38:837–847.

[89]Haller C, Holzner B, Mur E, Günther V. The impact of life events on patients with rheumatoid arthritis: A psychological myth? *Clin Exp Rheum.* 1997;15:175–179.

[90]Pietrini P, Guazzelli M. Life events in the course of chronic diseases: A psychological myth or a psycho-neuro-biochemical loop? *Clin Exp Rheum.* 1997;15:125–128.

[91]Wallace DJ, Metzger A. Can an earthquake cause flares of rheumatoid arthritis or lupus nephritis? *Arthritis Rheum.* 1994;37: 1826–1828.

[92]Yoshino S, Fujimori J, Kohda M. Effects of mirthful laughter on neuroendocrine and immune systems in patients with rheumatoid arthritis. *J Rheumatol.* 1996;23:793–794.

[93]Smedstad LM, Kvien TK, Moum T, Vaglum P. Life events, psychosocial factors, and demographic variables in early rheumatoid arthritis: Relations to one-year changes in functional disability. *J Rheumatol.* 1995;22:2218–2225.

[94]Baker PRA, Groh JD, Kraag GR, Tugwell P, Wells GA, Bolsvert D. Impact of patient with patient interaction on perceived rheumatoid arthritis overall disease status. *Scand J Rheumatol.* 1996;25: 207–212.

[95]James WH. Life events and the onset of rheumatoid arthritis (letter; comment). *J Psychsom Res.* 1995;39:507–508.

[96]Senecal J-L, Uthman I, Beauregard H. Cushing's disease-induced remission of severe rheumatoid arthritis. *Arthritis Rheum.* 1994;37: 1826–1828.

[97]Hall J, Morand EF, Medbak S, *et al.* Abnormal hypothalamic-pituitary-adrenal axis function in rheumatoid arthritis. *Arthritis Rheum.* 1994;37:1132–1137.

[98]Gare BA. Epidemiology of rheumatic disease in children. *Curr Opin Rheumatol.* 1996;8:449–454.

[99]Feldman BM, Birdi N, Boone JE, Dent PB, Duffy CM. Seasonal onset of systemic-onset juvenile rheumatoid arthritis. *J Pediatr.* 1996;129:513–518.

[100]Sampalis JS, Medsger TA, Fries JF, et al. Risk factors for adult Still's disease. *J Rheumatol.* 1996;23:2049–2054.

[101]MacMahon B, Trichopoulos D. *Epidemiology: Principles and Methods.* 2nd edition. Boston: Little, Brown and Company, 1996; 208–210.

[102]Rothman KJ. *Modern Epidemiology.* Boston; Little, Brown and Company, 1986.

[103]Kwaw KT, Tazuke S, Barrett-Connor E. Cigarette smoking and levels of adrenal androgens in postmenopausal women. *N Engl J Med.* 1988;318:1705–1709.

[104]Symmons DPM, Bankhead CR, Harrison BJ, *et al.* Blood transfusion, smoking and obesity are risk factors for the development of rheumatoid arthritis: Results from a primary care-based incident case-control study in Norfolk. *Arthritis Rheum.* 1997;40:1955–1961.

[105]Twisk JWR, Kemper HCG, van Mechelen W, Post Gb. Tracking of risk factors for coronary heart disease over a 14-year period: A comparison between lifestyle and biologic risk factors with data from the Amsterdam Growth and Health Study. *Am J Epidemiol.* 1997;145:888–898.

[106]Isomaki HA, Hakulinen T, Joutsenlahti U. Excess risk of lymphomas, leukemia and myeloma in patients with rheumatoid arthritis. *J Chronic Dis.* 1978;31:691–696.

[107]Allebeck P. Increased mortality in rheumatoid arthritis. *Scand J Rheumatol.* 1982;11:81–86.

[108]Katusic S, Beard CM, Kurland LT, *et al.* Occurrence of malignant neoplasms in the Rochester, Minnesota rheumatoid arthritis cohort. *Am J Med.* 1985;78:50–55.

[109]Gridley G, McLaughlin JK, Ekbom A, *et al.* Incidence of cancer among patients with rheumatoid arthritis. *J Natl Cancer Inst.* 1993;85:307–311.

[110]Prior P. Cancer and rheumatoid arthritis: Epidemiologic considerations. *Am J Med.* 1985;78:15–21.

[111]Laakso M, Mutru O, Isomaki H, *et al.* Cancer mortality in patients with rheumatoid arthritis. *J Rheumatol.* 1986;13:522–526.

[112]Helmers R, Galvin J, Hunninghake GW. Pulmonary manifestations associated with rheumatoid arthritis. *Chest.* 1991;100:235–238.

[113]Field AE, Colditz GA, Willett WC, *et al.* The relation of smoking, age, relative weight, and dietary intake to serum adrenal steroids, sex hormones, and sex hormone-binding globulin in middle-aged men. *J Clin Endocrinol Metab.* 1994;79:1310–1316.

[114]Deighton CM, Watson M, Walker DJ. RA sex ratios, HLA-DR, and testosterone. *Ann Rheum Dis.* 1993;52:244.

[115]Ollier W, Spector T, Silman A, *et al.* Are certain HLA haplotypes responsible for low testosterone levels in males? *Dis Markers.* 1989;7:139–143.

[116]Jaraquemada D, Ollier W, Awad J, *et al.* HLA and rheumatoid arthritis: A combined analysis of 440 British patients. *Ann Rheum Dis.* 1986;45:627–636.

[117]McVeigh GE, Lemay L, Morgan D, Cohn JN. Effects of long-term cigarette smoking on endothelium-dependent responses in humans. *Am J Cardiol.* 1996;78:668–672.

[118]*The Health Consequences of Smoking—Cardiovascular Disease: A Report of the Surgeon General.* Rockville, MD: US Dept of Health and Human Services, Public Health Service, Office on Smoking and Health, 1983.

[119]Willett WC, Green A, Stampfer MJ, *et al.* Relative and absolute excess risks of coronary heart disease among women who smoke cigarettes. *N Engl J Med.* 1987;317:1303–1309.

[120]Powel JT, Higman DJ. Smoking, nitric oxide and the endothelium. *Brit J Surg.* 1994;81:785–787.

[121]Seddon JM, Willett WC, Speizer FE, Hankinson SE. A prospective study of cigarette smoking and age-related macular degeneration in women. *JAMA.* 1996;276:1141–1146.

[122]Christen WG, Glynn RJ, Manson JE, Ajani UA, Buring JE. A prospective study of cigarette smoking and risk of age-related macular degeneration in men. *JAMA.* 1996;276:1147–1151.

[123]Sooranna SR, Morris NH, Steer PJ. Placental nitric oxide metabolism. *Reprod Fertil Dev.* 1995;7:1525–1531.

[124]Cohen RA. The role of nitric oxide and other endothelium-derived vasoactive substances in vascular disease. *Prog Cardiovasc Dis.* 1995;38:105–128.

[125]Moncada S. The L-arginine:nitric oxide pathway. *Acta Physiol Scand.* 1992;145:201–227.

[126]Moncada S, Higgs A. The L-arginine-nitric oxide pathway. *N Engl J Med.* 1993;329:2002–2012.

[127]Farrell AJ, Blake DR. Nitric oxide. *Ann Rheum Dis.* 1996;55: 7–20.

[128]Felson DT, Anderson JJ, Naimark A, Hannan MT, Kannel WB, Meenan RF. Does smoking protect against osteoarthritis? *Arthritis Rheum.* 1989;32:166–172.

[129]National Center for Health Statistics. *Health, United States, 1995.* Hyattsville, MD. Public Health Service, 1996;Table 63, p. 173.

[130]Lawrence RC, Hochberg MC, Kelsey JL, *et al.* Estimates of the prevalence of selected arthritic and musculoskeletal diseases in the United States. *J Rheumatol.* 1989;16:427–441.

[131]Yelin E. The costs of rheumatoid arthritis: Absolute, incremental, and marginal estimates. *J Rheumatol.* 1996;(suppl 44)23:47–51.

[132]Greenland S, Robbins JM. Conceptual problems in the definition and interpretation of attributable fractions. *Am J Epidemiol.* 1988;128:1185–1197.

[133]Coughlin SS, Benichou J, Weed DL. Attributable risk estimation in case-control studies. *Epidemiol Rev.* 1994;16:51–64.

[134]Swedler W, Wallman J, Froelich CJ, Teodorescu M. Routine measurement of IgM, IgG, and IgA rheumatoid factors: High sensitivity, specificity, and predictive value for rheumatoid arthritis. *J Rheumatol.* 1997;24:1037–1044.

[135]Jonsson T, Valdimarsson H. Clinical significance of rheumatoid factor isotypes in seropositive arthritis. *Rheumatol Int.* 1992;12: 111–113.

[136]Jonsson T, Thorsteinsson J, Kolbeinsson A, *et al.* Population study of the importance of rheumatoid factor isotypes in adults. *Ann Rheum Dis.* 1992;51:863–868.

[137]Jonsson T, Valdimarsson H. Is measurement of rheumatoid factor isotypes clinically useful? *Ann Rheum Dis.* 1993;52:161–164.

[138]McDonagh JE, Walker DJ. Smoking and rheumatoid arthritis—observations from a multicase family study: Comment on the article by Silman *et al.* (letter). *Arthritis Rheum.* 1997;40:594.

[139]Walker DJ, Pound JD, Griffiths ID, Powell RJ. Rheumatoid factor tests in the diagnosis and prediction of rheumatoid arthritis. *Ann Rheum Dis.* 1986;45:684–690.

[140]Silman AJ, Ollier WER, Mageed RA. Rheumatoid factor detection in the unaffected first-degree relatives in families with multicase rheumatoid arthritis. *J Rheumatol.* 1991;18:512–514.

[141]MacGregor AJ, Ollier WER, Venkovsky J, Mageed RA, Carthy D, Silman AJ. Rheumatoid factor isotypes in monozygotic and dizygotic twins discordant for rheumatoid arthritis. *J Rheumatol.* 1995;22:2203–2207.

[142]Vischer TL. HLA-DR4 does not predispose to higher amounts of rheumatoid factor in healthy persons. *Ann Rheum Dis.* 1983;42: 702.

[143]Vaughan JH. Pathogenetic concepts and origins of rheumatoid factor in rheumatoid arthritis. *Arthritis Rheum.* 1993;36:1–6.

[144]Struthers GR, Scott DL, Delamere JP, Sheppeard H, Kitt M. Smoking and rheumatoid vasculitis. *Rheumatol Int.* 1981;1:145–146.

[145]Voskuyl AE, Zwinderman AH, Breedveld FC, Hazes JMW. Smoking and the risk of vasculitis in rheumatoid arthritis. *Br J Rheum.* 1997;36(suppl 1):164.

[146]Masi AT, Fecht T, Aldag JC, Malamet RL, Hazes JM. Smoking and rheumatoid arthritis: comment on the letter by McDonagh and Walker. *Arthritis Rheum.* 1998 Jan;41(1):184–185.

[147]Masi AT, Aldag JC, Fecht T, Teodorescu M, Sipe JD, Agopian MS, Lin H-C, Malamet RL: Rheumatoid factor positively (RF+) and current cigarette smoking (CCS+) of 30+ daily are independent long-term predictors of RA. *Arthritis Rheum.* 1997;40:S 312.

11

Drug, Alcohol, Diet-Induced and Saturnine Gout

Marina Rull and H. Ralph Schumacher, Jr.

Gout has a multifactorial origin with genetic and environmental contributions. To the genetic background are added well-known environmental factors which are implicated in the pathogenesis of gout and must always be considered for diagnosis and treatment. Environmental factors include diet, alcohol and drugs, as well as general environmental factors such as lead. All of them can affect formation and/or excretion of uric acid.

HISTORY

It is not only folklore that has linked gout to overindulgence in food and drink. Support of these associations is also found in a rich compilation of texts from Hippocrates to Sydenham and, of course, in the current literature. Physical inactivity, gluttony and especially reckless drinking are all believed to favor the appearance of gout. In *Poor Richard's Almanac* (1734) Benjamin Franklin provided the following advice: "Be temperate in wine, in eating, girls and sloth, or the gout will seize you and plague you both."[1-3]

Two thousand years ago, radial nerve palsy associated with abdominal cramps and constipation was described in the Roman literature. These manifestations and the mental deterioration of Claudius, Caligula, Nero and other Roman dignitares were related to chronic lead poisoning.[4] The term "saturnine gout" was introduced by Musgrave (1723) in his book on the relationship between chronic lead intoxication and gout. In 1859 Alfred Baring Garrod considered that lead intoxication from alcoholic drinks and paints accounted for one in four of his cases of gout. Lead contaminating alcohol in drinks caused an epidemic of lead intoxication in the eighteenth century. In the 1960s in the United States, saturnine gout was reported in consumers of homemade "moonshine" whisky which had been contaminated with lead.[5,6]

Therefore, the role of environmental factors has been known ever since gout, "the king of diseases" and "the disease of kings," has been described. More recently, this role has been firmly established for dietary factors, alcohol and drugs, opening doors to understanding the pathogenesis and improving the therapy of gout.

EPIDEMIOLOGY

Epidemiologic studies of gout and hyperuricemia have been widely performed and support the role of environmental factors. Caucasians, African-Americans, Hispanic, Asian, Indian and European populations have been studied.[7-9] Although epidemiologic studies of gout suffer from deficiencies or bias, the environment is unquestionably important in the pathogenesis of gout and hyperuricemia.[10] Studies of Filipinos are the best example of a dietary environmental influence in gout. Hyperuricemia and an increased frequency of gout were noted in Filipinos living in the continental United States and Hawaii compared to those living in the Philippines. It has been suggested that Filipinos have a genetic predisposition to hyperuricemia, with an increased frequency of underexcretion of uric acid that becomes manifest only if the environment is changed. A prominent environmental difference between Filipinos living in the Philippines and those living in the United States is the change to a Western diet with a higher purine content.[11,12]

An association between alcohol and gout has been observed for centuries. Lieber and coworkers found that the serum uric acid levels in a group of men admitted to the hospital in an intoxicated state were elevated and that these returned to a normal range once the consumption of alcohol was discontinued.[13] Gout patients have been noted to consume alcohol more frequently compared to patients with other rheumatic diseases. Beer has been noted to be a particular source of alcohol in many gout sufferers and contains guanosine, which is probably the most readily absorbed dietary purine.[14]

The incidence of gout has been changing in some populations with time. Although increased consumption of purines from diet, caloric intake and alcohol are important factors, drugs are currently the most common cause of hyperuricemia. Diuretics are the major trigger. A study from Finland has clearly confirmed the importance of diuretic-induced hyperuricemia in older patients,[15] and a survey of gout in general practice in the United Kingdom estimated that about 10% of cases could be attributed to thiazide diuretics.[16] In 1984 it was observed that recipients of cadaveric renal allografts receiving cyclosporine had higher serum uric acid levels than those receiving azathioprine and steroids. Subsequent reports have confirmed this observation.[17-20] For other drugs implicated with gout, only case reports and observations rather than epidemiological studies are available.

It has been estimated that saturnine gout accounts for less than 5% of all cases of gout.[21] Since the prevalence of gout in the United States is estimated to be 0.2 to 1.5%, saturnine gout is an uncommon but important consideration among individuals with gout. At highest risk are workers who manufacture storage batteries, persons who cut and weld lead panels, workers with lead-containing paints, lead metallurgists and potters. In the 1960s saturnine gout was reported in consumers of homemade "moonshine" whisky contaminated by lead in illicit stills.[5,6,22,23] The potential important role of urban pollution of the air, drinking water and vegetation with tetraethyl lead from gasoline and petrol has not yet been studied.[24] Although exposure to lead is important, the incidence of saturnine gout may be decreasing, as judged by the number of publications in this area.

GOUT AND THE METABOLISM AND EXCRETION OF URIC ACID

Gout is the consequence of deposition in joints and other connective tissue of monosodium urate (MSU) crystals. It is important to keep in mind that not all patients with hyperuricemia have gout, and not all patients with gout have hyperuricemia.[25] Different clinical manifestations or phases must be distinguished, including: 1) Asymptomatic hyperuricemia with an increased risk of gout; and 2) Gout represented by a heterogenous group of manifestations such as a) recurrent attacks of characteristic acute arthritis, in which MSU crystals are demonstrable in synovial fluid, b) tophi, which represent aggregated deposits of MSU in and around joints, c) renal disease involving glomerular, tubular and interstitial tissues and blood vessels, and d) uric acid nephrolithiasis. All the manifestations can occur in different combinations.[26]

Uric acid is the end product of the catabolism of purines. Any derangement in this process can lead to hyperuricemia and gout. Purines are derived exogenously from diet or endogenously from the turnover of nucleotide pools in tissues, or by *de novo* synthesis. The first step in purine synthesis is the conversion of 5-phosphoribosyl 1-pyrophosphate (PRPP) to 5-phosphoribosylamine. The availability of PRPP appears to be the main regulator of *de novo* purine biosynthesis, which leads to the formation of inosinic acid. Uric acid is formed from inosinic acid via oxidation to inosine, hypoxanthine and xanthine. The last two steps are mediated by the xanthine oxidase (see Figure 11-1).[27]

Since humans lack uricase, they excrete uric acid. Less than one third of uric acid is excreted through the gastrointestinal tract, where it is oxidized by bacterial uricase. The remainder of uric acid is eliminated by the kidney. All plasma uric acid is filtered at the glomerulus, and more than 95% of the filtered load undergoes proximal tubular reabsorption. Finally, urinary uric acid is derived from proximal tubular secretion.[28] Evidence for active tubular secretion is the paradoxical effect of salicylates and other uricosuric agents, which reduce urate excretion in low doses but enhance it when given in higher doses.[29] This can be explained by inhibition of secretion alone at low doses but inhibition of both secretion and absorption at higher doses. Although bidirectional tubular transport of uric acid is well established, details of its components remain to be clarified. The exact sites of this transport system within the nephron are unknown, and they may coexist throughout the proximal tubule.[30]

Environmental factors, including diet, alcohol, drugs and lead exposure, can produce hyperuricemia and gout by acting on various sites in the above pathways, resulting in increased production or decreased excretion of uric acid (see Table 12-1).

DIET AND ALCOHOL

With the advent of uricosuric drugs and allopurinol, less emphasis has been placed upon the role of diet and alcohol in the pathogenesis of gout and hyperuricemia. However, many studies have demonstrated an association between body weight, obesity and serum uric acid levels.[31-33] Patients with a history of gout are more often obese than healthy controls.[34,35]

Detailed studies of diet and alcohol have established their participation in the pathogenesis of gout. In gouty patients, absorption of dietary purines causes a steeper rise in serum uric acid levels than equivalent quantities in normouricemic individuals.[36,37] This reflects the relative impairment of renal uric acid clearance among the majority of patients with gout.[12] Substitution of an entirely purine-free diet over a period of days reduces the blood uric acid of healthy men from an average of 5.08 mg/dl to 3.05 mg/dl.[38]

Several studies have provided support to the observation of an association between overindulgence in alcohol and gout. Acute oral or intravenous administration of alcohol

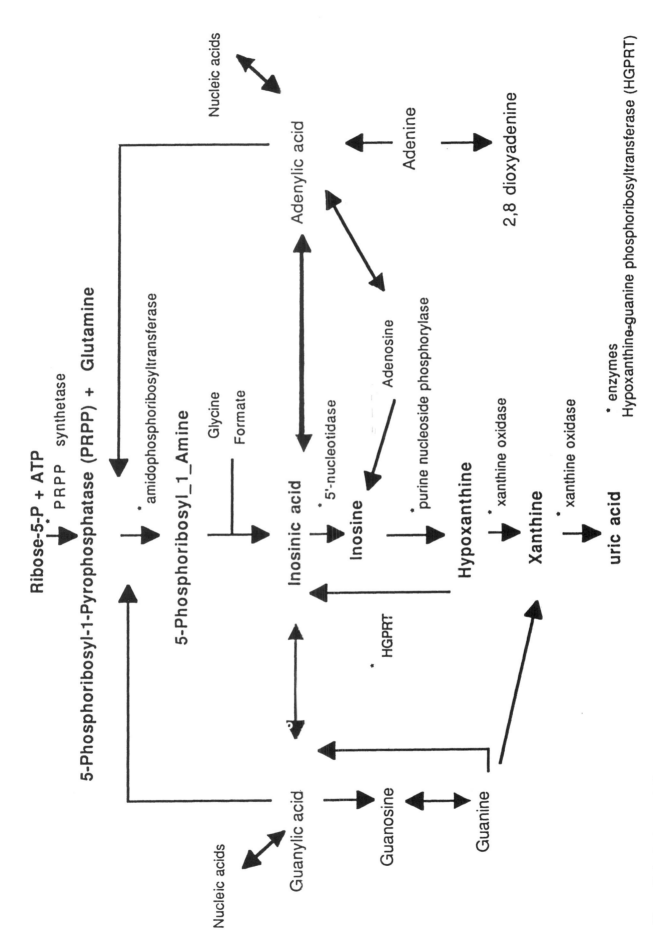

Figure 11-1 Purine metabolism.

Table 11-1 Classification of environmental factors associated with gout and hyperuricemia

---

A. Factors associated with increased production of uric acid
　Diet
　Cytotoxic agents
　Fructose
　Vitamin A
B. Factors associated with diminished excretion of uric acid
　Diuretics
　Cyclosporine
　Salicylates
　Pyrazinamide
　Ethambutol
C. Factors associated with both production and excretion
　Alcohol
　Nicotinic acid
　Lead
D. Unknown mechanism
　Omeprazole
　Gemfibrozil
　Erythropoietin
　Nitroglycerine

---

produces hyperuricemia associated with lactic acidemia and ketosis. Hyperuricemia results from suppression of the renal tubular secretion of uric acid.[39,40] In addition, Faller and Fox demonstrated that during long-term oral administration of alcohol, serum and urinary uric acid concentrations rise, as do urinary oxypurines and uric acid turnover.[41] Thus, alcohol increases uric acid synthesis by enhancing the turnover of adenosine nucleotides. The effect of beer on uric acid levels showed an increased excretion and clearance of uric acid in controls as well as individuals with gout despite an increase in serum lactate.[42] The former was attributed to the high purine content of the beer rather than a direct effect upon purine synthesis. Therefore, beer may be a greater risk factor for gout than other alcoholic beverages.

DRUGS ASSOCIATED WITH UNDEREXCRETION OF URIC ACID

Diuretics

Diuretics are among the most commonly prescribed medications for the elderly.[43] Prolonged use of benzthiazides and related compounds is associated with hyperuricemia and gout. The same is true for loop diuretics such as ethacrynic acid and furosemide, and the carbonic anhydrase inhibitor acetazolamide.[44]

Diuretics can cause hyperuricemia indirectly by volume depletion and directly by affecting renal tubular uric acid secretion and absorption. The role of volume depletion was demonstrated in a study utilizing parenterally administered furosemide and ethacrynic acid to normal subjects.[45] Following the intravenous administration of the diuretic, uric acid excretion initially increased, but during the second hour it decreased simultaneously with contraction of the extracellular fluid volume. If urinary loss was replaced with isotonic saline solution, excretion of uric acid remained normal. It was postulated that the stimulatory and suppressive effects of both diuretics on uric acid secretion could be mediated indirectly through altered renal blood flow and angiotensin release. It has also been demonstrated that volume depletion and prerenal azotemia due to a variety of conditions can cause severe hyperuricemia, and that serum uric acid levels return to normal levels following rehydration.[46] A direct effect of diuretics upon tubular transport has also been demonstrated. A paradoxical dosage effect can be observed, as low doses cause retention of uric acid, and high doses promote uricosuria by suppressing secretion and absorption as described with salicylates.[47,48]

When evaluating a patient with gout who is using a diuretic, it is important to search for the presence of other factors that might contribute to hyperuricemia. One of the most commonly associated factors is impaired glomerular filtration.[49] In addition, hypertension itself may predispose to hyperuricemia. It has been observed that 18% to 38% of untreated patients with hypertension had hyperuricemia, although the prevalence rises to 58% to 67% when hypertension is treated.[50,51] A family history of gout or the presence of other diseases, such as myeloproliferative and thyroid disorders, should be considered.

Although the classical presentation of gout occurs in an overweight middle-aged man with hypertension, hyperlipidemia and alcohol intake, one should be aware of the atypical findings in older women with Heberden's nodes who have been taking diuretics for years.[52] The incidence of gout in women is increasing. The typical presentation is acute podagra. In some patients, subacute polyarticular disease may be misdiagnosed as rheumatoid arthritis or osteoarthritis. Another common presentation in women is the development of tophi without prior acute attacks. The tophaceous deposits tend to localize on Heberden's nodes, sometimes drain spontaneously, and thus may be diagnosed as infections.[53–55]

Management of diuretic-induced gout should balance the severity of articular disease and the indication for treatment. Acute attacks can be treated, as in other cases, with nonsteroidal anti-inflammatory drugs (NSAIDs), colchine or prednisone, depending upon the clinical setting. If there is a need to control serum uric acid levels, this may be achieved with uricosuric agents or allopurinol. The most important step is to review the indications for diuretic treatment. Not all diuretics predispose to hyperuricemia. Organomercurials and the potassium-sparing diuretics triamterene,[56] amiloride and spironolactone are less likely to increase serum uric acid levels.[57,58] Phenoxyacetic acid compounds, tienilic acid and indacrinone, which are not available in the United States, are uricosuric.[59]

Cyclosporine

Cyclosporine, a neutral hydrophobic cyclic peptide composed of eleven amino acids, is widely used for immunosuppression after organ transplantation and as an alternative treatment for autoimmune disease. Its use is complicated by many side effects, including hyperuricemia. Cyclosporine-induced hyperuricemia and gout are a challenge for the clinician treating patients with organ transplants. Hyperuricemia occurs independently of overt nephrotoxicity in 30% to 84% of patients with renal transplants, and gouty arthritis develops in 7% to 28% of all cyclosporine-treated patients. Among heart transplant patients, hyperuricemia develops in 72% of males and 81% of females treated with cyclosporine, and 10% of men develop gout.[60,61]

Varying degrees of renal insufficiency and the use of diuretics contribute to cyclosporine-associated hyperuricemia in transplanted patients, but an independent effect of cyclosporine upon renal transport is very likely. Markers of renal tubular function other than uric acid have been shown to be generally normal during cyclosporine therapy, suggesting that hyperuricemia is not the result of nonspecific tubular dysfunction.[18,62] A specific cyclosporine-induced tubular defect has been suggested, with significant reduction of uric acid clearance in cyclosporine-treated renal transplant recipients compared with patients receiving azathioprine.[63] It has also been demonstrated that for a given level of serum creatinine, serum uric acid levels are higher in cyclosporine-treated patients than in those receiving azathioprine.[60] It has been postulated that intrarenal vasoconstriction and decreased glomerular ultrafiltration due to acute cyclosporine nephrotoxicity causes enhanced tubular reabsorption of uric acid, whereas the reduced renal mass associated with chronic cyclosporine nephrotoxicity eventually lead to a reduction in uric acid secretion.[17,64]

Cyclosporine accelerates the course of gout among transplanted patients. The onset of acute arthritis occurs after a mean of less than 1.5 years of asymptomatic hyperuricemia, with progression to polyarticular tophaceous gout in nearly half of the patients within less than three to five years after the first episode of gout.[65] Other factors leading to gout must also be considered. Patients taking cyclosporine who had episodes of gout were predominantly men, taking diuretics and with more advanced renal dysfunction than those who had hyperuricemia without gout.

Preexisting gout is not a contraindication to transplantation and should be treated aggressively in the pretransplant period. After transplantation, reversible renal insufficiency associated with NSAIDs is common; these drugs can be avoided. Some NSAIDs, such as diclofenac, may also increase cyclosporine levels.[66] Uricosuric agents are generally ineffective when the glomerular filtration rate is less than 50 ml per minute. Renal insufficiency increases the risk of bone marrow and neuromuscular toxicity from colchicine and hypersensitivity reactions to allopurinol. The combination of allopurinol and azathioprine may result in life-threatening leukopenia. Nevertheless, low doses of allopurinol may be added to azathioprine with a 50% to 75% reduction in the azathioprine dose or can be used with another immunosuppressive drug, such as thioguanine.[66]

Salicylates

Salicylates have contributed greatly to the knowledge of renal handling of uric acid because of their paradoxical effect on renal tubular function.[29] Other drugs, such as phenylbutazone and probenecid, have been shown to have the same property.[67] Yu and Gutman found that salicylates in low doses inhibit the renal tubular secretion of uric acid, whereas in higher doses they inhibit both secretion and reabsorption.[29] Because of the high dosage necessary to inhibit both tubular secretion and reabsorption, salicylates have not been accepted as useful uricosuric agents. However, greater than 4 grams of aspirin per day, as used to treat some patients with rheumatoid arthritis, can produce dramatic hypouricemia. The very small doses of aspirin given to patients with arterial disease to prevent thrombotic episodes have not been associated with reports of gout, although this has not been carefully evaluated. Another important effect of salicylates is to block probenecid.

Pyrazinamide and Ethambutol

The antituberculous drug pyrazinamide is a powerful uric-acid-retaining agent. The most common toxic effects of pyrazinamide are hepatotoxicity and polyarthralgia related to the elevation of serum uric acid concentrations.[68] Acute gout attacks are well documented among patients taking pyrazinamide.[69] Pyrazinamide acts by reducing renal uric acid clearance by over 80%.[70] It was thought that this effect resulted from suppression of tubular secretion, but it has been demonstrated that very large doses of pyrazinamide produce uricosuria in animals,[71] suggesting that pyrazinamide may also affect tubular reabsorption.

Another antituberculous drug capable of causing hyperuricemia and gout is ethambutol.[72–74] The renal effect of ethambutol is less pronounced and less constant than that of pyrazinamide.

DRUGS ASSOCIATED WITH AN INCREASED PRODUCTION OF URIC ACID

Cytotoxic Agents

Radiotherapy and cytotoxic drugs such as vincristine, busulphan, thiotepa, cytarabine, 6-mercaptopurine and chlorambucil, especially when used for hematologic malignancies, can cause severe hyperuricemia. This results in the excretion of massive amounts of uric acid, causing acute uric acid nephropathy and urinary obstruction due to deposition of uric acid crystals in the collecting ducts, pelvis and ureters. These drugs cause breakdown of nucleoproteins, resulting in increased production of uric acid. Fortunately, the renal toxicity can be prevented by allopurinol. Treatment with allopurinol should be commenced before cytotoxic therapy is started, to cover the period of maximum tissue breakdown.[75,76]

An experimental cytotoxic drug, 2-ethylamino-1,3,4-thia-diazole, produces an increase in serum uric acid levels and urinary uric acid excretion by increasing hepatic cell levels of PRPP and inducing activity of hepatic xanthine oxidase.[77]

Fructose

Phosphorylation of fructose is associated with ATP consumption and a reduction in total adenyl nucleotides through conversion of adenosine monophosphate (AMP) to IMP and further catabolic products. It may also act by stimulating *de novo* purine biosynthesis, probably by reducing hepatic adenosine diphosphate, which is thought to be an important inhibitor of PRPP synthesis.[78] Intravenous infusion of fructose leads to increases in serum and urinary concentrations of uric acid within the first half-hour. However, chronic ingestion of fructose does not significantly affect serum uric acid levels.

DRUGS ASSOCIATED WITH UNDEREXCRETION AND OVERPRODUCTION OF URIC ACID

Nicotinic Acid

Nicotinic acid is used for treating schizophrenia and hypercholesterolemia. Its toxic effects include hyperuricemia and occasionally gout.[79] Two mechanisms have been implicated: impaired excretion of uric acid with a 75% decrease in clearance following the administration of nicotinic acid in a daily dose of 4.5 g,[80] and stimulation of *de novo* purine synthesis. The latter mechanism has been demonstrated in animals and is due to increased production of ribose phosphate. Nicotinic acid is converted to its ribonucleotide by a reaction which consumes PRPP, and it is possible that there is both increased formation and consumption of the compound.[81,82]

OTHER DRUGS

From time to time, reports of drugs causing hyperuricemia and gout are published. It is important to be aware of these associations, although most have not been studied systematically.

Nitroglycerine has been reported to cause hyperuricemia and acute gout during intravenous therapy for unstable angina. It was speculated that the alcohol content in intravenous nitroglycerine preparations may alter serum uric acid levels and precipitate acute gouty flares in patients who are at increased risk for gout.[83] One case of vasculitis and acute gout attributed to erythropoietin has been reported.[84] Fibric acid derivatives, such as fenofibrate, clofibrate and halofenate, have been reported to be uricosuric. Gemfibrozil has not been studied, but one report described acute gout involving the acromioclavicular joint following treatment.[85] Two cases of acute gout during therapy with omeprazole have been reported.[86] A number of cases of hyperuricemia and two cases of podagra have been reported following the use of isotretinoin (13-cis-retinoic acid), a synthetic derivative of vitamin A, for severe acne.[87]

SATURNINE GOUT

Kidney disease and hypertension are among the most common consequences of lead intoxication, particularly as a result of chronic low-level exposure. The causative role of lead is clearly proven in saturnine gout.

Lead has been used by humans for 8000 years. Poisoning from occupational exposure was believed to have been eliminated by the introduction of modern occupational safety standards. Nevertheless, our civilization remains heavily polluted with lead. Industrial lead exposure remains a significant problem. Weeden and colleagues,[88] in 1975, reported detailed studies of renal function in eight lead workers, six of whom were asymptomatic and four of whom had renal disease. This study was extended to a larger population with similar results.[89] A common source of urban pollution is tetraethyl lead, which is found in gasoline and petrol. This causes pollution not only of the air but also of drinking water and vegetation.[90]

Lead Physiology and Toxicity

Lead, which has no known biological use, is classified as an aphysiological toxic trace element. The daily intake of lead derived from food and drinking water is between 100 to 500 μg, although only 10% is absorbed. One to 120 μg of lead is inhaled daily and 40% is absorbed. The average daily lead absorption has been estimated as 35 μg. According to World Health Organization standards, 45 μg of lead is the maximum allowable daily intake.[91]

Lead is primarily bound to red blood cells and is mainly excreted by glomerular filtration, with smaller amounts across the gastrointestinal tract and in sweat. The excreted amount of lead is less than the ingested amount, resulting in accumulation of 5 to 7 μg of lead per day. As a result, the lead content of the body gradually increases, and 20 to 500 μg can accumulate during the life of an individual.[92] The largest amount of absorbed lead accumulates in the bones and is tightly bound to hydroxyapatite. Lead in bone is excreted slowly over years. Lead also accumulates in nails, hair, aorta and, less often, in the liver, kidneys, spleen and lungs.

The toxicity of lead is due to its interaction with sulphydryl groups of different enzymes and cell membrane proteins. It can block, in a dose dependent manner, the activities of these enzymes and special transport processes of membranes.

Lead Toxicity and Saturnine Gout

It was initially suggested that lead accelerated nucleoprotein turnover. Recent studies have confirmed that lead primarily inhibits tubular urate excretion.[93] The fact that saturnine gout is frequently associated with renal failure supports a renal mechanism.[94,95] Complexes of lead and urate have been observed in the serum of patients with saturnine gout. It was suggested that this complex promoted urate nucleation and crystallization.[96] Electron microscopy and electron probe elemental analysis to search for lead in crystals from synovial fluids of patients with saturnine gout was negative (Schumacher *et al.*, unpublished observations).

Clinical Presentation

As in other forms of gout, factors such as heredity, obesity, alcohol and hypertension may be involved.[97] Saturnine gout is usually preceded by other symptoms of lead toxicity such as colic, constipation, nerve palsies, anemia due to disturbance in porphyrin synthesis and renal damage. Gout is usually the result of renal involvement but might develop without evidence of renal failure.[98] One of the clues in differentiating primary from saturnine gout is that renal failure occurs late in the first but frequently precedes the onset of articular manifestations in the second. Polyarticular acute saturnine gout with recurrent attacks is not uncommon and tends to affect the knees. Acute gouty attacks become less severe as the chronic tophaceous stage is reached. The serum uric acid concentrations are usually higher in saturnine gout than in primary gout, but urinary uric acid excretion is significantly lower, and renal calculi are rare in saturnine gout.[99,100]

Diagnosis

The diagnosis of saturnine gout should rest on the verification of the presence of gout, confirmation of lead exposure prior to the onset of gout and exclusion of other causes. In acute gouty arthritis due to lead intoxication, MSU crystals are also found.[101] The following parameters should be measured to confirm excess exposure to lead:[102]

1) δ-aminolaevulinic acid dehydratase concentration in blood normally lower than 80U/ml. This is the earliest biochemical abnormality indicating lead toxicity. The levels of this enzyme and of lead in serum and urine promptly return to normal when exposure to lead ceases.

2) Lead concentration in blood in excess of 80 μg/100 ml and baseline urinary excretion in excess of 80 μg/24 hours.

3) Urinary δ-aminolaevulinic acid concentration higher than 600 μg/100 ml. This persists for a longer period after exposure to lead.

4) Prior lead exposure, occurring some years earlier, can only be confirmed by calcium disodium edetate or X-ray fluorescence analysis. Lead excretion is in excess of 650 μg/24 hours following parenteral administration of one gram of calcium disodium edetate.

Treatment

Treatment of saturnine gout consists of elimination of lead from the body and therapy specifically for gout. Gout should be treated as primary gout; however, renal failure is frequent, requiring a reduction in the doses of allopurinol or colchicine because of their prolonged half-lives with renal impairment. Serious toxic effects of allopurinol, including fever, skin rash, progressive renal failure, eosinophilia and hepatitis, occur more often in patients with renal failure.

Removal of lead from the body can be achieved by calcium disodium edetate, which acts by forming highly stable chelates with lead which are excreted by the kidneys.[103] Dimercaprol, another chelating agent, and D-penicillamine are also effective. Calcium disodium edetate must be administered parenterally. One gram in 200 ml to 500 ml of 5% glucose solution is given slowly by intravenous infusion over a period of an hour during two courses daily for three to five days and repeated after two and 14 days. Alternatively, it can be administered intramuscularly, giving one gram one to three times a week over a period of six to 50 months. Complications of calcium disodium edetate treatment include renal toxicity, histamine-like reaction, anemia, glycosuria, prolongation of the prothrombin time, dermatitis and transient mild hypotension. Dimercaprol is administered intramuscularly in a dose of 4 mg/kg every four hours for 48 hours, then every six hours for 48 hours and finally every six to 12 hours for an additional week. The combination of calcium disodium edetate and dimercaprol is more effective than either alone. D-penicillamine is administered orally in a dose of 250 mg four times a day for five days. With chronic administration the dose should not exceed 40 mg/kg per day.[22,104] There is no evidence that removal of lead improves gout, but this has not been systematically evaluated.

REFERENCES

[1]Talbott JH. History. In: Talbott JH, Yu TF. *Gout and Uric Acid Metabolism.* New York: Stratton Intercontinental Medical Book Corp, 1976;1–25.

[2]Rodnan GP. Invitation to gout. A consideration of the role of various predisposing and provocative factors in the genesis of acute gout arthritis. *Transactions and Studies of the College of Physicians of Philadelphia.* 1967;35:47–62.

[3]Appelboom T, Bennett JC. Gout of the rich and famous. *J Rheumatol.* 1986;13:618–622.

[4]Nriagu JO. Saturnine gout among Roman aristocrats: Did lead poisoning contribute to the fall of the empire? *N Engl J Med.* 1983;308:660–663.

[5]Emmerson BT. The clinical differentiation of lead gout from primary gout. *Arthritis Rheum.* 1968;11:623–634.

[6]Reynolds PP, Knapp MJ, Baraf HS, Holmes EW. Moonshine and lead: Relationship to the pathogenesis of hyperuricemia in gout. *Arthritis Rheum.* 1983;26:1057–1064.

[7]Hochberg MC, Thomas J, Thomas DJ, Mead L, Levine DM, Klag MJ. Racial differences in the incidence of gout. The role of hypertension. *Arthritis Rheum.* 1995;38:628–632.

[8]Zalokar J, Lellouch J, Claude JR, Kuntz D. Epidemiology of serum uric acid and gout in Frenchmen. *J Chronic Dis.* 1974;27:59–75.

[9]Talbott JH. It happened on the way to the XIII international congress on rheumatology in Kyoto and after I had arrived. *Arthritis Rheum.* 1975;18:699–707.

[10]Acheson RM. Epidemiology of serum uric acid and gout: An example of the complexities of multifactorial causation. *Proc Roy Soc Med.* 1970;63:193–197.

[11]Healey LA. Epidemiology of hyperuricemia. *Arthritis Rheum.* 1975;18:709–712.

[12]Healey LA, Skeith MD, Decker JL, Bayani-Sioson P. Hyperuricemia in Filipinos: Interaction of heredity and environment. *Am J Hum Genet.* 1967;19:81–85.

[13]Lieber CS, Jones DP, Lasowsky MS, Davidson CS. Interrelation of uric acid and ethanol metabolism in man. *J Clin Invest.* 1962;41:1380.

[14]Eastmond CJ, Garton M, Robins S, Riddoch S. The effects of alcoholic beverages on urate metabolism in gout sufferers. *Br J Rheum* 1995;34:756–759.

[15]Takala J, Attila S, Gref CG, Isomaki H. Diuretics and hyperuricemia in the elderly. *Scand J Rheumatol.* 1988;17:155–160.

[16]Currie WJ. Prevalence and incidence of the diagnosis of gout in Great Britain. *Ann Rheum Dis.* 1979;38:101–106.

[17]Palestine AG, Nussenblatt RB, Chan CC. Side effects of systemic cyclosporine in patients not undergoing transplantation. *Am J Med.* 1984;77:652–656.

[18]Calne RY, Wood AJ. Cyclosporine in cadaveric renal transplantation: Three-year follow up of a European multicenter trial. *Lancet.* 1985;2:549–555.

[19]Lin HY, Rocher LL, McQuillan M, Schmaltz S, Palella TD, Fox IH. Cyclosporine-induced hyperuricemia and gout. *N Eng J Med.* 1989;321:287–292.

[20]West C, Carpenter BJ, Hakala TR. The incidence of gout in renal transplant recipients. *Am J Kidney Dis.* 1987;10:369–372.

[21]Hallal JT, Ball GV. Saturnine gout: A review of 42 patients. *Semin Arthritis Rheum.* 1982;11:307–314.

[22]Peitzman SJ, Bodison W, Ellis I. Moonshine drinking among hypertensive veterans in Philadelphia. *Arch Intern Med.* 1985;145:632–634.

[23]Wright LF, Saylor RP, Cecere FA. Occult lead intoxication with gout and kidney disease. *J Rheumatol.* 1984;11:517–520.

[24]Poor G, Mituszova M. Saturnine gout. *Baillieres Clin Rheumatol.* 1989;3:51–61.

[25]McCarty D. Gout without hyperuricemia. *JAMA.* 1994;271:302–303.

[26]Kelley WN, Schumacher HR. Crystal-associated synovitis. In: Kelley WN, Harris E, *et al.* eds. *Textbook of Rheumatology.* Philadelphia: W.B. Saunders Company, 1993;1291–1336.

[27]Terkeltaub R. Epidemiology, pathology, and pathogenesis. In: Schumacher HR, ed. *Primer on the Rheumatic Diseases.* Atlanta: Arthritis Foundation, 1993;209–212.

[28]Steele TH. Control of uric acid excretion. *N Engl J Med.* 1969;284:1193–1196.

[29]Yu TF, Gutman AB. Study of the paradoxical effect of salicylate in low, intermediate and high dosage on the renal mechanism for excretion of urate in man. *J Clin Invest.* 1959;38:1298.

[30]Weiner JM. Urate transport in the nephron. *Am J Physiology.* 1979;237:85–92.

[31]Krizek V. Serum uric acid in relation to body weight. *Ann Rheum Dis.* 1966;25:456–458.

[32]Acheson RM, Chan YK. New Haven survey of joint diseases. The prediction of serum uric acid in a general population. *J Chronic Dis.* 1969;21:543–553.

[33]Gibson T, Rodgers AV, Simmonds HA, Cant-Brown F, Todd E, Heilton V. A controlled study of diet in patients with gout. *Ann Rheum Dis.* 1983;42:123–127.

[34]Grahame R, Scott JT. Clinical survey of 354 patient with gout. *Ann Rheum Dis.* 1970;29:461–468.

[35]Gibson T, Grahame R. Gout and hyperlipidaemia. *Ann Rheum Dis.* 1974;33:298–303.

[36]Zollner N, Griebsch A. Diet and gout. *Adv Exp Med Biol.* 1974;41B:435–442.

[37]Clifford AJ, Riumallo JA, Young VR, Scrimshaw NS. Effect of oral purines on serum and urinary uric acid of normal, hyperuricaemic and gouty humans. *J Nutr.* 1976;106:428–450.

[38]Griebsch A, Zoller N. Effect of ribomononucleotides given orally on uric acid production in man. *Adv Exp Med Biol.* 1974;41B;435–442.

[39]Yu TSF, Sirota JH, Berger L, *et al.* Effect of sodium lactate infusion on urate clearance in man. *Proc Soc Exp Biol Med.* 1957;96:809–813.

[40]MacLachlan MJ, Rodnan GP. Effects of food, fast and alcohol on serum uric acid and acute attacks of gout. *Am J Med.* 1967;2:38–57.

[41]Faller J, Fox IH. Ethanol-induced hyperuricemia. Evidence for increased urate production by activation of adenine nucleotide turnover. *N Engl J Med.* 1982;307:27–30.

[42]Gibson T, Rodger AV, Simmonds HA, Toseland P. Beer drinking and its effect on uric acid. *Br J Rheumatol.* 1984;23:203–209.

[43]Williamson J, Chopin JM. Adverse reactions to prescribed drugs for the elderly: A multicenter investigation. *Age and Ageing.* 1980;9:73–80.

[44]Scott JT. Drug-induced gout. *Baillieres Clin Rheumatol.* 1991; 5:39–60.

[45]Steel TH, Oppenheimer S. Factors affecting urate excretion following diuretic administration in man. *Am J Med.* 1969;47:564–574.

[46]Feinstein EI, Quion-Verde H, Kaptein EM, Massry SG. Severe hyperuricemia in patients with volume depletion. *Am J Nephrol.* 1984;4:77–80.

[47]Demartini FE. Hyperuricemia induced by drugs. *Arthritis Rheum.* 1965;8:823–829.

[48]Bryant JH, Yu TF, Berger L, *et al.* Hyperuricemia induced by the administration of chlorthalidone and other sulphonamide diuretics. *Am J Med.* 1962;33:408–420.

[49]Scott JT, Higgens CS. Diuretic-induced gout: A multifactorial condition. *Ann Rheum Dis.* 1992;51:259–261.

[50]Breckenridge A. Hyperuricemia and hypertension. *Lancet.* 1966; 1;15–18.

[51]Cannon PJ, Stason WB, Demartini Fe, *et al.* Hyperuricemia in primary and renal hypertension. *N Engl J Med.* 1966;275:457–464.

[52]Macfarlane DG, Dieppe PA. Diuretic-induced gout in elderly women. *Br J Rheumatol.* 1985;24:155–157.

[53]Wordsworth BP, Mowat AG. Rapid development of gouty tophi after diuretic therapy. *J Rheumatol.* 1985;12:376–377.

[54]Simkin PA, Campbell PM, Larson EB. Gout in Heberden's nodes. *Arthritis Rheum.* 1983;26:94–97.

[55]Macfarlane D, Dieppe P. Changing pattern of hospital gout. *Ann Rheum Dis.* 1983;42:219.

[56]Walker Br, Hoppe RC, Alexander F. Effect of triamterine on the renal clearance of calcium, phosphate and uric acid in man. *Clin Pharmacol Ther.* 1972;13:245–250.

[57]Paterson JW, Dollery CT, Haslam RM. Amiloride hydrochloride in hypertensive patients. *BMJ.* 1968;1:422–423.

[58]Schersten B, Thulin T, Kuylenstierna J, *et al.* Clinical and biochemical effects of spironolactone administered once daily in primary hypertension. *Hypertension.* 1980;2:672–679.

[59]Reardon JA, Scott JT. Controlled in-patient study of tielinic acid in treatment of gout and hypertension. *Ann Rheum Dis.* 1980;39:367–372.

[60]Lin H, Rocher LL, McOuillan MA, Schmaltz S, Palella T, Fox I. Cyclosporine-induced hyperuricemia and gout. *N Engl J Med.* 1989;321:287–292.

[61]Burack DA, Griffith BP, Thompson ME, Kahl LE. Hyperuricemia and gout among heart transplant recipients receiving cyclosporine. *Am J Med.* 1992;92:141–146.

[62]Palestine AG, Austin HA, Nussenblatt RB. Renal tubular function in cyclosporine-treated patients. *Am J Med.* 1986;81:419–424.

[63]Noordzji TC, Leunissen KML, Van Hoof JP. Cyclosporine-induced hyperuricemia in gout. *N Engl J Med.* 1990;322:335.

[64]Chapman JR, Harding NGL, Griffiths D, Morris PJ. Reversibility of cyclosporine nephrotoxicity after three months treatment. *Lancet.* 1985;1:128–130.

[65]Baethge BA, Work J, Landreneau MD, McDonald JC. Tophaceous gout in patients with renal transplants treated with cyclosporine A. *J Rheumatol.* 1993;20:718–720.

[66]George T, Mandell BF. Gout in the transplant patient. *J Clin Rheumatol.* 1995;1:328–334.

[67]Yu TF, Gutman AB. Paradoxical retention of uric acid by uricosuric drugs in low dosage. *Proc Soc Exp Biol Med.* 1955;90:542–547.

[68]Girling DJ. Adverse effects of antituberculosis drugs. *Drugs.* 1982;23:56–74.

[69]Amodio MI, Bengualid V, Lowy FD. Development of acute gout secondary to pyrazinamide in a patient without a prior history of gout. *Ann Pharmacother.* 1990;24:115–116.

[70]Gutman AB, Yu TF, Berger L. Renal function in gout. III. Estimation of tubular secretion and reabsorbtion of uric acid by use of pyrazinamide (pyrazinoic acid). *Am J Med.* 1969;47:575–592.

[71]Weiner AM, Tinker JP. Pharmacology of pyrazinamide: Metabolic and renal function studies related to the mechanism of drug-induced urate retention. *J Pharmacol Exp Ther.* 1972;180:411–434.

[72]Self TH, Fountain FF, Taylor WJ, Stucclif WD. Acute gouty arthritis associated with the use of ethambutol. *Chest.* 1977;71:561–562.

[73]Postlethwaite AE, Bartel AG, Kelley WN. Hyperuricemia induced by ethambutol. *Adv Exp Med Biol.* 1974;41B:763–767.

[74]Khanna BK. Acute gouty arthritis following ethambutol therapy. *Br J Dis Chest.* 1980;74:409–410.

[75]Kjesllstrand CM, Campbell Dc, Von Hartiztch B, Buselmier J. Hyperuricemic acute renal failure. *Arch Intern Med.* 1974;133:349–359.

[76]Watts RWE, Watkins PJ, Matthias JQ, Gibbs DA. Allopurinol and acute uric acid nephropathy. *Br Med J.* 1966;1:205–208.

[77]Lalanne M, Henderson JF. Effects of hormones and drugs on phosphoribosylpyrophosphate concentrations in mouse liver. *Biochem Cell Biol.* 1975;53:394–399.

[78]Kelley WN, Fox IH, Wyngaarden JB. Essential role of phosphoribosylpyrophosphate (PRPP) in regulation of purine biosynthesis in cultural human fibroblasts. *Clin Res.* 1970;18:457 (abstract).

[79]Parsons WB. Studies of nicotinic acid: Use in hypercholesterolemia. *Arch Int Med.* 1961;107:653–667.

[80]Gau ZN, Pocelinko R, Solomon HM, Thomas GB. Oral glucose tolerance, plasma insulin and uric acid excretion in man during chronic administration of nicotinic acid. *Metab Clin Exp.* 1971;20:1031–1035.

[81]Becker MA, Raivio KO, Meyer LJ, Seegmiller JE. Effects of nicotinic acid on human purine metabolism. *Clin Res.* 1973;21:616–621.

[82]Shuster L, Abraham G. The effect of nicotinamide on incorporation in vivo of formate-C17. *J Biol Chem.* 1959;234:129–133.

[83]Shergy WJ, Gilkenson GS, German DC. Acute gouty arthritis and intravenous nitroglycerine. *Arch Intern Med.* 1988;148:2505–2507.

[84]Buchbinder A, Adler H, Ballard H. An unusual and unreported toxicity to erythropoietin. *Am J Hematol.* 1993;42:412–413.

[85]Miller-Blair D, White R, Greenspan A. Acute gout involving the acromioclavicular joint following treatment with gemfibrozil. *J Rheumatol.* 1992;19:166–168.

[86]Kraus A, Flores LF. Acute gout associated with omeprazole. *Lancet.* 1995;345:461–462.

[87]Mawson AR, Onor GI. Gout and vitamin A intoxication: Is there a connection? *Sem Arthritis Rheum.* 1991;20:297–304.

[88]Weeden RP, Maesaka JK, Weiner B, Lipat GA, Lyons MM, Vitale LF, Joselow MM. Occupational lead nephropathy. *Am J Med.* 1975;59:630–641.

[89]Weeden RP, Mallik DK, Batuman V. Detection and treatment of occupational lead nephropathy. *Arch Intern Med.* 1979;139:53–57.

[90]Nolan CV, Shaikh ZA. Lead nephrotoxicity and associated disorders: Biochemical mechanisms. *Toxicology.* 1992;73:127–146.

[91]Schroeder HA, Bratleboro VT, Tipton IH. The human body burden of lead. *Arch Env Health.* 1968;17:965–978.

[92]Rabinowitz MB, Wetherill GW, Kopple JD. Kinetic analysis of lead metabolism in healthy humans. *J Clin Invest.* 1976:58:260–270.

[93]Ball GV, Sorensen LB. Pathogenesis of hyperuricemia in saturnine gout. *N Engl J Med.* 1968;280:1199–2002.

[94]Batuman V, Maesaka JK, Haddad B, Tepper E, Landy E, Wedeen RR. The role of lead in gout nephropathy. *N Engl J Med.* 1981;304:520–523.

[95]Wright LF, Saylor RP, Cecere FA. Occult lead intoxication with gout and kidney disease. *J Rheumatol.* 1984;11:517–520.

[96]Tak HK, Wilcox WR, Cooper SM. The effect of lead upon urate nucleation. *Arthritis Rheum.* 1981;24:1291–1295.

[97]Reynolds PP, Knapp M, Baraf HS, *et al.* Moonshine and lead. Relationship to the pathogenesis of hyperuricemia in gout. *Arthritis Rheum.* 1983;26:1057–1064.

[98]Campbell BC, Moore MR, Goldberg A. Subclinical lead exposure: A possible cause of gout. *BMJ.* 1978;18:1403.

[99]Yu TF. Lead nephropathy and gout. *Am J Kidney Dis.* 1983;2:555–559.

[100]Craswell PW, Price J, Boyle PD, Heazlewood VJ, Baddeley H, Lloyd MM, Thomas BJ. Chronic renal failure with gout: A marker of chronic lead poisoning. *Kidney Internat.* 1984;26:319–323.

[101]Malawista SE, Gordon W, Atkins E, Cheung HS, McCarty DJ. Crystal-induced endogenous pyrogen production, a further look at gout inflammation. *Arthritis Rheum.* 1985;28:1039–1046.

[102]Morgan JM, Burch HB. Comparative tests for diagnosis of lead poisoning. *Arch Intern Med.* 1972;130:335–340.

[103]Chisholm JJ. Treatment of acute lead intoxication—choice of chelating agents and supportive therapeutic measures. *Clin Toxicol.* 1970;3:527–540.

[104]Batuman V. Lead nephropathy, gout and hypertension. *Am J Med Sci.* 1993;305:241–246.

12

Hazards Associated with Biologic Therapies

John J. Cush

INTRODUCTION

In the past two decades, there has been an increasing effort therapeutically to manipulate aberrant immune responses associated with neoplastic or autoimmune disorders. Biopharmaceuticals have entered the clinical arena during an era of escalating knowledge of disease pathogenesis, advances in biotechnology (especially monoclonal antibody and peptide engineering) and the success realized in animal models of human disease. "Biologic" agents are a diverse group of naturally occurring compounds that are primarily manufactured by a burgeoning biotechnology industry and include recombinant vaccines (for example, hepatitis B vaccine) and blood products (for example, erythropoietin), cytokines, growth factors, thrombolytics (for example, recombinant TPA), monoclonal antibodies and gene therapies, to name a few.[1–3] Many of these new biologic therapies have the capacity to target specific immune responses and other effector mechanisms thought to be crucial to the pathogenesis of these disorders. Nonetheless, the development of biotherapeutics has not been without hazard. The value of any novel biologic therapy must be weighed against its clinical toxicity and potential immunotoxicity. This chapter intends to present the manifest and potential hazards associated with several biopharmaceutical agents utilized in the treatment of rheumatic, autoimmune and neoplastic disorders.

MONOCLONAL ANTIBODIES

Monoclonal antibody technology has been utilized specifically to target relevant antigens.[2,3] Typically, monoclonal antibodies (mAb) have been used to target cell-subset-specific antigens (for example, tumor cells, CD4+ T cells, CD19+ B cells), adhesion molecules and circulating and bound cytokines or their receptors. The effects of mAb therapy are dependant upon the characteristics of the targeted antigen (for example, cell surface density or tissue distribution) and of the mAb (for example, fine specificity, avidity, heavy chain isotype). Mechanisms by which therapeutic mAb exert their effects have not been elucidated and may vary depending on the mAb used.[2] Such mechanisms may also be responsible for some of the toxicities associated with mAb therapy. These biologic effects may include: 1) blocking the function of the target antigen; 2) modulation of cellular function; 3) opsonization and removal of immunoreactive cells by the reticuloendothelial system; 4) induction of complement-mediated cytotoxicity; or 5) direct cytotoxicity by delivery of bound toxin (for example, ricin A-chain) to the cytosol (see below). A variety of mAb preparations have been tested therapeutically and include murine, chimeric and humanized mAb.

Murine mAb

Although there has been a great deal of experience with murine mAb, they have limited applicability because of their short serum half-life, uniform immunogenicity (manifest as human antimouse antibodies [HAMA]) and potential interference by HAMA or anti-idiotypic antibodies. For instance, the murine mAb OKT3, an anti-CD3 mAb, has been extensively used in the treatment of transplant rejection.[4,5]

Chimeric and Humanized mAb

The immunogenicity and other problems posed by the use of murine mAb have resulted in the development of less immunogenic chimeric and humanized mAb. Chimeric mAb have been created by combining murine mAb variable regions (Fab portion) with the constant region of a human antibody.[2] Chimeric antibodies are thus less immunogenic. A more refined construct utilizes only the hypervariable or complementary determining regions (CDR) from the murine mAb. This "humanized" or "CDR engrafted" mAb is even less immunogenic than the chimeric mAb. Nonetheless, the host is still capable of making anti-idiotypic antibodies to these mAb.

Toxicities Associated with mAb Therapy

A variety of mAb have been utilized as immunomodulatory agents in the treatment of infectious, autoimmune and neoplastic conditions. Minor adverse reactions, recognizable clinical syndromes and major toxicities have been reported and are a consequence of either the host's immune response to the mAb (or immunoconjugate) or the natural sequelae of antibody-mediated cellular activation and cytokine release (Table 12-1). Minor adverse reactions associated with mAb therapies include fever, rash, malaise, nausea and other constitutional manifestations. Often patients complain of a "flu-like" syndrome following the administration of mAb.[1,2]

The use of OKT3 in treating allograft rejection is often limited by associated toxicities.[4,5] The administration of this anti-CD3 mAb may result in the "cytokine release syndrome" (Table 12-1) characterized by flulike symptoms, including fever, chills, headache, malaise, myalgia and nausea. In these instances, it has been suggested that mAb-mediated activation of T cells leads to the systemic release of cytokines, especially tumor necrosis factor alpha (TNFα), interferon gamma (IFNγ), interleukin 6 (IL-6) and possibly IL-2.[1,6] For most, symptoms are seldom serious, usually self-limited, and can be prevented by using analgesics or corticosteroids. The cytokine release syndrome is not unique to anti-CD3 mAb and has been reported with other mAb (anti-CD4, -CD7 and -CD52, and an anti-CD5 immunotoxin) therapies.[2] This syndrome may relate to the particular mAb utilized and may not occur with all mAb preparations.[7]

A less common but more ominous occurrence is the "capillary leak syndrome" (Table 12-1) characterized by hypoalbumineria, weight gain, edema, and, less commonly, hypotension, wheezing, congestive heart failure or pulmonary edema.[8–11] The capillary leak syndrome has been observed with numerous mAb, immunotoxins and cytokine therapies (Table 12-2).

Table 12-1 Common events associated with monoclonal antibody therapy*

Cytokine Release Syndrome	Capillary Leak Syndrome
Flulike symptoms	Hypoalbuminemia
Fever	Edema
Chills	Weight gain
Headache	Wheezing
Nausea/vomiting	Hypotension
Fatigue/malaise	Congestive heart failure
Myalgia	Pulmonary edema

*modified from Cush, Kavanaugh.[2]

Table 12-2 Toxicities associated with biologic therapies*

Symptom/Sign	Causative Biologic Agent
Cytokine release syndrome	αCD3, αCD4, αCD7, αCD52, αCD5IT
Capillary leak syndrome	IL-1, IL-2, IL-3, IL-4, GM-CSF, ricin, αCD3, αCD5IT, αCD22IT, αCD19IT, αCD25IT
Flulike syndrome	IFN-γ, IFN-α, IFN-β, αCD5IT, αCD52, αCD4
Fever, chills	IL-1, IL-2, IL-3, IL-6, rTNF, GM-CSF, IFN-γ, IFN-β, IFN-α, αCD4, αCD5IT, αCD7, αCD52, αCD25IT
Leukopenia	IL-2, rTNF, IFN-γ, IFN-β, IFN-α, αCD4, αCD52
Thrombocytopenia	IL-2, IL-3, rTNF, M-CSF, IFN-α, αCD19IT, αCD30IT
Hepatic dysfunction	IL-2, IL-4, IFN-γ, IFN-α, ricin, diptheria toxin, αCD19IT
Proteinuria/renal dysfunction	IL-2, IL-4, IFN-γ
Mental status changes	IL-1, IL-2, IL-4, IFN-γ, IFN-α
Neuropathy	IT, IFN-α, IFN-β
Thyroid disease	IFN-β, IFN-α, IL-2
Injection site reactions	IL-1ra, IL-3, IFN-γ, IFN-β, IFN-α, G-CSF
Cardiac dysfunction**	IFN-γ, IL-2, rTNF
Pulmonary congestion	IL-2, IL-4, αCD5IT, αCD52
Opportunistic infections	αCD4? αCD52? IL-1ra? αTNF?

*modified from Thomas[1] and Vial, Descotes.[22]
α = mAb directed against.
IT = immunotoxin.
**frequently results in those with preexisting ischemic heart disease.
? There is no reliable statistically sound data to judge whether these agents render the patient at risk for opportunistic infection. Their inclusion here is based on single case reports or conjecture.

Immunologic Sequelae to mAb Therapy

Biologic therapies are administered with the hope of favorably influencing immune responses. However, past experience has revealed potential detrimental immunological and clinical sequelae. The immunological sequelae result from the direct effect of mAb administration, the immune response to administered mAb or the indirect effects associated with mAb therapy.

Antibodies, peptides, growth factors and toxins are all capable of inducing an immunogenic response. Such responses vary widely depending on the preparation, but are likely to increase with repeated or continued use. A majority of patients treated with murine or chimeric mAb will develop HAMA or human anti-chimeric antibodies (HACA). Titers of HAMA and HACA appear to rise and tend to be dramatically higher with repeated courses of therapy.[12–15] Nevertheless, clinical manifestations or allergic reactions related to their presence are quite infrequent. It does however, appear that the development of HAMA or HACA may interfere with circulating levels, tissue penetration and the pharmacokinetics of the administered biopharmaceutical. Thus it may be more difficult to achieve therapeutic circulating or tissue levels of mAb with repeated or chronic mAb administration. Moreover, the concomitant use of other pharmacologic immunosuppressives (for example, azathioprine, methotrexate) does not appear to abrogate these immunologic responses.[1] In most mAb trials, an increased risk of toxicity or severity of toxicity has not been observed with repeated use of mAb.[1,12,16] Furthermore, some trials have demonstrated that the development that the development of HAMA may be associated with less toxicity and, possibly, greater efficacy.[6] The development of anti-idiotypic antibodies may also confound the therapeutic effect by blocking the binding of the original mAb. Such "blocking antibodies" may, in some instances, serve to potentiate the action of the original mAb.[16] These events underscore the need to assess the biologic and pharmacokinetic effects of biologics administered in clinical trials in order better to understand the mechanisms underlying their success or failure.

In many mAb trials, a biologic effect may manifest as a reduction in target cell number or an associated functional alteration. For example, the administration of a chimeric anti-CD4 mAb to patients with rheumatoid arthritis leads to a prompt and dramatic decline in circulating CD4+ T cells.[15] Moreover, this has been associated with a decline in T cell responses to mitogens *in vitro*.[14,17] Whether such changes render the host "immunosuppressed" is dependent upon the duration of mAb effect and the nature of the underlying disorder. Infrequently, there have been reports of opportunistic infections following treatment with mAb therapies (Table 12-2). However, the limited size of such trials does not allow for the reliable interpretation of such events. Moreover, the recent introduction of biologic therapies has provided information regarding their short-term, rather than long-term, benefits and hazards.

Lastly, several mAb preparations, especially the anti-CD4 and anti-CD52 mAb, have been associated with profound and persistent depletion of T cells, especially CD4+ T cells.[13,15] Some of these trials have been marred by life-threatening infectious events. Moreover, mechanisms underlying persistent cytopenias are unclear but seem to relate to the suppressive effects of particular mAb on marrow precursors and the inability of adults to regenerate marrow T cells.

IMMUNOTOXINS

Immunotoxins or immunoconjugates are defined as biologically active compounds comprised of a tissue-specific, cell-binding ligand that is covalently linked to a cytotoxin capable of producing cell death.[8–12,18,19] The most commonly utilized ligands are target-specific mAb, although hormones and growth factors have also been used. Monoclonal antibodies are often selected on the basis of their tissue specificity, low cross-reactivity, binding affinity for

cell receptor, the ability to deliver the linked toxin to the cytosol and its *in vitro* cellular effects. The biologic effects of mAb and immunoconjugates are not cell-cycle-specific but are, rather, tissue-specific and are, therefore, capable of eliminating or interfering with both resting and dividing cells.

Immunotoxins have been widely used in cancer trials during the past decade and have also been applied to patients with graft-versus-host disease (GVHD) and a variety of autoimmune conditions, including rheumatoid arthritis.[12] A variety of toxin moieties have been used in immunoconjugates and are derived from plant (ricin, abrin, gelonin), bacterial (diptheria toxin, pseudomonas exotoxin A) or fungal (α-saracin) sources. Among these, the most extensively studied and utilized has been ricin.

Ricin is a 65kD heterodimeric glycoprotein from the plant *Ricinus communis* and is composed of an A-chain and B-chain. The A-chain is a ribosome inactivating protein that is specific for ribosomal RNA. The B-chain of ricin mediates the binding of the toxin to terminal galactose residues on the cell surface and it also facilitates the translocation of the A-chain to the cytoplasm. Once ricin A-chain is endocytosed, it is routed to the cytoplasm where it acts upon ribosomal RNA and inhibits protein synthesis, leading to cell death *in vitro*.[8–12,18] The use of ricin has resulted in an unacceptable degree of nonspecific toxicity, as numerous organs are rich in lectin-binding sites, including the liver, spleen and, possibly, muscle. For these reasons, many investigators have chosen to substitute other binding molecules for the B-chain (for example, mAb) with the hope of less toxicity and enhanced tissue-specificity.

Ricin immunotoxins have been generated against a variety of cell types and have been used in the treatment of autoimmune diseases (rheumatoid arthritis), lymphomas, leukemias, solid tumors (breast, colorectal, ovarian cancer), osseous sarcomas and melanoma. Despite the impressive tissue specificity of many immunoconjugates, it is unknown how effective these agents are at delivering the toxin to the targeted cell or tissue. Immunotoxins have been most successful when treating readily accessible targets or highly vascular disorders such as lymphohematopoetic disorders (for example, B and T cell lymphoma, B cell leukemias, Hodgkin's disease), GVHD and, possibly, rheumatoid arthritis. This contrasts the lack of success in less vascular solid tumors (breast, ovarian and so on). The fate of ricin in the circulation is determined by the stability of the conjugate. Ricin immunotoxins are rapidly cleared by the reticuloendothelial system, as the intact moiety has numerous lectin residues facilitating its uptake by the liver.

Toxicities Associated with Ricin Immunoconjugates

The most common and clinically important toxicities associated with the use of immunoconjugates are listed in Table 12-3.[10–12] These events are due to the toxin alone or to the

Table 12-3 Common and clinically important adverse events associated with immunotoxin therapies*

Common	Uncommon/Rare
Flulike symptoms	Hepatitis
Cytokine release syndrome	Hypotension
Capillary leak syndrome	Congestive heart failure
Rash/urticaria	Pulmonary edema
Pruritus	Anaphylactoid reaction
	Vasculitis
	Palpable purpura
	Synovitis
	Chest "tightness"
	Pericardial effusion
	Neuropathy
	CPK elevation
	Myopathy
	Rhabdomyolysis

*modified from Cush.[12]

host's immune response to the tissue-specific ligand (for example, murine mAb), toxin or both (immunoconjugate). In a variety of phase I and II clinical trials with solid tumors or GVHD, a majority of the individuals developed minor, short-lived toxicities including fever, anorexia, malaise, myalgia and fatigue. In clinical trials using an anti-CD5 ricin A-chain immunoconjugate for rheumatoid arthritis, a similar "flulike syndrome" was commonly observed.[12,20]

Major toxicities are uncommon and most are the direct consequence of ricin exposure to the endothelium and other tissues (for example, liver, muscle). Ricin has been shown to bind and disrupt vascular endothelium.[21] This has occasionally lead *In vivo* to the development of the "capillary leak syndrome" similar to that observed with other biologic therapies (Table 12-2).[1,2] The etiology of the capillary leak syndrome is unclear in those instances where ricin has not been employed. One report suggests that increased vascular permeability may result from IL-2-induced suppression of endothelin-1, local release of TNF and neutrophil activation or IL-2-induced complement activation.[22]

Lastly, uptake of ricin A by Kupffer cells may result in hepatotoxicity.[8-12] Hepatotoxicity has also been observed in patients receiving blocked immunotoxins[19] or diphtheria and other bacterial toxins that are taken up by the liver. Myalgia is commonly observed in patients treated with immunotoxin. Mechanisms underlying these manifestations have not been elucidated. Neurotoxicity has been reported in several immunotoxin trials.[8,23] In such instances, it is thought that cross-reactivity of the mAb with neural tissues, rather than toxin effect on nerve, was responsible. Other uncommon events associated with immunotoxin administration include reports of anaphylactoid reactions, palpable purpura, vasculitis, immune-complex-mediated phenomenon (for example, acute postinfusion synovitis, urticaria and chest tightness), myopathy and rhabdomyolysis (Table 12-3).

CYTOKINE-DIRECTED THERAPY

As the secreted products of activated cells, cytokines function as endocrine, paracrine or autocrine effector molecules in the course of normal and pathologic immune responses.[24] Disorders such as rheumatoid arthritis, multiple sclerosis and Hodgkin's disease often demonstrate patterns of immune dysregulation typified by distinctive cytokine alterations.[6,24] Understanding of the complex networks in which various cytokines function is incomplete. Moreover, the apparent redundancy in cytokine action suggests that the elimination or enhancement of any individual cytokine may not achieve the desired biological or clinical effects.

IL-1

A considerable body of literature has documented the pivotal role of IL-1 as a proinflammatory molecule with significant physiologic and metabolic effects.[24] Moreover, IL-1 is involved in the regulation of hematopoiesis, has potent effects on vascular endothelium, and has shown significant antitumor activity alone or in combination with various chemotherapeutic agents.[24-29] IL-1β has also been shown to reduce mortality from infection in animal models. For these reasons IL-1 has been employed in several cancer trials. Patients have received IL-1α or IL-1β alone or in combination with other chemotherapeutic regimens in the treatment of a variety of disorders, including bone marrow transplantation, idiopathic aplastic anemia, metastatic renal cell carcinoma, Hodgkin's disease, non-Hodgkin's lymphoma and chronic myeloid leukemia. In these trials, IL-1 has demonstrated limited efficacy as adjunctive antitumor therapy, but has been useful in replenishing marrow elements damaged by neoplasia or chemotherapeutic agents.

Toxicities associated with recombinant IL-1 are common but tend to be moderate and non-life-threatening.[25-29] Postadministration symptoms commonly include fever, chills, rigors, hypertension or hypotension, fatigue, headache and weight gain. Neurologic toxicity has been observed and may manifest as somnolence or seizures. The majority of patients demonstrate an acute, transient increase in neutrophil and platelet counts. There have been no reports of rheumatological or serological sequelae. Nonetheless, IL-1 is capable of potentiating or abrogating the development of type II collagen induced arthritis in rats,[30] and injection of IL-1 into the joints of experimental animals has been shown to cause inflammatory arthritis.[31]

Numerous inflammatory disorders are characterized by the excess production of IL-1, and several methods have been proposed to nullify its effects.[31] The naturally occurring IL-1 receptor antagonist (IL-1ra) binds to the IL-1 receptor on various target cells but transduces no signal, and thereby acts as a competitive inhibitor of endogenous IL-1. IL-1ra has therefore been effectively utilized to inhibit IL-1-mediated events *in vitro* and *in vivo*. IL-1ra has been utilized in a limited number of studies and has been shown to be effective in a dose-dependent manner. A recently reported multicenter, multidose trial of IL-1ra in patients with rheumatoid arthritis demonstrated the safety and possible efficacy of IL-1ra. Most common side effects included injection site reactions, rash, headache, nausea, paraesthesia and fatigue.[32] Serious events included a vasovagal episode and two patients with serious infections. It is unknown if these infections were related to the underlying disorder or the administration of IL-1ra.

TNF

Like IL-1, TNF plays an important role in the pathophysiology of autoimmune and neoplastic disorders, based upon its spectrum of effects as an immunoregulatory, antitumor and proinflammatory molecule.

The administration of a chimeric anti-TNF mAb to patients with rheumatoid arthritis has demonstrated significant clinical improvement with a parallel reduction in acute phase reactants (for example, C-reactive protein) and IL-6 levels.[33,34] Infusion-related side effects are uncommon (headache, nausea, fever). While it appears that many patients will develop HACA, retreatment is possible but may be associated with tachyphylaxis. Sporadic reports of ANA and anti-dsDNA positivity following treatment with anti-TNF-α mAb are of uncertain clinical significance.

Recombinant TNF (rTNF) has been used in cancer trials because of its ability to induce tumor necrosis. Symptoms due to rTNF may be severe and correlate with the known biologic effects of TNF. These include features of endotoxic shock, cachexia, resorption of cartilage and bone, hypercalcemia, hypophosphatemia, myocardial dysfunction and arthritis.[1,35]

IL-2

IL-2 is a potential target for immunomodulation of T-cell-mediated diseases. IL-2 is produced exclusively by activated T cells, and mediates its effects by binding specific high-affinity receptors (IL-2 receptor or CD25) expressed on activated T cells. IL-2 is capable of promoting T cell growth and enhancing natural killer cell and antigen-specific cytotoxic T cell activities. IL-2 also induces proliferation of lymphokine-activated killer cells which lyse tumor cells *in vitro*. IL-2 may be a useful target in the treatment of rheumatoid arthritis and psoriasis as it has been shown that T cells within the rheumatoid synovium or psoriatic skin are activated and express CD25. Moreover, the inhibition of IL-2 production by cyclosporine and the established utility of cyclosporine in rheumatoid arthritis and patients with psoriasis offers additional support for a role of IL-2 in these disorders.[7] The anti-

CD25 mAb campath-6 has been used to target CD25+ cells with little clinical benefit and with previously observed mAb-associated toxicity (Table 12-1).[2] IL-2 has also been genetically fused with the toxic domain of diphtheria toxin to form an IL-2 fusion toxin.[2] This has been administered to patients with rheumatoid arthritis and psoriasis with variable clinical success. Short-term toxicity was limited to cutaneous reactions (rash, pruritus, and so on) and hepatotoxicity. There were no instances of profound immunosuppression, infection or other remote sequelae.

IL-2 has also been used to treat tumors such as melanoma and renal cell carcinoma. Exogenous IL-2 is administered in excess with the hope of inducing host immune responsiveness against neoplastic cells. Recombinant IL-2 has also been used with some success in the treatment of malignancies refractory to standard agents.[1,22,36,37]

Toxicity associated with IL-2 administration is common, dose-limiting and usually due to the induction of secondary cytokines (TNF-α, IFN-γ and IL-6). Symptoms include nausea, diarrhea, fever, chills, fatigue, skin rash (for example, exfoliative dermatitis), hypotension, disorientation, renal insufficiency, hyperbilirubinemia, anemia and thrombocytopenia. Moreover, high-dose IL-2 has been associated with the induction of autoimmune disorders and/or autoantibodies in nearly 15% of patients.[36,37] Autoimmune thyroiditis is most common, but pemphigus, vitiligo, anti-insulin antibodies, antinuclear antibodies (ANA) vasculitis, and exacerbations of psoriasis, Crohn's disease, reactive arthritis and rheumatoid arthritis have also been reported.[22,37] Musculoskeletal manifestations are uncommon but include reports of rheumatoid-like arthritis, arthralgia, myalgia and fibromyalgia.

IL-3

IL-3 is capable of promoting the growth of multipotential progenitor cells to platelets, neutrophils, eosinophils, monocytes and lymphocytes.[1] It is therefore not surprising that such an agent may be useful in treating disorders of marrow depletion or arrest (aplastic anemia, myelodysplasia and so on). Toxicity associated with IL-3 administration includes fever, chills, bone pain, headache, stiff neck, injection-site erythema and thrombocytopenia.[1]

IL-6

IL-6 is a potent inducer of inflammation and the acute phase response, and provides help to B cell growth and immunoglobulin synthesis. IL-6 has therefore become an attractive candidate for further study. A murine mAb against IL-6 has been administered to patients with rheumatoid arthritis, multiple myeloma and non-Hodgkin's lymphoma and to AIDS patients with large-cell lymphoma.[38–40] Clinical benefits were greater in rheumatoid arthritis patients, and toxicity was mild. The most common adverse effects were reductions in circulating neutrophil and platelet counts.

Recombinant IL-6 has been used in the treatment of thrombocytopenia and metastatic tumor.[41] *In vitro* studies have shown that IL-6 is important in the proliferation and maturation of multipotential hematopoietic progenitor cells and induces the maturation of megakaryocytes. Animal studies have also shown that IL-6 is capable of mediating regression of metastatic tumors. Early trials in humans with advanced malignancies have demonstrated that fever, chills and fatigue were common following IL-6 administration. Therapy was effective at producing thrombocytosis, a normochromic-normocytic anemia and a marked decrease in serum iron but had no effect on peripheral leukocyte counts. Mild elevations of hepatic enzymes and hypoalbuminemia were often seen. Features of the capillary leak syndrome have not been seen with IL-6 therapy.

IL-10

IL-10 is a 35-kD heterodimeric peptide and was previously called the "cytokine synthesis inhibitory factor" because of its ability to inhibit the production of IL-2 and IFN-γ by TH1 CD4+ T cells. Like other cytokines, IL-10 has numerous biologic effects and tends to inhibit or counteract the effects of other proinflammatory cytokines. Thus, IL-10 is capable of inhibiting macrophage-dependent T cell proliferation and the production of IL-2 and IFN-γ *in vitro*. It is also capable of inhibiting macrophage production of IL-1, TNF-α, IL-6, IL-8, G-CSF and nitric oxide. Lastly, IL-10 tends to promote B cell growth and immunoglobulin synthesis. Because of its "anti-inflammatory" effects, it has been postulated that IL-10 may be useful in the treatment of sepsis, chronic arthritis or inflammatory bowel disease.

Although there are no data available on the use of IL-10 in these disorders, a phase I, dose-escalating, double-blind, placebo-controlled trial of IL-10 has been completed. In this trial, 17 normal volunteers received either placebo or three different doses of IL-10 (1 μg/kg, 10 μg/kg, or 25 μg/kg) as a single intravenous bolus. Subjects were carefully monitored for 96 hours, and no "clinically significant" adverse symptoms or signs were noted. Laboratory tests did reveal a transient but significant neutrophilia, monocytosis and pan-T-cell lymphopenia. Moreover, there was a dose-dependent inhibition of TNF-α and IL-1β production.[42]

Colony Stimulating Factors (CSF)

CSF are secreted products that stimulate the proliferation and differentiation of marrow precursors, such as granulocytes. These agents have been available as recombinant products for several years and have been used largely in the treatment of myelodysplasia or pancytopenia related to infection, drugs or malignancy. CSF have also been used successfully in the treatment of Felty syndrome.[1,43,44] Granulocyte CSF (G-CSF), also known as filgrastim, has been FDA-approved for use during bone marrow transplantation and myelosuppressive chemotherapy. Granulocyte macrophage-CSF (GM-CSF), also known as sargramostim, has also been used for myeloid reconstitution following bone marrow transplantation. The use of G-CSF has been associated with little toxicity that can be ascribed to the agent alone. Most common are reports of nausea, hypertension, rash and peritonitis. Cutaneous reactions have included a nonspecific rash, local injection-site reactions (when administered subcutaneously) and facial flushing. Musculoskeletal manifestations are common. Up to 20% of patients experience short-lived medullary bone pain that responds to narcotic analgesics. Arthralgia and myalgia usually occur in the two-to-three day period prior to the rise in peripheral blood cell counts.[1] There have been sporadic reports of G-CSF exacerbating cutaneous psoriasis, vasculitis and rheumatoid arthritis.[22,43,44] GM-CSF has been noted to induce fever, capillary leak syndrome and autoantibodies.[1] In general, G-CSF is less toxic than GM-CSF.

Recombinant macrophage-CSF (M-CSF) has undergone limited use as antitumor therapy in those patients resistant to conventional measures. In limited number of phase I patients, the relative safety of this agent was demonstrated. Reported toxicities included thrombocytopenia, splenomegaly, monocytosis, iritis, episcleritis and fatigue.[45]

IFN

In general, the interferons are cytokines produced by TH1 helper T cells and tend to exhibit antiviral and antiproliferative effects. IFN-γ is a T-cell-derived cytokine which has profound effects upon the immunoregulatory function of antigen-presenting cells as well as other cell types. It has been shown to have both enhancing as well as inhibitory effects on the immune response, depending upon the system investigated. Whereas IFN-γ has antiviral effects similar to IFN-α and IFN-β, IFN-γ is a potent inducer of macrophage function, inducing the release of oxygen radicals and the expression of class II MHC antigens. IFN-γ has been utilized in the treatment of chronic granulomatous disease and rheumatoid arthritis.[1,22]

Recombinant IFN-γ is commonly administered by subcutaneous injection. The most common toxicities include subcutaneous injection site reactions (erythema and tenderness) and flulike manifestations such as fever, chills, headache, rash, nausea, vomiting and fatigue. Laboratory abnormalities may include leukopenia, elevated levels of hepatic enzymes, proteinuria and hypertriglyceridemia.[1,22] The incidence of musculoskeletal manifestations ranges from 2% to 10% and includes myalgia (10%), back pain (3%), arthralgia (2% to

3%) and arthritis (less than 1%). Between 5% and 17% of patients may develop ANA positivity following IFN-γ therapy.[22] There have been reports of symmetric polyarthritis and worsening of dermatomyositis following the use of IFN-γ.[22,46] Doses of more than 250 mcg/m² per day may exacerbate preexisting cardiac disease (for example, ischemic heart disease, heart failure, arrhythmia) or induce central nervous system manifestations (dizziness, altered mental status, gait disturbances).[22,46]

IFN-β possesses immunoregulatory and antiviral properties. Recombinant IFN-β has been used in the treatment of multiple sclerosis, AIDS, Kaposi's sarcoma, malignant melanoma and acute non-A/non-B hepatitis. The mechanism of action in disorders such as multiple sclerosis is unclear. The toxicities are similar to IFN-γ. Most pronounced is a flulike syndrome which has been observed in nearly half of the treated patients, especially at the start of therapy.[46] Other side effects include injection site reactions, abdominal pain, photosensitivity, goiter, leukopenia and lymphopenia.[46] Myalgia is the most common musculoskeletal manifestation.[46] Arthritis, bursitis, tenosynovitis and myositis have been reported less frequently.[46]

Recombinant IFN-α is similar to IFN-β, with comparable immunoregulatory and antiviral activities. It has been used in the treatment of chronic non-A/non-B/C hepatitis, hairy cell leukemia, condylomata acuminata and AIDS-related Kaposi's sarcoma. It is administered as an intramuscular, subcutaneous or intralesional injection. Common adverse reactions include flulike symptoms such as fever, chills and headache; myalgia or arthralgias; alopecia; sore throat; confusion; hepatic dysfunction; hyper- or hypothyroidism; leukopenia and thrombocytopenia. Apart from myalgia, other rheumatic complaints are uncommon (less than 10%) and include arthritis, bone pain, leg cramps and muscle weakness. There have also been occasional reports of Raynaud phenomenon vasculitis, ANA and rheumatoid factor positivity.[22,47] There have also been anecdotal reports of IFN-α therapy inducing systemic lupus erythematosus.[22] Such patients differed from cases of drug-induced lupus by manifesting renal disease, depressed serum complement levels and antibodies against dsDNA.

CONSEQUENCES OF IMMUNOSUPPRESSION

The potential for untoward remote effects resulting from the manipulation of the immune response is difficult to ascertain with biopharmaceutical agents. Most clinical trials thus far have been careful to document the short-term immunotoxicity and identify regimens that may be overly immunosuppressive. Lessons learned from the use of nonspecific immunosuppressive regimens (for example, cyclophosphamide, leukapheresis, IV gammaglobulin) suggest that as the specificity of biologic intervention decreases, the theoretical potential for untoward consequences may increase.[2] The use of more biospecific therapy may therefore lessen

these risks. Unfortunately, the specificity of current therapies is not as refined as one would hope and in many instances the precise mechanism(s) of action for these agents has not been elucidated.[2] Theoretical consequences, such as the increased risk of infection or neoplasia, are of grave concern when administering agents that may result in the loss of normal immunoregulatory function.

Treatment with the mAb OKT3 may be associated with the remote development of secondary neoplasia. It has been postulated that such sequelae may result from the loss of T cell regulatory control, thereby permitting the proliferation of EBV-infected B cells with the resultant emergence of secondary lymphomas.[4] Alternatively, the loss of T cells involved in normal immunosurveillance may permit the growth of neoplastic cells. There have been several reports claiming an increased risk of lymphoproliferative disorders (for example, non-Hodgkin's lymphoma) in transplant recipients treated with the immunosuppressive OKT3 mAb.[4] The data is most convincing for patients treated with OKT3 and cyclosporine or antithymocyte globulin. Current recommendations suggest that the use of this mAb is safe when administered at the recommended doses or duration of therapy. Until similar long-term immunotoxicity data is available, such concerns need to be addressed during drug development and clinical testing of new agents.

SUMMARY

This chapter has reviewed the rationale for the use of biologic agents and has detailed some of the many untoward effects associated with the use of biologic therapies. The

Table 12-4 Musculoskeletal manifestations due to biologic therapies

Symptom/Sign	Causative Biologic Agent
Myalgia	IL-2, IFN-γ, IFN-β, IFN-α, ricin, αCD22IT, mAb (in general)
Myopathy/weakness	IFN-α, αCD5IT
Myositis	IFN-β, αCD5IT
Rhabdomyolysis	IFN-α, αCD5IT, αCD22IT
Arthralgia	IL-2, IFN-γ, IFN-β, IFN-α
Arthritis	IL-1, IL-2, rTNF, IFN-γ, IFN-β, IFN-α, αCD5IT
Rheumatoid arthritis	IL-2, IFN-β, IFN-α
Bone pain	IL-3, IFN-α, G-CSF, GM-CSF
Lupuslike disease	IFN-α, IFN-γ
Back pain	IFN-γ
Bursitis	IFN-β
Raynaud phenomenon	IFN-α
Vasculitis	IL-2, IFN-α, αCD5IT
Serological Abnormalities	
ANA positivity	IL-2, αTNF, IFN-α, IFN-γ, GM-CSF
dsDNA positivity	TNF, IFN-α, IFN-γ

scope and magnitude of these adverse events ranges from localized to systemic and mild to life-threatening. The systemic nature of these agents often results in recognizable syndromes or patterns of disease (Table 12-2) that may limit their future use. Not surprisingly, the manipulation of the immune response with biologic response modifers may promote rather than control immune dysregulation. Thus the appearance of numerous musculoskeletal and autoimmune manifestations of biologic toxicity (Table 12-4) tends to highlight the immunologic mechanisms responsible for these commonly seen features. Efficacy and toxicity data accrued from these biologic trials suggest that the experimental use of such agents will not only add new therapeutic interventions, but will also provide new and valuable information regarding the underlying pathogenesis of autoimmune and rheumatologic disorders.

REFERENCES

[1]Thomas JA. Recent developments and perspectives of biotechnology-derived products. *Toxicology.* 1995;105:7–22.

[2]Cush JJ, Kavanaugh AF. Biologic interventions in rheumatoid arthritis. *Rheum Dis Clin N Am.* 1995;21:797–816.

[3]Cavagnaro JA. Immunotoxicity assessment of biotechnology products: A regulatory point of view. *Toxicology.* 1995;105:1–6.

[4]Sgro C. Side-effects of a monoclonal antibody, muromonab CD3/orthoclone OKT3: Bibliographic review. *Toxicology.* 1995;105:23–29.

[5]Chatenoud L, Bach J-F. Monoclonal antibodies to CD3 as immunosuppressants. *Semin Immunol.* 1990;2:437–447.

[6]Moreau T, Coles A, Wing M, et al. Transient increase in symptoms associated with cytokine release in patients with multiple sclerosis. *Brain.* 1996;119:225–237.

[7]Kavanaugh AF, Lipsky PE. The application of biotechnological advances to the treatment of rheumatoid arthritis. In: Wolfe F, Pincus T, eds. *Rheumatoid Arthritis: Pathogenesis, Assessment, Outcome, and Treatment.* New York: Marcel Dekker, 1994;373.

[8]Gottstein C, Winkler U, Bohlen H, Diehl V, Engert A. Immunotoxins: Is there a clinical value? *Ann Oncol.* 1994;5(Suppl 1):S97–S103.

[9]Hertler AA, Frankel AE. Immunotoxins: A clinical review of their use in the treatment of malignancies. *J Clin Oncol.* 1989;7:1932–1942.

[10]Vitetta ES, Thorpe PE, Uhr JW. Immunotoxins: Magic bullets or misguided missiles? *Immunol Today.* 1993;14:252–259.

[11]Vallera DA. Immunotoxins: Will their clinical promise be fulfilled? *Blood.* 1994;83:309–316.

[12]Cush JJ. Anti-CD5/Ricin A chain immunoconjugate therapy in rheumatoid arthritis. In: *Novel Therapeutic Agents for the Treatment of Autoimmune Diseases.* Strand V, et al., eds. New York: Marcel Decker Inc., 1997;11–24.

[13]Weinblatt ME, Maddison PJ, Bulpitt KJ, et al. Campath-1-H, a humanized monoclonal antibody in refractory rheumatoid arthritis. *Arthritis Rheum.* 1995;38:1589–1594.

[14]Horneff G, Emmrich F, Burmester GR. Advances in immunotherapy in rheumatoid arthritis: Clinical and immunological findings following treatment with anti-CD4 antibodies. *Br J Rheumatol.* 1993;32(suppl 4):39–47.

[15]Moreland LW, Pratt PW, Mayes MD, et al. Double-blind, placebo-controlled multicenter trial using chimeric monoclonal anti-CD4 antibody, cM-T412, in rheumatoid arthritis patients receiving methotrexate. *Arthritis Rheum.* 1995;38:1581–1588.

[16]Frodin JE, Lefvert AK, Mellstedt H. The clinical significance of HAMA in patients treated with mouse monoclonal antibodies. *Cell Biophysics.* 1992;21:153–165.

[17]Fishwild DM, Strand V. Administration of an anti-CD5 immunoconjugate to patients with rheumatoid arthritis: Effect of peripheral blood mononuclear cells and in vitro immune function. *J Rheumatol.* 1994;21:596–604.

[18]Fishwild DM, Staskawicz MO, Wu HM, Carroll SF. Cytotoxicity against human peripheral blood mononuclear cells and T cell lines mediated by anti-T cell immunotoxins in the absence of added potentiator. *Clin Exp Immunol.* 1991;86:506–513.

[19]Collinson AR, Lambert JM, Liu Y, et al. Anti-CD6-blocked ricin: An anti-pan T-cell immunotoxin. *Int J Immunopharmacol.* 1994;16:37–49.

[20]Strand V, Lipsky PE, Cannon GW, et al. The CD5 Plus Rheumatoid Arthritis Investigators Group. *Arthritis Rheum.* 1993;36:620–630.

[21]Soler-Rodriguez AM, Ghettie MA, Oppenheimer-Marks N, Uhr JW, Vitetta ES. Ricin A-chain and ricin A-chain immunotoxins rapidly damage human endothelial cells: Implications for vascular leak syndrome. *Exper Cell Res.* 1993;206:227–234.

[22]Vial T, Descotes J. Immune-mediated side-effects of cytokines in humans. *Toxicology.* 1995;105:31–57.

[23]Ilercil O, Laske DW, Walbridge S, Muaszko K, Oldfield EH, Youle RJ. Neurotoxicity and immunotoxins. *Molecular Chem Neuropathol.* 1994;21:279–286.

[24]Lipsky PE, Davis LS, Cush JJ, et al. The role of cytokines in the pathogenesis of rheumatoid arthritis. *Springer Semin Immunopathol.* 1989;11:123–162.

[25]Nemunaitis J, Ross M, Meisenberg B, et al. Phase I study of recombinant human interleukin-1 beta (rhIL-1 beta) in patients with bone marrow failure. *Bone Marrow Transplantation.* 1994;14:583–588.

[26]Redman BG, Abubakr Y, Cou T, Esper P, Flaherty LE. Phase II trial of recombinant interleukin-1 beta in patients with metastatic renal cell carcinoma. *J Immunotherapy with Emphasis on Tumor Immunology.* 1994;16:211–215.

[27]Weisdorf D, Katsanis E, Verfaillie C, et al. Interleukin-1 alpha administered after autologous transplantation: A phase I/II clinical trial. *Blood.* 1994;84:2044–2049.

[28]Nemunaitis J, Appelbaum FR, Lilleby K, et al. Phase I study of recombinant interleukin-1 beta in patients undergoing autologous bone marrow transplant for acute myelogenous leukemia. *Blood.* 1994;83:3473–3479.

[29]Jonson CS. Modulation of chemotherapy antineoplastic agents with biologic agents: Enhancement of antitumor activities by interleukin-1. *Curr Opinion Oncol.* 1992;4:1108–1115.

[30]Lrelon E, Gillet P, Muller N, et al. Pro- and anti-inflammatory properties of human recombinant IL-1 beta during experimental arthritis in rats: 2. Period-dependent effect. *Life Sciences.* 1993;53:1709–1717.

[31]Arend WP, Dayer JM. Inhibition of the production and effects of interleukin-1 and tumor necrosis factor α in rheumatoid arthritis. *Arthritis Rheum.* 1995;38:151–160.

[32]Campion GV, Lebsack ME, Lookabaugh J, Gordon G, Catalano M. The IL-1Ra Arthritis Study Group. *Arthritis Rheum.* 1996;39:1092–1101.

[33]Elliott MJ, Maini RN, Feldmann M, *et al.* Treatment of rheumatoid arthritis with chimeric monoclonal antibodies to tumor necrosis factor α. *Arthritis Rheum.* 1993;36:1681–1690.

[34]Elliott MJ, Maini RN, Feldmann M, *et al.* Randomized double-blind comparison of chimeric monoclonal antibody to tumor necrosis factor α (cA2) versus placebo in rheumatoid arthritis. *Lancet.* 1994;344:1105–1110.

[35]Mavligit GM. Zukiwski AA, Chamsangavej C, Carrsco CH, Wallace S, Gutterman JU. Regional biologic therapy. Hepatic arterial infusion of recombinant tumor necrosis factor in patients with liver metastases. *Cancer.* 1992;69:557–561.

[36]Massarotti EM. Chronic inflammatory arthritis after treatment with high dose interleukin-2. *Am J Med.* 1992;92:693–697.

[37]Rosenberg SA, Yang JC, Topalian SL, *et al.* Treatment of 283 consecutive patients with metastatic melanoma or renal cell cancer using high-dose bolus interleukin 2. *JAMA.* 1994;271:907–913.

[38]Wendling D, Racadot E, Wijdenes J. Treatment of severe rheumatoid arthritis by anti-interleukin-6 monoclonal antibody. *J Rheumatol.* 1993;20:259–262.

[39]Emilie D, Wijdenes J, Gisselbrecht C, *et al.* Administration of an anti-interleukin-6 monoclonal antibody to patients with acquired immunodeficiency syndrome and lymphoma: Effect of lymphoma growth and on B clinical symptoms. *Blood.* 1994;84:2472–2479.

[40]Brochier J, Legcuffe E, Liautard J, *et al.* Immunomodulating IL-6 activity by murine monoclonal antibodies. *Int J Immunopharmacol.* 1995;17:41–48.

[41]Kammuller ME. Recombinant human interleukin-6: Safety issues of a pleiotrophic growth factor. *Toxicology.* 1995;105:91–107.

[42]Chernoff AE, Granowitz EV, Shapiro L, *et al.* A randomized, controlled trial of IL-10 in humans. *J Immunol.* 1995;154:5492–5499.

[43]Hayat SQ, Hearth-Holmes M, Wolf RE. Flare of arthritis with successful treatment of Felty's syndrome. *Clin Rheumatol.* 1995;14:211–212.

[44]Kelly R, Marsden RA, Bevan D. Exacerbation of psoriasis with GM-CSF therapy. *Br J Dermatol.* 1993;128:468–469.

[45]Bukowski RM, Budd GT, Gibbons JA, *et al.* Phase I trial of subcutaneous recombinant macrophage colony-stimulating factor: Clinical and immunomodulatory effects. *J Clin Oncol.* 1994;12:97–106.

[46]Vial T, Descotes J. Clinical toxicity of the interferons. *Drug Safety.* 1994;10:115–150.

[47]Kiely PDW, Bruckner FE. Acute arthritis following interferon α therapy. *Br J Rhematol.* 1994;33:502–503.

13

Silicone-Related Rheumatic Disorders

Lori A. Love and John Varga

INTRODUCTION

Since their development in the 1930s, the use of silicones has become pervasive in modern society.[1-5] Silicone is a generic term for synthetic polymers containing a repeating silicon oxide backbone and some organic side chain group.[3,4,6] Depending upon the length and composition of the chain, and the degree of cross-linking, silicones can be produced as liquids (fluids, gels) or solids (elastomers, rubbers). One of the most commonly produced silicones, poly-dimethylsiloxane (PDMS), has a repeating $(CH_3)_2SiO$ unit. Beyond their many industrial uses, silicones are ingredients in many cosmetics, foods, drugs and medical devices. Originally believed to be biologically inert, silicones were first used medically as waterproof wound dressings.[3] The first silicone-gel-filled breast implant procedure was performed in the U.S. in 1962.[3] By the mid-1960s silicone was used for reconstructive face surgery, and other medical uses soon became widespread. There were few reported complications associated with these early procedures. Local adverse events including local hemorrhage, infection and capsular contraction were recognized.[7,8] "Capsule" formation around the implant, which could be accompanied by granulomatous inflammation, was thought to be part of the "normal" healing process associated with various implants of silicone.[3,8] The capsule appeared to wall off the implant from the rest of the body and it was therefore thought to limit cellular interactions with silicone.

Since the published reports in the early 1980s describing a syndrome that resembled connective tissue disorders and was associated with silicone breast injections or implants,[9-14] there has been an explosion of information regarding potential local and systemic complications associated with implanted silicone devices.[3,4,8,15-17] At the same time, there has been an increase in our understanding of the potential biological effects of silicones and the pathogenetic mechanisms involved.

Diverse types of information are now available to evaluate critically possible associations between exposure to silicone and subsequent clinical syndromes. The information includes data from human, animal and *in vitro* studies. Human data include published case reports or series, retrospective cohort or population-based studies and prospective clinical studies. These human studies, as well as studies with animal models or *in vitro* techniques, have well-recognized limitations in their ability to provide definitive information concerning potential risks associated with environmental exposures. However, when examined and evaluated in their totality, the data yield useful information concerning potential etiological agents, disease susceptibility and pathogenesis, therapeutic considerations and prognosis. This chapter will summarize these data and provide a basis upon which to evaluate potential associations between silicone implants and human illnesses.

INFLAMMATORY AND IMMUNE RESPONSES TO SILICONE

Evidence for Local Immune Reactions to Silicone

Results from a number of human studies and investigations in animals suggest that silicones, in a variety of forms, can induce local activation of the immune system, sustain immune responses and establish immunologic memory.[5,17,18] The observations from these studies are supported further by several lines of evidence (summarized in Table 13-1): histopathological, immunohistochemical and molecular findings from capsules surrounding injected silicone or implants in both humans and animals[19-22]; functional *in vitro* assays that demonstrate the adjuvant activity of certain silicones[23-29] and their capacity to activate or otherwise modulate subsets of mononuclear cells[30-34]; evidence for the development of antibodies to silicone or complexes of silicone and pro-

Table 13-1   Immunological sequelae reported with exposure to silicones

Local Immunological Effects Reported with Silicone Injection or Silicone Implants[5,17,18]	
Acute and chronic inflammatory responses:	Fibrous capsule formation[1,41,42]
	Activated mononuclear cells[19-21]
	Restricted T cell receptor V-gene expression[22]

Systemic Immunological Effects	
Humoral mediated immunity:	
Adjuvant effects of silicones	[23-29]
Altered immunoglobulin levels	[48-51]
Antisilicone antibodies	[35-39]
Autoantibodies	ANA, DS-DNA, RNP, RF, centromere,[30,48,50-59] collagen[79-81]
Alterations in cell mediated immunity:	Alterations in mononuclear cell phenotypes[30-34]
	Alterations in cytokine release
	Delayed type hypersensitivity responses to polydimethylsiloxane in animal studies[40]
Rheumatic/connective tissue disorders:	(see Table 13.2 for details)
Role in tumor formation:	Plasmacytomas in susceptible mouse strains[66,82,83]
	Possible multiple myeloma and monoclonal gammopathy in women with silicone breast implants[84-86]
	Possible lymphomas in silicone breast implant recipients[38,87,88]

teins[35-39]; and recent studies with *in vitro* T cell stimulations.[40]

Early experiments in animals demonstrated that injection or implantation of silicones can induce a local immune response. This response was characterized primarily by granulomatous inflammation involving macrophages, multinucleated giant cells, mononuclear cells and other cell types.[21] Similar pathological changes have been described in capsules of silicone breast implants (SBI).[1,41-43] Although these silicone implant capsules vary from person to person in thickness and cellular composition, in general they have a layer of vacuolated pallisading pseudosynovial cells at the surface that adjoins the implant. This is surrounded by a vascular layer of tissue containing activated macrophages, T lymphocytes and B lymphocytes surrounding what appear to be silicone vacuoles.[22] A dense collagenous layer forms the outermost surface of the capsule.

It remains unclear what stimuli trigger the immune system in individuals with silicone implants and what the pathogenetic mechanisms are that result in capsule formation. The exact functions of the capsule are likewise unknown. Silicone is known to diffuse or "bleed" even through intact silicone elastomer envelopes.[8] It has been postulated that the implant capsule develops in order to isolate and process silicone at the implant surface, thereby limiting exposure to silicone.[43,44] It is probable that components of silicone implants either alone or more likely complexed to proteins, may directly stimulate immunocytes and other cells to migrate to and surround the implant and/or free silicone.[43]

Immunocytes, upon phagocytosis of silicone that diffuses or "bleeds" from a silicone-gel-filled implant, can move to other parts of the body.[41,45-47] In cases of implant rupture, silicone itself migrates to distant sites in the body, resulting in the development of regional lymphadenopathy with pain, tenderness and occasionally severe local tissue destruction.[8] In these circumstances, a systemic immune response may be initiated, inducing cytokine networks that sustain or amplify the response.[43] This may account for the reduction of the number of circulating NK cells in animals[33,34] and in women with silicone implants,[30] and their return towards normal levels following explantation in women.[31] Significant alterations have also been reported in other circulating lymphocyte subpopulations, including both elevated or depressed T helper/suppressor ratios, and differences have been found in various lymphocyte functional assays in women with silicone breast implants.[30]

Animal studies clearly demonstrate that certain polydimethylsiloxanes, especially low-molecular-weight compounds, such as D4, can act as powerful adjuvants, enhancing antibody responses to coadministered foreign proteins.[23,40] Elevated levels of immunoglobulins,[48-51] antinuclear and other autoantibodies,[30,48,50-59] and possibly other antibodies[35-39] are detected in humans with silicone implants compared to normal (laboratory) control values. Furthermore, serum levels of silicone-binding immunoglobulins have been reported by certain investigators to be higher in women who have ruptured breast implants compared to those without implants or with intact implants.[37,50] Several studies in humans[60,61] and animals[32] have examined the capacity of T cells to be stimulated by silicone or silica compounds following prior exposure to silicone. This may be the laboratory corollary of reports of DTH responses to silastic tubing and other silicone materials in some patients.[39,62] An interesting preliminary study examined T cell receptor (TCR) usage in lymphocytes from explanted implant capsules.[22] A common restriction in TCR expression in different parts of the same implant capsule was observed. This same restricted TCR repertoire was found even in tissue from the contralateral capsule when bilateral explantation occurred.[22] Taken together with immunogenetic associations with certain immune response (HLA) genes in women who develop myositis after silicone implants[63] or those who have CTD symptoms,[64,65] the findings of limited TCR repertoire suggest that genetically determined susceptibility to antigen-driven immune responses to silicone may influence whether a localized immune response following silicone implantation evolves into a more systemic one. (See Chapter 4 "Genetics of Environmentally Associated Rheumatic Disorders" for a more complete discussion.)

Several studies have explored the capacity of silicone gels to induce activation and uncontrolled growth of lymphocytes and other cells. In a murine model, intraperitoneal placement of silicone gel from SBIs, but not PDMSs of different sizes, induced the development of B lymphocyte-derived plasmacytomas.[66] The plasmacytomas were found only in genetically susceptible mouse strains. Because plasmacytomas developed many months after the inflammatory response was initiated and occurred only in certain strains, it may not be surprising that earlier animal studies, which were predominately of short duration, had not detected this complication of silicone gel. Long-term exposure to silicone gel has also been shown to induce fibrosarcoma formation in rats.[67]

Localized Adverse Events Following Exposure to Silicone

Complications associated with silicone implants can be grouped broadly into those that are limited to local or regional manifestations and those that are systemic in nature (Table 13-2). Localized manifestations are relatively frequent fol-

lowing silicone implantation,[8] but reliable information about their prevalence and natural history is not available. The most common local disorders are implant failure (that is, rupture of the prothesis), local diffusion of silicone through an intact elastomer envelope (gel bleed) and capsular contraction. Both rupture and bleed of the implant result in the release of substantial quantities of silicone into surrounding tissues. Associated clinical manifestations include nodules (silicomas), changes in breast size and symmetry, and local pain and tenderness. Other local complications include infections, rashes, formation of hematoma and nipple discharge, including galactorrhea (Table 13-2). Local injury or trauma, including that related to capsulectomy or mammography, has been implicated in implant rupture. Because some of these complications appear to increase in frequency with the duration of the implant, biodegradation of the implant and its components may also be related to these local complications. Implant duration and degradation of the implant and its components may also be important factors associated with systemic disorders following silicone exposure.

Evidence for Systemic Disorders Following Exposure to Silicone

A variety of clinical disorders has been reported to be associated with silicone implants (Table 13-2). Although a small proportion of individuals develops well-defined connective tissue disorders (CTD) following silicone implantation (SI), most persons with implant-related complications develop an ill-defined set of symptoms and signs that, in aggregate, fail to meet established criteria for a CTD. These syndromes are characterized clinically by a combination of fatigue, malaise, fever, lymphadenopathy, arthralgia and myalgia. These manifestations may be accompanied by lab-

Table 13-2 Disorders reported following silicone implants

Local Disorders/Complications[7,8]	Rheumatic/Connective Tissue Disorders[8,15,16,71,89]	Other Disorders
Capsular contraction	Scleroderma	Monoclonal gammopathy and multiple myeloma[84,86]
Implant bleed	Lupus eryue	Lymphoma[87,88,90]
Implant rupture	Mixed connective tissue disorders	Lymphadenopathy[91-93]
Delayed wound healing	Inflammatory myopathy	Acute pneumonitis[94,95]
Lymphadenopathy	Rheumatoid arthritis	Toxic shock syndrome[96]
Rashes	Sjögren syndrome	Granulomatous hepatitis[38]
Infections	Fibromyalgia	Primary biliary cirrhosis
Pain	Inflammatory synovitis	Multiple sclerosis[97]
Breast asymmetry	Atypical connective tissue disorder	Neurological/neurocognitive dysfunction[48]
Nipple discharge (galactorrhea)		Chest wall syndrome[98]
Hematoma		Embolism (pulmonary)[94,99]
Seratoma		Sarcoidosis[100]
Altered sensation		Carpal or tarsal tunnel syndrome[101]
Local extension and tissue destruction		

oratory abnormalities, including elevated erythrocyte sedimentation rate, anemia, abnormal serum lipids, elevated levels of immunoglobulins and serological evidence of autoimmunity. A myriad of names has been proposed to describe these syndromes: human adjuvant disease,[68] silicone reactive disorder,[69] silicone-induced immune dysfunction syndrome,[70] silicone allergy,[62] atypical connective tissue disease[51] and others.[16]

Several investigations have attempted to define the incidence and patterns of disorders following silicone implantation, most of which occur in association with breast implants. An in-depth review of published studies is beyond the scope of this chapter, and several recent reviews are available.[8,15,16] Population-based epidemiologic surveys to date have mainly been studies of convenience. Such studies utilize databases established for other purposes, include only few subjects evaluated consistently by rheumatologists, and consequently have major limitations. To date, no prospective epidemiological studies with sufficient power to exclude silicone implants as a risk factor for development of systemic CTD have been published.

In recent years several relatively large observational studies have been published.[71,72,73] The results from these studies may be interpreted as excluding the presence of large risk of developing a CTD following silicone breast implantation. However, these studies have been underpowered (study groups contain an inadequate sample size) to assess small or medium degrees of risk associated with SBI. The definition of a large risk versus small or medium risk is also a source of debate. Furthermore, the question of atypical rheumatic or connective tissue manifestations, which appear to be the most prevalent clinical findings among persons with silicone implants, has not been addressed adequately by any of these studies. Studies of a retrospective design are hampered by other limitations, including the lack of appropriate control groups, the absence of consistent evaluations or appropriate follow-up of study participants (data obtained by questionnaire or chart review only) and the use of inappropriate or inadequate diagnostic criteria.

Information from several extensive population-based investigations of silicone implants and CTD is summarized in Table 13-3. The largest study published to date examined the prevalence of silicone breast implants in the Women's Health Professions retrospective cohort study.[71] This study evaluated the responses of 395,543 female health care professionals between the ages of 18 and 99 years who completed and returned questionnaires for participation in the prospective Womens Health Study, a randomized, placebo-controlled trial to evaluate the risks/benefits of low-dose aspirin, beta carotene and vitamin E in the primary prevention of cardiovascular disease and cancer. As in the majority of other observational studies, analyses was limited to data available prior to 1992 in order to avoid potential reporting bias due to widespread publicity regarding the potential health risks associated with silicone breast implants. The

results indicated the presence of a small but statistically significant increase in the risk of developing any CTD (rheumatoid arthritis [RA], systemic lupus erythematosus [SLE], Sjögren's disorder [SS], systemic sclerosis [SSc], polymyositis/dermatomyositis [PM/DM] and others) among women who reported SBI (RR = 1.24, 95% CI: 1.08–1.141, p = 0.0015). Other studies are summarized in Table 13-3.

Taken together, the results from these epidemiologic studies rule out the presence of a large increase in the risk for development of classic CTDs following silicone breast implantation. None of these studies, however, adequately address the issue of atypical rheumatic syndromes. Furthermore, all of these studies suffer from methodological imperfections that limit their ability to provide clinically meaningful information about the medical risks associated with exposure to silicone.

Limitations in Studies of Silicones

Several factors have influenced the ability to conduct and publish credible scientific studies examining potential silicone-related rheumatic disorders. These factors include:

1) The lack of adequate information concerning the true exposure of the individual to silicones (implants and other sources);

2) Variation in implant composition and surgical location;

3) Lack of validated criteria for definition of potentially silicone-related clinical syndromes;

4) Inadequate sample size and control groups to evaluate rare outcomes in epidemiologic studies;

5) Inadequate duration of follow-up;

6) Medicolegal issues which may impair the ability to collect unbiased data and potentially influence the ability to fund certain investigations.

The number of persons in the U.S. with silicone implants is unknown, because there are no systems to monitor this information. It is estimated that approximately one million women have SBIs with the prevalence of implants approximately eight to ten per 1000 women per year.[74–76] The majority of women receiving implants are white and undergo implantation for cosmetic reasons. There are also geographical differences in the rates of silicone breast implantation. The prevalence of other types of silicone implants is thought to be much lower than that of breast implants although reliable data do not exist for these other types of implants either. The majority of implanted silicone devices are silicone-gel-filled breast prostheses. However, this is a heterogeneous category, since various widely used types of breast implants differ from each other in chemical composition and thickness of the solid silastic envelope and the exact chemical composition of the gel.

In addition to the uncertainties associated with determining the duration and nature of exposure to silicone implants, definition of what constitutes a "case" for a particular epidemiologic study is also problematic. The majority of persons who develop medical problems following silicone implantation manifest nonspecific symptoms and signs which are often difficult to evaluate and characterize. Epidemiologic studies that limit definition of a case to those persons who develop a classic CTD following exposure to silicone must deal with the fact that only crude estimates of prevalence and incidence of CTDs exist. Additionally, human studies are hampered by lack of adequate systems to collect and evaluate reports of adverse effects associated with silicone implants. Even with the widespread publicity that silicone implants have received, the true scope of medical problems potentially associated with silicone implants may be underrecognized and underreported. Legal issues arising from the litigation of potential cases (for example, control of medical records) may also inhibit participation of subjects in scientific studies.

It is unlikely that prospective epidemiologic studies will be able adequately to address questions related to the potential causal association between silicone implants and rheumatic disorders. Some of the reasons include the imprecision of incidence and prevalence estimates of CTD, the rarity of CTDs in the general population and the multiplicity of factors associated with the host (immunogenetics) or the device (type, materials, location, duration of implant, presence of infectious agents, implant rupture and leakage) that may influence the rate, nature and severity of subsequent disorders. The restricted availability of certain types of silicone implants also influences the ability to conduct prospective studies in this area. A prospective study with sufficient power to address each of the many variables that could influence the risk of development of disease following silicone implant exposure would be inordinately expensive, as a very large number of subjects (tens of thousands) and long period of follow-up (up to ten years) to account for latency effects would be required.[73] In light of constraints on clinical research and current mandates for cost containment in health care, the prospects for such definitive studies are bleak. The possibility that atypical clinical disorders may be related to SI adds further complexity to these studies.

APPROACHES TO DETERMINING BIOMEDICAL COMPLICATIONS OF SI THAT OVERCOME CURRENT LIMITATIONS

When sufficient amounts of information can be gathered, epidemiological data are useful in evaluating the risk of developing a disease or condition associated with a variable such as silicone breast implants. In contrast, such data are not useful in defining the risk to a particular individual. What, then, is needed to advance our understanding in this area, and

how do we deal with the constraints posed by decreasing support and funding for clinical studies? A combined approach integrating epidemiologic, clinical and laboratory studies is essential to grasp the full biomedical implication of silicone implantation. One such approach is to target carefully defined subsets of subjects to ascertain host and other factors that may modulate the rate, pathogenesis, severity and natural history of a disorder associated with exposure to environmental agents. Such factors are listed in Table 13-4. This approach has been used successfully to study illnesses associated with certain drugs, including those recognized as causes of drug-related lupus (reviewed in[101,102] and Chapter 9). These studies have shown that persons who develop drug-related lupus differ from those with the idiopathic disease in a number of important variables. For instance, patients with drug-related lupus display distinct types and specificities of autoantibodies, immunogenetic backgrounds and clinical manifestations.[77,78] A combined serologic, immunogenetic and clinical approach has been applied to a preliminary study of silicone-implant-associated inflammatory myopathy which compared the characteristics of women developing myositis following silicone implants to those women with idiopathic inflammatory myopathy.[63] Preliminary results indicated that women who developed myositis following silicone implantation and women with idiopathic myositis had different immunogenetic backgrounds, autoantibodies and clinical manifestations. These findings parallel similar differences described in subjects who develop drug-related lupus compared to those with idiopathic systemic lupus erythematosus.

Additional coordinated approaches are necessary to address the questions surrounding the potential biological effects of silicones. It is essential to establish and validate adequate criteria for definition and classification of atypical disorders. Experimental animal models, including transgenic models which may more closely approximate the human immune system, and well-designed clinical studies are necessary to evaluate disease pathogenesis and immune-mediated effects resulting from exposure to silicone. These efforts will require collaboration among scientists from academia, government and industry.

SUMMARY

Certain kinds of silicone can induce specific and nonspecific immune responses in both animals and humans. Local complications are known to result from silicone breast implantation, but the incidence and risk factors for these complications are not known. Currently there are inadequate data to assess if implantation of silicone devices is associated with the development of well-defined clinical systemic syndromes. Most individuals with symptoms following silicone implants do not meet criteria for diagnosis of a defined rheumatic/connective tissue disorder but, rather, appear to

Table 13-3 Population-based investigations evaluating connective tissue disorders following silicone breast implantation

Study Name and Type (Reference)	Study Methodology	Study Results and Conclusions	Comments/Design Issues
Women's Health Professionals Retrospective observational cohort[71] (published 2/96)	- return of questionnaire - data analyzed from 1962–91 - self-reported diagnoses and exposure - data stratified by duration of BI exposure	395,843 evaluable questionnaires 10,830 women with SBI 11,805 women with CTD 24% increased or ↑ risk comparing SBI to NBI (RR = 1.24, p = 0.0015) |	SBI	NBI	RR	P | |---|---|---|---|---| | any CTD | | | 1.24 | 0.0015 | | RA | | | 1.18 | 0.096 | | SLE | | | 1.15 | 0.44 | | SS | | | 1.49 | 0.067 | | PM/DM | | | 1.52 | 0.68 | | SSc | | | 1.84 | 0.06 | | MCTD/Other | | | 1.30 | 0.017 |	- no information on type of BI, reason for procedure, complications associated with procedure - no definition of what constitutes "other CTD" - only classical CTD considered, no evaluation of atypical rheumatic/CTD (no questions on fatigue, myalgia, cognitive dysfunction, sicca symptoms) - data limited to questionnaire; no attempts to validate data (subjects not examined, nor medical records evaluated to verify information) - large background rate of CTD in control group compared to typical reported prevalence in US - 30% of women with CTD excluded because date of diagnosis not provided
Harvard Nurses Health Study Retrospective observation cohort[72,102] Sanchez-Guerrero (published 6/95)	- original cohort of nurses from 11 states (CA, CT, FL, MD, MA, MI, NJ, NY, OH, PA and TX) - 1992 biennial questionnaire returned by 88,153 who answered questions related to SI exposure - data analyzed from 06/76 to 05/90 - chart analysis only	Total eligible cohort 87,501 women (1,181,244 person-yr f/u) 1183 with any type of BI (170 saline, 1013 silicone gel), 9.9 y mean f/u, 11,170 person-yr f/u 516 with definitive CTD no increased risk for defined CTD |	SBI	NBI	RR | |---|---|---|---| | any CTD (self reported) | 17 | 1277 | 1.5 | | def CTD | 4 | 513 | 0.3 | | SSx CTD | 6 | 898 | 0.7 | - 88,153 of 92 questionnaire responded to questions related to SI exposure - supplemental questionnaire returned by 1809/1861 women reporting any type of BI or injections of silicone, paraffin or collagen, of these 1183 with confirmed BI in May 90, or earlier - chart review validation attempted on 100 randomly chosen women (67 medical records reviewed),	- inadequate sample size to detect rare diseases (only 1183 women with implants) - short duration of f/u for diseases that may be associated with long latency periods - ascertainment of implant status incomplete and possibly inaccurate (implants claimed prior to 1960) - diagnoses based on chart review without verification - atypical symptomology purportedly evaluated, but questionnaire sent to few women with implants (to receive questionnaire, self-reported classical CTD prior to 06/10/90; prior to 1992 none of the questionnaires asked about SS, SSc, ACTD, PM/DM or other forms of arthritis; fibromyalgia excluded from all questionnaires) - data on implant rupture not analyzed - no data collection on 5514 women in cohort who died

| Mayo Clinic Study
Retrospective cohort/medical record database[73] Gabriel (published 6/94)
Women in Olmsted County, MN | - cases: received a SBI between 01/01/64 and 12/31/91
- 2 age matched controls per case
- medical record (in- and out-patient) review for occurrence of CTD (RA, SLE, SS, PM/DM, SSc, AS, PA, PMR, VAS, arthritis assoc w/ IBD, polychondritis), other disorders thought to have autoimmune pathogenesis (Hashimotos, PBC, sarcoidosis, lymphoproliferative disorders) and cancer other than breast
- cases categorized as to reason for implant | - general agreement found with self-reported data
- chart review of all reported CTD, with positive questionnaires
- 749 women with BI identified (7.8 y mean f/u), matched with 1498 community controls (8.3 y follow up)
- total of 1006 surgical procedures majority had 1 (572) or 2 (124) procedures, 83% bilateral BI 78% SBI, 5 saline BI, 10% polyurethane, 7% silicone + saline BI
- no increased risk for "defined" CTD | - lacked power (inadequate sample size) to detect an increased risk of rare CTD which the study acknowledges (calculated that 6200 women with SBI, and 12,400 without followed for an average of 10 y necessary to detect doubling of risk of scleroderma (assuming 1.6 cases of SSc/100,000 women); in reality this study lacked the power to detect anything less than a 10X increase risk for most CTD, except possibly RA)
- f/u too short for diseases that may be associated with long latency periods such as SSc
- data not stratified by duration of exposure
- diagnosis based on chart review without verification by examination; (no uniform H&P, laboratory evaluation); laboratory data presented on minority of women (27/1498 controls, 11/749 SBI) = incomplete ascertainment of critical data
- included a number of diseases never reported as associated with SBI in analysis, possibly obscuring linkage of SBI to any one disease |

	SBI	NBI	RR
any CTD*	5 (8.6)	10 (8.1)	1.06
*(SBI = 2 PMR)			
(NBI = 3 AS, 2 RA, 2 SLE, 1 PA, 1 PMR, 1 SS)			
SSx: any arthritis	25 (42.8)	39 (31.6)	1.35
morning stiffness	30 (51.3)	35 (28.3)	1.81 (SS)
sicca	33 (56.4)	50 (40.5)	1.39
salivary gland enlargement	2 (3.4)	3 (2.4)	1.42
serositis	18 (30.8)	21 (17)	1.81

Abbreviations:

ACTD = atypical connective tissue disorders
AS = ankylosing spondylitis
BI = breast implant
CTD = connective tissue disorder
Dx = diagnosis
f/u = follow up
H&P = history and physical
IBD = inflammatory bowel disease
MCTD = mixed connective tissue disorders
NBI = no breast implant
PA = polyarteritis
PBC = primary biliary cirrhosis

PM/DM = polymyositis/dermatomyositis
PMR = polymyalgia rheumatica
SSc = systemic sclerosis
RA = rheumatoid arthritis
RR = relative risk
SBI = silicone breast implant
SI = silicone implant
SLE = systemic lupus erythematosus
SS = Sjögren syndrome
SSx = signs and symptoms
VAS = vasculitis

Table 13-4 Factors possibly important in the development of silicone-related disorders

Implant-Related Factors	
Local complications of implantation	
acute:	hemorrhage, infection
chronic:	infection, inflammation, capsule formation, capsular contraction, implant rupture
Type of implant:	breast
	other
Composition of implant:	silicone gel
	saline
	composite
	polyurethane
	other
Size (volume) of implant	
Location of implant:	breast
	pectoral
	calf
	testicular
	joint
	other
Duration since implant	
Local trauma	

Host-Related Factors	
Immunogenetics	
Gender	
Endocrine status	
Race	
Preexisting conditions	
Other environmental exposures:	talc (from surgical procedures)
	other

have signs and symptoms suggestive of rheumatic disease, including chronic fatigue, fevers, polymyalgia, polyarthralgia, neurocognitive dysfunction, rashes, sicca syndrome and neurological disturbances.

Recent studies suggest the possibility that a nonrandom occurrence of certain CTDs exists in the population exposed to silicone implants. In this group, scleroderma is overrepresented and rheumatoid arthritis underrepresented when compared to U.S. prevalence rates for these diseases.

Reporting biases are driven by publicity of results from investigations that are frequently preliminary in nature or that have major limitations because of study methodology and conduct. Further politicitized by the controversy surrounding this area, these biases hamper research and polarize the scientific and medical community. In spite of the many shortcomings of studies reviewed above, the evolving scientific literature does indicate the possibility that silicones may play a role in the pathogenesis of localized and possibly systemic disorders in susceptible individuals. Carefully designed studies are now needed to evaluate which individu-

als are at risk of developing medical problems following silicone implantation, to determine the pathophysiological events mediating the risk, and to determine how to treat these individuals.

Finally, the development of a standardized approach to investigate and define possible environmental triggers for rheumatic disorders is needed to avoid repeating the difficulties associated with the silicone story as concerns emerge regarding new environmental agents. These investigations will require coordinated efforts involving academic, government and industry resources to establish criteria for case definitions, to conduct epidemiologic investigations and to design appropriate human and animal studies to further our knowledge in this area.

The views expressed herein are solely the professional opinions of the authors, and do not necessarily reflect those of the institutions that they represent.

The authors thank Gary Solomon, M.D., for useful discussions and comments on these issues and Frederick W. Miller, M.D., Ph.D., for critical review of this paper.

REFERENCES

[1] Kossovsky N, Freiman CJ. Silicone breast implant pathology. Clinical data and immunologic consequences. *Arch Pathol Lab Med.* 1994;118:686–693.

[2] Kossovsky N, Freiman CJ. Immunology of silicone breast implants. *J Biomater Appl.* 1994;8:237–246.

[3] Bridges AJ, Vasey FB. Silicone breast implants. History, safety, and potential complications. *Arch Intern Med.* 1993;153:2638–2644.

[4] Yoshida SH, Chang CC, Teuber SS, Gershwin ME. Silicon and silicone: Theoretical and clinical implications of breast implants. *Regul Toxicol Pharmacol.* 1993;17:3–18.

[5] Yoshida SH, Teuber SS, German JB, Gershwin ME. Immunotoxicity of silicone: Implications of oxidant balance towards adjuvant activity. *Food Chem Toxicol.* 1994;32:1089–1100.

[6] Duffy DM. Silicone: A critical review. *Adv Dermatol.* 1990;5:93–107.

[7] Burkhardt BR. Complication of augmentation mammaplasty. In: Georgiade NG, Georgiade GS, Riefkohl R, eds. *Aesthetic Surgery of the Breast.* Philadelphia: W.B. Saunders Company, 1990; 121–132.

[8] Silverman BG, Brown SL, Bright RA, Kaczmarek RG, Arrowsmith-Lowe JB, Kessler DA. Reported complication of silicone gel-breast implants: An epidemiologic review. *Ann Intern Med.* 1996; 124:744–756.

[9] van Nunen SA, Gatenby PA, Basten A. Post-mammoplasty connective tissue disease. *Arthritis Rheum.* 1982;25:694–697.

[10] Baldwin CM Jr, Kaplan EN. Silicone-induced human adjuvant disease? *Ann Plast Surg.* 1983;10:270–273.

[11] Byron MA, Venning VA, Mowat AG. Post-mammoplasty human adjuvant disease. *Br J Rheumatol.* 1984;23:227–229.

[12]Kumagai Y, Shiokawa Y, Medsger TA Jr, Rodnan GP. Clinical spectrum of connective tissue disease after cosmetic surgery. Observations on eighteen patients and a review of the Japanese literature. *Arthritis Rheum.* 1984;27:1–12.

[13]Fock KM, Feng PH. Connective tissue disease after augmentation mammoplasty (letter). *Arthritis Rheum.* 1984;27:1440.

[14]Fock KM, Feng PH, Tey BH. Autoimmune disease developing after augmentation mammoplasty: Report of 3 cases. *J Rheumatol.* 1984;11:98–100.

[15]Bridges AJ. Rheumatic disorders in patients with silicone implants: A critical review. *J Biomater Sci Polym Ed.* 1995;7:147–157.

[16]Sanchez-Guerrero J, Schur PH, Sergent JS, Liang MH. Silicone breast implants and rheumatic disease. Clinical, immunologic, and epidemiologic studies. *Arthritis Rheum.* 1994;37:158–168.

[17]Teuber SS, Yoshida SH, Gershwin ME. Immunopathologic effects of silicone breast implants. *West J Med.* 1995;162:418–425.

[18]Tang L, Eaton JW. Inflammatory responses to biomaterials. *Am J Clin Pathol.* 1995;103:466–471.

[19]Allieu Y, Lussiez B, Martin B. Long-term results of the Swanson implant for the treatment of basal joint arthrosis [in French]. *Rev Chir Orthop Reparatrice Appar Mot.* 1990;76:437–441.

[20]Shanklin DR, Smalley DL. Microscopic techniques and histologic findings in silicone mammary implant capsules and regional paranodal tissues. *Curr Top Microbiol Immunol.* 1996;210:253–261.

[21]Shanklin DR, Smalley DL. Quantitative aspects of cellular responses to silicone. *Int J Occup Med Toxicol.* 1995;4:99–111.

[22]O'Hanlon TP, Okada S, Love LA, Dick G, Young VL, Miller FW. Immunohistopathology and T cell receptor gene expression in capsules surrounding silicone breast implants. *Curr Top Microbiol Immunol.* 1996;210:237–242.

[23]Naim JO, Lanzafame RJ, van Oss CJ. The adjuvant effect of silicone-gel on antibody formation in rats. *Immunol Invest.* 1993;22:151–161.

[24]Naim JO, Ippolito KM, Lanzafame RJ, van Oss CJ. Induction of type II collagen arthritis in the DA rat using silicone gels and oils as adjuvant. *J Autoimmun.* 1995;8:751–761.

[25]Naim JO, Ippolito KM, Lanzafame RJ, van Oss CJ. Induction of type II collagen arthritis in the DA rat using silicone gel as adjuvant. *Curr Top Microbiol Immunol.* 1996;210:103–111.

[26]Nicholson JJ III, Wong GE, Frondoza CG, Rose NR. Silicone gel and octamethylcyclotetrasiloxane potentiate antibody production to bovine serum albumin in mice. *Curr Top Microbiol Immunol.* 1996;210:139–144.

[27]Klykken PC, White KL Jr. The adjuvancy of silicones: dependency on compartmentalization. *Curr Top Microbiol Immunol.* 1996;210:113–121.

[28]Chang YH. Adjuvanticity and arthritogenicity of silicone. *Plast Reconstr Surg.* 1993;92:469–473.

[29]Naim JO, Ippolito KM, Lanzafame RJ. The effect of molecular weight and gel preparation on humoral adjuvancy of silicone oils and silicone gels. *Immunol Invest.* 1995;24:537–547.

[30]Vojdani A, Campbell A, Brautbar N. Immune functional impairment in patients with clinical abnormalities and silicone breast implants. *Toxicol Ind Health.* 1992;8:415–429.

[31]Campbell A, Brautbar N, Vojdani A. Suppressed natural killer cell activity in patients with silicone breast implants: Reversal upon explanation. *Toxicol Ind Health.* 1994;10:149–154.

[32]McDonald AH, Weir K, Sanger JR. Silicone-induced T cell proliferation in mice. *Curr Top Microbiol Immunol.* 1996;210:189–198.

[33]Wilson SD, Munson AE. Silicone-induced modulation of natural killer cell activity. *Curr Top Microbiol Immunol.* 1996;210:199–208.

[34]Bradley SG, White KL Jr, McCay JA, et al. Immunotoxicity of 180-day exposure to polydimethylsiloxane (silicone) fluid, gel and elastomer and polyurethane disks in female B6C3F1 mice. *Drug Chem Toxicol.* 1994;17:221–269.

[35]Vojdani A, Brautbar N, Campbell AW. Antibody to silicone and native macromolecules in women with silicone breast implants. *Immunopharmacol Immunotoxicol.* 1994;16:497–523.

[36]Kossovsky N, Conway D, Kossowsky R, Petrovich D. Novel anti-silicone surface-associated antigen antibodies (anti-SSAA(x)) may help differentiate symptomatic patients with silicone breast implants from patients with classical rheumatological disease. *Curr Top Microbiol Immunol.* 1996;210:327–336.

[37]Wolf LE, Lappe M, Peterson RD, Ezrailson EG. Human immune response to polydimethylsiloxane (silicone): Screening studies in a breast implant population. *FASEB J.* 1993;7:1265–1268.

[38]Kossovsky N, Gornbein JA, Zeidler M, et al. Self-reported signs and symptoms in breast implant patients with novel antibodies to silicone surface associated antigens [anti-SSAA(x)]. *J Appl Biomater.* 1995;6:153–160.

[39]Goldblum RM, Pelley RP, O'Donell AA, Pyron D, Heggers JP. Antibodies to silicone elastomers and reactions to ventriculoperitoneal shunts. *Lancet.* 1992;340:510–513.

[40]Naim JO, Lanzafame RJ, van Oss CJ. The effect of silicone-gel on the immune response. *J Biomater Sci Polym Ed.* 1995;7:123–132.

[41]Kasper CS. Histologic features of breast capsules reflect surface configuration and composition of silicone bag implants. *Am J Clin Pathol.* 1994;102:655–659.

[42]Hameed MR, Erlandson R, Rosen PP. Capsular synovial-like hyperplasia around mammary implants similar to detritic synovitis. A morphologic and immunohistochemical study of 15 cases. *Am J Surg Pathol.* 1995;19:433–438

[43]Hardt NS, Emery JA, LaTorre G, Batich C, Winter WE. Macrophage-silicone interactions in women with breast prostheses. *Curr Top Microbiol Immunol.* 1996;210:245–252.

[44]Kossovsky N, Freiman CJ. Physicochemical and immunological basis of silicone pathophysiology. *J Biomater Sci Polym Ed.* 1995;7:101–113.

[45]Garrido L, Bogdanova A, Cheng LL, et al. Detection of silicone migration and biodegradation with NMR. *Curr Top Microbiol Immunol.* 1996;210:49–58.

[46]Pfleiderer B, Garrido L. Migration and accumulation of silicone in the liver of women with silicone gel-filled breast implants. *Magn Reson Med.* 1995;33:8–17.

[47]Pfleiderer B, Ackerman JL, Garrido L. Migration and biodegradation of free silicone from silicone gel-filled implants after long-term implantation. *Magn Reson Med.* 1993;30:534–543.

[48]Shoaib BO, Patten BM, Calkins DS. Adjuvant breast disease: An evaluation of 100 symptomatic women with breast implants or silicone fluid injections. *Keio J Med.* 1994;43:79–87.

[49]Henderson J, Culkin D, Mata J, Wilson M, Venable D. Analysis of immunological alterations associated with testicular prostheses. *J Urol.* 1995;154:1748–1751.

[50]Lewy RI, Ezrailson E. Laboratory studies in breast implant patients: ANA positivity, gammaglobulin levels, and other autoantibodies. *Curr Top Microbiol Immunol.* 1996;210:337–353.

[51]Bridges AJ, Conley C, Wang G, Burns DE, Vasey FB. A clinical and immunologic evaluation of women with silicone breast implants and symptoms of rheumatic disease. *Ann Intern Med.* 1993;118:929–936.

[52]Bridges AJ, Anderson JD, Burns DE, Kemple K, Kaplan JD, Lorden T. Autoantibodies in patients with silicone implants. *Curr Top Microbiol Immunol.* 1996;210:277–282.

[53]Tan EM, Ochs RL, Kumagai Y, Cuellar ML, Espinoza LR. Re-evaluation of autoantibodies and clinical overview of silicone-related disorders. *Curr Top Microbiol Immunol.* 1996;210:291–298.

[54]Cuellar ML, Scopelitis E, Tenenbaum SA, *et al.* Serum antinuclear antibodies in women with silicone breast implants. *J Rheumatol.* 1995;22:236–240.

[55]Claman HN, Robertson AD. Antinuclear antibodies and breast implants. *West J Med.* 1994;160:225–228.

[56]Claman HN, Robertson AD. Antinuclear antibodies in apparently healthy women with breast implants. *Curr Top Microbiol Immunol.* 1996;210:265–268.

[57]Press RI, Peebles CL, Kumagai Y, Ochs RL, Tan EM. Antinuclear autoantibodies in women with silicone breast implants. *Lancet.* 1992;340:1304–1307.

[58]Bar-Meir E, Teuber SS, Lin HC, *et al.* Multiple autoantibodies in patients with silicone breast implants. *J Autoimmun.* 1995;8:267–277.

[59]Smith HR. Do silicone breast implants cause autoimmune rheumatic diseases? *J Biomater Sci Polym Ed.* 1995;7:115–121.

[60]Smalley DL, Shanklin DR, Hall MF, Stevens MV, Hanissian A. Immunologic stimulation of T lymphocytes by silica after use of silicone mammary implants. *FASEB J.* 1995;9:424–427.

[61]Shanklin DR, Smalley DL, Hall MF, Stevens MV. T cell-mediated immune response to silica in silicone breast implant patients. *Curr Top Microbiol Immunol.* 1996;210:227–236.

[62]Jimenez DF, Keating R, Goodrich JT. Silicone allergy in ventriculoperitoneal shunts. *Childs Nerv Syst.* 1994;10:59–63.

[63]Love LA, Weiner SR, Vasey FB, *et al.* Clinical and immunogenetic features of womes who develop myositis after silicone implant (MASI). *Arthritis Rheum.* 1992;9(suppl):S66:187(abstract).

[64]Young VL, Nemecek JR, Schwartz BD, Phelan DL, Schorr MW. HLA typing in women with and without silicone gel-filled breast implants. *Curr Top Microbiol Immunol.* 1996;210:209–225.

[65]Young VL, Nemecek JR, Schwartz BD, Phelan DL, Schorr MW. HLA typing in women with breast implants. *Plast Reconstr Surg.* 1995;96:1497–1519.

[66]Potter M, Morrison S, Wiener F, Zhang XK, Miller FW. Induction of plasmacytomas with silicone gel in genetically susceptible strains of mice. *JNCI.* 1994;86:1058–1065.

[67]Hatanaka S, Oneda S, Okazaki K, *et al.* Induction of malignant fibrous histiocytoma in female Fisher rats by implantation of cyanoacrylate, zironia, polyvinyl chloride or silicone. *In Vivo.* 1993;7:111–115.

[68]Spiera RF, Gibofsky A, Spiera H. Silicone gel filled breast implants and connective tissue disease: An overview. *J Rheumatol.* 1994;21:239–245.

[69]Lappe MA. Silicone-reactive disorder: A new autoimmune disease caused by immunostimulation and superantigens. *Med Hypotheses.* 1993;41:348–352.

[70]Campbell A, Brautbar N. Norplant: Systemic immunological complications—case report. *Toxicol Ind Health.* 1995;11:41–47.

[71]Hennekens CH, Lee IM, Cook NR, *et al.* Self-reported breast implants and connective-tissue diseases in female health professionals. A retrospective cohort study. *JAMA.* 1996;275:616–621.

[72]Sanchez-Guerrero J, Colditz GA, Karlson EW, Hunter DJ, Speizer FE, Liang MH. Silicone breast implants and the risk of connective-tissue diseases and symptoms. *N Engl J Med.* 1995;332:1666–1670.

[73]Gabriel SE, O'Fallon WM, Kurland LT, Beard CM, Woods JE, Melton LJ III. Risk of connective-tissue diseases and other disorders after breast implantation. *N Engl J Med.* 1994;330:1697–1702.

[74]Cook RR, Perkins LL. The prevalence of breast implants among women in the United States. *Curr Top Microbiol Immunol.* 1996;210:419–425.

[75]Cook RR, Delongchamp RR, Woodbury M, Perkins LL, Harrison MC. The prevalence of women with breast implants in the United States—1989. *J Clin Epidemiol.* 1995;48:519–525.

[76]Gabriel SE, O'Fallon WM, Beard CM, Kurland LT, Woods JE, Melton LJ III. Trends in the utilization of silicone breast implants, 1964–1991, and methodology for a population-based study of outcomes. *J Clin Epidemiol.* 1995;48:527–537.

[77]Adams LE, Hess EV. Drug-related lupus. Incidence, mechanisms and clinical implications. *Drug Saf.* 1991;6:431–449.

[78]Yung RL, Richardson BC. Drug-induced lupus. *Rheum Dis Clin North Am.* 1994;20:61–86.

[79]Rowley MJ, Cook AD, Mackay IR, Teuber SS, Gershwin ME. Comparative epitope mapping of antibodies to collagen in women with silicone breast implants, systemic lupus erythematosus and rheumatoid arthritis. *Curr Top Microbiol Immunol.* 1996;210:307–316.

[80]Teuber SS, Rowley MJ, Yoshida SH, Ansari AA, Gershwin ME. Anti-collagen autoantibodies are found in women with silicone breast implants. *J Autoimmun.* 1993;6:367–377.

[81]Rowley MJ, Cook AD, Teuber SS, Gershwin ME. Antibodies to collagen: Comparative epitope mapping in women with silicone breast implants, systemic lupus erythematosus and rheumatoid arthritis. *J Autoimmun.* 1994;7:775–789.

[82]Potter M, Morrison S, Miller F. Induction of plasmacytomas in genetically susceptible mice with silicone gels. *Curr Top Microbiol Immunol.* 1995;194:83–91.

[83]Potter M, Morrison S. Plasmacytoma development in mice injected with silicone gels. *Curr Top Microbiol Immunol.* 1996;210:397–407.

[84]Silverman S, Vescio R, Silver D, Renner S, Weiner S, Berenson J. Silicone gel implants and monoclonal gammopathies: Three cases of multiple myeloma and the prevalence of multiple myeloma and

monoclonal gammopathy of undetermined significance. *Curr Top Microbiol Immunol.* 1996;210:367–374.

[85]Rabkin CS, Silverman S, Tricot G, Garland LL, Ballester O, Potter M. The National Cancer Institute Silicone Implant/Multiple Myeloma Registry. *Curr Top Microbiol Immunol.* 1996;210:385–387.

[86]Garland LL, Ballester OF, Vasey FB, *et al.* Multiple myeloma in women with silicone breast implants. Serum immunoglobulin and interleukin-6 studies in women at risk. *Curr Top Microbiol Immunol.* 1996;210:361–366.

[87]Duvic M, Moore D, Menter A, Vonderheid EC. Cutaneous T-cell lymphoma in association with silicone breast implants. *J Am Acad Dermatol.* 1995;32:939–942.

[88]Cook PD, Osborne BM, Connor RL, Strauss JF. Follicular lymphoma adjacent to foreign body granulomatous inflammation and fibrosis surrounding silicone breast prosthesis. *Am J Surg Pathol.* 1995;19:712–717.

[89]Edelman DA, Grant S, van Os WA. Autoimmune disease following the use of silicone gel-filled breast implants: A review of the clinical literature. *Semin Arthritis Rheum.* 1994;24:183–189.

[90]Murakata LA, Rangwala AF. Silicone lymphadenopathy with concomitant malignant lymphoma. *J Rheumatol.* 1989;16:1480–1483.

[91]Rivero MA, Schwartz DS, Mies C. Silicone lymphadenopathy involving intramammary lymph nodes: A new complication of silicone mammaplasty. *AJR Am J Roentgenol.* 1994;162:1089–1090.

[92]Rogers LA, Longtine JA, Garnick MB, Pinkus GS. Silicone lymphadenopathy in a long distance runner: Complication of a silastic prosthesis. *Hum Pathol.* 1988;19:1237–1239.

[93]Lazaro MA, Garcia Morteo D, de Benyacar MA, *et al.* Lymphadenopathy secondary to silicone hand joint prostheses. *Clin Exp Rheumatol.* 1990;8:17–22.

[94]Matsuba T, Sujiura T, Irei M, *et al.* Acute pneumonitis presumed to be silicone embolism. *Intern Med.* 1994;33:481–483.

[95]Lai YF, Chao TY, Wong SL. Acute pneumonitis after subcutaneous injections of silicone for augmentation mammaplasty. *Chest.* 1994;106:1152–1155.

[96]Moser N, Hood C, Ervin D. Toxic shock syndrome in a patient using bilateral silicone nasal splints. *Otolaryngol Head Neck Surg.* 1995;113:632–633.

[97]Shoaib BO, Patten BM. Human adjuvant disease: Presentation as a multiple sclerosis-like syndrome. *South Med J.* 1996;89:179–188.

[98]Lu LB, Shoaib BO, Patten BM. Atypical chest pain syndrome in patients with breast implants. *South Med J.* 1994;87:978–984.

[99]Preiss G, Brunner P, Tulusan AH. Pulmonal silicone-embolism. Light microscopic, electron microscopic and enzymehistochemical investigations in the rabbit lung. *Virchows Arch A Pathol Anat.* 1977;373:55–65.

[100]Teuber SS, Howell LP, Yoshida SH, Gershwin ME. Remission of sarcoidosis following removal of silicone gel breast implant. *Int Arch Allergy Immunol.* 1994;105:404–407.

[101]Frey C, Naritoku W, Kerr R, Halikus N. Tarsal tunnel syndrome secondary to cosmetic silicone injections. *Foot Ankle.* 1993;14:407–410.

[102]Karlson EW, Sanchez-Guerrero J, Wright EA, *et al.* A connective tissue disease screening questionnaire for population studies. *Ann Epidemiol.* 1995;5:297–302.

14

Environmental Factors in Fibromyalgia and Chronic Fatigue Syndrome

Frederick Wolfe, Dean A. Pollina and Lauren B. Krupp

FIBROMYALGIA

Fibromyalgia is a disorder of decreased pain threshold and widespread pain. Associated characteristic symptoms include fatigue, sleep disturbance, morning stiffness, headaches, irritable bowel syndrome, paresthesia and, often, psychological distress (Table 14-1). The syndrome is 10 times more common in women than men, and has a peak age of about 50 years of age.[1] Fibromyalgia is diagnosed when most of the symptoms and physical findings listed above are identified. Increasingly, the American College of Rheumatology (ACR) 1990 Criteria for the Classification of Fibromyalgia[3] are applied in diagnosis. The ACR criteria are satisfied when the patient has widespread pain and reports pain on palpation in 11 of 18 specified tender-point sites.

Geographic Distribution and Societal Factors

Fibromyalgia is a common disorder in industrialized societies, where its prevalence is estimated at 1% to 4.5% of the adult population.[1-4] Less developed forms of the syndrome have been observed in nonindustrialized communities. In one study of 1102 persons in a rural South African community, few subjects complained of widespread pain, although in 3.2% tender points were found.[5] In another study, no persons were identified satisfying the tender-point criterion among a population of Pima Indians.[6]

Psychosocial Factors

Fibromyalgia occurs more commonly among smokers, obese individuals, those who have been divorced and those who do not complete formal education.[1] Individuals with the syndrome report increased rates of childhood sexual abuse[7,8] and come from families where alcoholism is common.[9] These observations suggest that psychosocial disruption and stress may be factors leading to the development of the syndrome. Further evidence in support of a role for psychosocial factors comes from a series of studies identifying current and previous depression in patients with fibromyalgia.[10-15]

Effect of Climate and Daylight

Certain aspects of fibromyalgia suggest that some patients might have seasonal affective disorders (SAD). In this condition, depression occurs in the dark months, is associated with carbohydrate craving, and remits in light months. Moldofsky studied fibromyalgia patients, patients with RA, and controls, using a SAD questionnaire.[16] Those with fibromyalgia reported feeling worse in the dark winter months and best during long days of the lighter months. Forty-three percent of fibromyalgia patients rated mood impairment equivalent to seasonal affective disorder, compared with 25% of controls and 16% of RA patients. Hawley and Wolfe, however, studied the pain and depression scores in fibromyalgia patients during paired light- and dark-month clinic visits.[17] No discernible differences were noted in depression and pain related to season in patients with fibromyalgia, depressed patients with fibromyalgia, or in patients with other rheumatic disorders.

Environmental Disturbances of Sleep

More than two decades ago, Moldofsky showed that patients with fibromyalgia had disturbed Stage IV non-REM sleep.[18-20] This observation has been confirmed by others[21] but is not specific for fibromyalgia and may occur in a number of medical conditions.[22-27] Moldofsky also showed that disruption of sleep in healthy volunteers was associated with the development or increase of musculoskeletal symptoms.[19] In addition, clinical sleep abnormalities ("poor sleep" or awakening "unrefreshed") is a complaint found in more than

Table 14-1 Prevalence of pain and symptoms in the 1990 American College of Rheumatology study of criteria for the classification of fibromyalgia

Criterion	% Positive	Classification Accuracy
Pain Symptoms		
Pain posterior thorax	72.3	73.9
15+ painful sites	55.6	70.6
Neck pain	85.3	67.5
Low back pain	78.8	66.6
Widespread pain	97.6	65.9
Symptoms		
Sleep disturbance	74.6	73.8
"Pain all over"	67.0	73.6
Fatigue	81.4	71.7
Morning stiffness >15 minutes	77.0	67.2
Paresthesias	62.8	63.6
Anxiety	47.8	62.9
Headache	52.8	62.3
Prior depression	31.5	58.0
Irritable bowel syndrome	29.6	57.1
Sicca symptoms	35.8	55.4
Urinary urgency	26.3	54.2
Dysmenorrhea history	40.6	53.4
Raynaud phenomenon	16.7	51.6
Modulating Factors		
Noise	24.0	68.5
Cold	79.3	66.6
Poor sleep	76.0	65.2
Anxiety	69.0	63.7
Humidity	59.6	63.6
Stress	63.0	60.4
Fatigue	76.7	60.3
Weather change	66.1	60.3
Warmth	78.0	50.8

Modified from Wolfe *et al.*[28] with permission.

75% of fibromyalgia patients.[28] A frequent anecdotal observation is that mothers with sick children or women with seriously ill family members, whose sleep is interrupted or must be "light," develop symptoms of fibromyalgia. Furthermore, there have been a few reports of the association of sleep apnea with fibromyalgia.[29,30] Persons living in areas of high environmental noise (airports, train stations, and so on) or those working alternating shift jobs could offer the ability to test the hypothesis that interference with sleep produces fibromyalgia. There are not enough data to establish if these or other sleep-disrupting factors are associated with the development of fibromyalgia.

Estrogen Abnormalities

It has been suggested that estrogen deprivation might predispose to the development of fibromyalgia.[31] Other evidence does not support such a hypothesis. Pain thresholds are lower in women than men regardless of menopausal status.[10,32–34] In addition, there are no studies of hormonal replacement in fibromyalgia, but anecdotal evidence does not suggest a favorable effect.

Allergies and Allergens

The prevalence of allergies is reported to be increased in fibromyalgia,[35] although there is no specific allergen or pattern of allergies. The striking number of allergic complaints among these individuals may be a reflection of the general increase in symptom reporting, or what has been referred to as the "irritable everything syndrome."[36]

Viruses

Fibromyalgia is sometimes reported to begin abruptly following a viral-like illness.[37] In an open-ended questionnaire, a postviral onset was elicited in 10%. When patients were asked directly: "Did your illness begin with a viral syndrome or an upper respiratory infection?" the rate increased to 55%.[37] However, no viral association with fibromyalgia has been demonstrated.[37–40]

Trauma and Fibromyalgia

Trauma through "overuse" or "repetitive strain" to a body region has been reported to be associated with fibromyalgia.[41] The reported prevalence of trauma as an initiating event has ranged from 11% to 24%. Although the association of trauma and fibromyalgia is a contentious medicolegal issue, no formal studies have examined this relationship.[42–54]

In the most common situation, the claimant is involved in a motor vehicle accident (MVA). Diffuse musculoskeletal complaints, medical testing and intervention follow, and fibromyalgia is subsequently diagnosed. In a second, common evolution, fibromyalgia develops following a local injury. This injury may be a tendonitis, a local "myofascial pain syndrome," an upper-extremity injury or "repetitive strain."[65,66] Although most such conditions resolve, a few continue and become more generalized. Table 14-2 describes a common set of findings associated with postinjury fibromyalgia.[43]

Several possible mechanisms have been suggested by which injuries might result in fibromyalgia. Changes within the central nervous system following injury (CNS plasticity)[55,56] could account for several of the clinical features. Support for this hypothesis comes from animal models wherein loose ligation of the sciatic nerve reproduces many of the manifestations of fibromyalgia including hyperalgesia, allodynia, spontaneous pain and dysesthesia.[57] Coderre

Table 14-2 Characteristic features of postinjury fibromyalgia

1. There is a discrete injury.
2. Pain spreads beyond the site of injury in a stepwise pattern.
3. Headache, bowel symptoms, paresthesias, sleep disturbance subsequently develop as the pain spreads.
4. There is allodynia, hyperesthesia and referred pain.
5. Pain threshold is decreased, but more so over initial pain
6. Pain is worsened by activities.
7. Conventional therapies (physical therapy, NSAIDs, analgesics) are of limited benefit.

and coworkers[56] noted that following tissue injury CNS sensitization occurs, leading to reduced thresholds and/or increased responsivity to afferent inputs, and prolonged after-discharges to repeated stimulation. Tissue injury is also associated with expansion of the peripheral receptive field of dorsal horn neurons. Such data from animal studies have possible relevance to fibromyalgia. Spreading hyperesthesia, allodynia and painful dysesthesia could be explained by changes in the CNS. In addition, prolonged after-discharges noted experimentally may have relevance to the postactivity increase in pain noted by those with fibromyalgia.[43]

In an alternate model implicating psychological and psychosocial factors, a relatively minor trauma is the trigger for a series of symptoms characteristic of fibromyalgia. The difficulties inherent in the adjudication of the fibromyalgia—trauma interaction have been summarized in a recent consensus report.[58]

Overall, then, data from the literature are insufficient to establish a causal relationship between trauma and fibromyalgia. The absence of evidence, however, does not mean that causality does not exist, but instead that appropriate studies have not been performed.

THE CHRONIC FATIGUE SYNDROME

Chronic fatigue syndrome (CFS) is a poorly understood illness that has been the subject of much controversy in the lay and medical community. It is characterized by subjective feelings of discomfort without a known etiology or consistent immunological, psychiatric or neuropsychological findings.

Defining CFS

The current definition for CFS used in the United States evolved from one initially designed for research purposes[59] to less restrictive criteria.[60] Both the original and current definitions define CFS as a condition of severe fatigue present for at least six months and not explained by other medical disorders. In 1992 the National Institutes of Health recommended modifications[61] which required that patients with specific psychiatric diagnoses postinfectious fatigue syndromes be excluded, while patients with selected confounding diagnoses be included.[62–65] This acknowledged that certain psychiatric disorders, as well as the fibromyalgia syndrome, overlap with CFS.[66] It was suggested that CFS patients with confounding diagnoses be stratified and analyzed separately for research purposes.[61] It was also recommended that the evaluation for CFS include tender-point examination[67] and routine screening for psychiatric distress (using a General Health questionnaire or a combination of self-report instruments).

In 1994 further changes simplified classification of fatigued patients who did or did not fulfill CFS criteria.[60] The recommended guidelines also further clarified the relationship between CFS and psychological disturbance. The current defining inclusion and exclusion criteria are as follows:

Inclusion criteria:

1) The fatigue must be of new onset (not be a lifelong problem), not be due to ongoing exertion, not be alleviated by rest, and result in substantial reduction of previous occupational, educational, social or personal activities. It is advised that the levels of fatigue are measured with a self-report instrument which assesses performance and subjective aspects.

2) There must be four or more of the following symptoms, all of which must have persisted or recurred during six or more consecutive months of illness and must not have predated the fatigue:

a) memory or concentration problems severe enough to interfere with day-to-day functioning;

b) sore throat;

c) tender cervical or axillary lymph nodes;

d) muscle pain;

e) polyarticular pain without joint swelling or redness;

f) headaches of a new type;

g) unrefreshing sleep;

h) postexertional malaise lasting more than 24 hours.

Specific exclusions:

1) Active medical disorders which can cause fatigue (such as untreated hypothyroidism, sleep apnea, medication side effects);

2) Incomplete resolution of past disorders which may cause chronic fatigue (treated malignancy, unresolved hepatitis B or C virus infection);

3) Past or current major depressive disorder with psychotic or melancholic features, bipolar affective disorders, schizophrenia of any subtype, delusional disorders of any subtype, dementias of any subtype, anorexia nervosa or bulimia nervosa;

4) Alcohol or substance abuse within two years before the onset of chronic fatigue and at any time thereafter.

Individuals who may be classified as CFS despite the presence of concurrent problems include those with:

1) Fibromyalgia;

2) Postinfectious fatigue:

a) Lyme disease with persistent fatigue after appropriate antibiotic therapy;

b) brucellosis with persistent fatigue after appropriate antibiotic therapy;

c) acute infectious mononucleosis (documented) followed by chronic debilitating fatigue;

d) acute cytomegalovirus infection;

e) acute toxoplasmosis (adequately treated).

3) Nonpsychotic and nonmelancholic depression;

4) Somatoform disorders;

5) Generalized anxiety disorder/panic disorder.

Epidemiology

Epidemiologic studies of fatigue suggest that there is a continuous spectrum of healthy normal fatigue at one extreme and the severe fatigue of CFS at the other.[68] The prevalence of CFS is significantly lower than the prevalence of prolonged fatigue not meeting full CFS criteria.[69]

Etiologies

Neuroimmune Features

The etiology of CFS was first considered to be viral infection. It subsequently became apparent that elevated antibody titers to a variety of viral agents were present in CFS patients, including antibodies to herpes virus, cytomegalovirus and measles virus. No single virus has been identified as the cause of CFS, and many individual agents have been excluded as an etiology, including retrovirus, human herpes virus-6, enterovirus and spumavirus.[70–73] Epstein Barr virus titers have no bearing on disease course, clinical presentation or laboratory abnormalities and do not distinguish CFS patients from healthy controls.[74] Despite the lack of a direct link between a specific viral agent and CFS, the finding of increased antibodies to a variety of viruses suggests that a generalized immunologic dysfunction might accompany CFS.[75]

Psychiatric Features

CFS has been associated with subjective reports of disturbances in multiple organs. The presence of these symptoms without objective laboratory evidence has suggested to some scientists and clinicians that these disorders should be classified as psychiatric illnesses.[76–78] Estimates of the frequency of current psychiatric illness in CFS range from 21% to 45% and are as high as 52% to 86% for lifetime psychiatric illness.[62–64,79,80] Depressions and/or somatization disorder are the most common psychiatric findings.[64,81] Many symptoms of the CFS are similar to those of anxiety and related disorders (for example, fatigue, tachycardia, dizziness).

Neurophysiological Findings

It has been proposed that hypothalamic-pituitary-adrenal (HPA) axis dysfunction might be responsible for both the physical and psychological symptoms of CFS.[82–84] Some investigators have suggested that a mild reduction in the adrenals' response to stress might contribute to the CFS disorder by causing a cortisol deficiency.[84] Hypothalamic dysfunction could explain many of the symptoms of CFS, including fatigue, appetite changes and fever. In one study, CFS patients demonstrated significant reductions in urinary free cortisol excretion and plasma glucocorticoid levels.[82] It has been speculated that the hypothalamic defect causes these observed cortisol reductions and might also promote enhanced antibody titers to viral antigens. Additional biologic hypotheses of the CFS disorder include a central motor control abnormality[85–87] and neurally mediated hypotension.[88,89]

Neuropsychological Findings

The results of neuropsychological testing indicate that CFS patients may have some mild memory impairment as well as possible deficits in the speed of information processing.[80,90–92] Mild memory disturbance has been associated with conceptual tasks involving encoding and retrieval.[91] Memory problems are not associated with specific measures of disease activity, laboratory abnormalities or physical findings, but have been associated with depressive symptoms.[80] A consistent behavioral finding in CFS is increased mean length of reaction time.[90,93] These reaction time changes occur across a relatively wide range of tasks requiring attention and mental speed.[91–94]

REFERENCES

[1] Wolfe F, Ross K, Anderson J, Russell IJ, Hebert L. The prevalence and characteristics of fibromyalgia in the general population. *Arthritis Rheum.* 1995;38:19–28.

[2] Croft P, Schollum J, Silman A. Population study of tender point counts and pain as evidence of fibromyalgia. *Br Med J.* 1994;309: 696–699.

[3]Schochat T, Croft P, Raspe H. The epidemiology of fibromyalgia—workshop of the Standing Committee on Epidemiology European League Against Rheumatism (EULAR), Bad-Sackingen, 19–21 November 1992. *Brit J Rheumatol.* 1994;33:783–786.

[4]Wolfe F. Aspects of the epidemiology of fibromyalgia. *J Musc Pain.* 1994;2:65–74.

[5]Lyddell C. The prevalence of fibromyalgia in a South African community. *Scand J Rheumatol.* 1992;94[Suppl]:S143(abstract).

[6]Jacobson L. Tender points are not found in Pima Indians. 1995;(abstract).

[7]Hudson JI, Pope HG Jr. Does childhood sexual abuse cause fibromyalgia? [editorial]. *Arthritis Rheum.* 1996;38:161–163 (abstract).

[8]Boisset-Pioro M, Esdaile JM, Fitzcharles MA. Sexual and physical abuse in women with fibromyalgia syndrome. *Arthritis Rheum.* 1996;38:235–241(abstract).

[9]Katz RS, Kravitz HM. Fibromyalgia, depression, and alcoholism: A family history study. *J Rheumatol.* 1996;23:149–154(abstract).

[10]Wolfe F, Ross K, Anderson J, Russell IJ. Aspects of fibromyalgia in the general population: Sex, pain threshold, and fibromyalgia symptoms. *J Rheumatol.* 1995;22:151–156.

[11]Buckelew SP, Parker JC, Keefe FJ, *et al.* Self-efficacy and pain behavior among subjects with fibromyalgia. *Pain.* 1994;59:377–384.

[12]Hudson JI, Pope HG. The concept of affective spectrum disorder: Relationship to fibromyalgia and other syndromes of chronic fatigue and chronic muscle pain. *Bailliere Clin Rheumatol.* 1994;8:839–856.

[13]Hawley DJ, Wolfe F. Depression is not more common in rheumatoid arthritis: A 10-year longitudinal study of 6,608 rheumatic disease patients. *J Rheumatol.* 1993;20:2025–2031.

[14]Wolfe F, Hawley DJ. Fibromyalgia. In: Kelley WN, Harris EDJ, Ruddy S, Sledge CB, eds. *Textbook of Rheumatology (Supplement).* 1993.

[15]Hudson JI, Goldenberg DL, Pope HGJ, Keck PEJ, Schlesinger L. Comorbidity of fibromyalgia with medical and psychiatric disorders. *Am J Med.* 1992;92:363–367.

[16]Moldofsky H. Chronobiological influences on fibromyalgia syndrome: Theoretical and therapeutic implications. *Bailliere Clin Rheumatol.* 1994;8:801–810.

[17]Hawley DJ, Wolfe F. Effect of light and season on pain and depression in subjects with rheumatic disorders. *Pain.* 1994;59:227–234.

[18]Smythe HA, Moldofsky H. Two contributions to understanding of the "fibrositis" syndrome. *Bull Rheum Dis.* 1977;28:928–931.

[19]Moldofsky H, Scarisbrick P. Induction of neurasthenic musculoskeletal pain syndrome by selective sleep stage deprivation. *Psychosom Med.* 1976;38:35–44.

[20]Moldofsky H, Scarisbrick P, England R, Smythe HA. Musculoskeletal symptoms and non-REM sleep disturbance in patients with "fibrositis syndrome" and healthy subjects. *Psychosom Med.* 1975;37:341–351.

[21]Drewes AM, Nielsen KD, Taagholt SJ, Bjerregard K, Svendsen L, Gade J. Sleep intensity in fibromyalgia: Focus on the microstructure of the sleep process. *Brit J Rheumatol.* 1995;34:629–635.

[22]Trojan DA, Cashman NR. Fibromyalgia is common in a postpoliomyelitis clinic. *Arch Neurol.* 1995;52:620–624.

[23]Hirsch M, Carlander B, Verge M, *et al.* Objective and subjective sleep disturbances in patients with rheumatoid arthritis—a reappraisal. *Arthritis Rheum.* 1994;37:41–49.

[24]Doherty M, Smith J. Elusive alpha-delta sleep in fibromyalgia and osteoarthritis. *Ann Rheum Dis.* 1993;52:245.

[25]Gudbjornsson B, Broman JE, Hetta J, Hallgren R. Sleep disturbances in patients with primary Sjögren's syndrome. *Brit J Rheumatol.* 1993;32:1072–1076.

[26]Moldofsky H. Sleep influences on regional and diffuse pain syndromes associated with osteoarthritis. *Semin Arthritis Rheum.* 1989;18:18–21.

[27]Moldofsky H. Nonrestorative sleep and symptoms after a febrile illness in patients with fibrositis and chronic fatigue syndromes. *J Rheumatol.* 1989;19[Suppl]:150–153.

[28]Wolfe F, Smythe HA, Yunus MB, *et al.* The American College of Rheumatology 1990 criteria for the classification of fibromyalgia: report of the Multicenter Criteria Committee. *Arthritis Rheum.* 1990;33:160–172.

[29]Molony RR, MacPeek DM, Schiffman PL, *et al.* Sleep, sleep apnea and the fibromyalgia syndrome. *J Rheumatol.* 1986;13:797–800.

[30]May KP, West SG, Baker MR, Everett DW. Sleep apnea in male patients with the fibromyalgia syndrome. *Am J Med.* 1993;94:505–508.

[31]Waxman J, Zatzkis SM. Fibromyalgia and menopause. Examination of the relationship. *Postgrad Med.* 1986;80:165–167,170–171.

[32]Scudds RA, Rollman GB, Harth M, McCain GA. Pain perception and personality measures as discriminators in the classification of fibrositis. *J Rheumatol.* 1987;14:563–569.

[33]Wolfe F, Ross K, Anderson J, Russell IJ. Aspects of fibromyalgia in the general population: Sex, pain threshold, and fibromyalgia symptoms. *J Rheumatol.* 1995;22:151–156.

[34]Tunks E, Crook J, Norman G, Kalaher S. Tender points in fibromyalgia. *Pain.* 1988;34:11–19.

[35]Cleveland CH Jr, Fisher RH, Brestel EP, Esinhart JD, Metzger WJ. Chronic rhinitis: An underrecognized association with fibromyalgia. *Allergy Proc.* 1992;13:263–267.

[36]Caro XJ, Kinsted NA, Russell IJ, Wolfe F. Increased sensitivity of health related questions with primary fibrositis syndrome. *Arthritis Rheum.* 1987;30:S63(abstract).

[37]Goldenberg DL. Fibromyalgia and other chronic fatigue syndromes: Is there evidence for chronic viral disease. *Semin Arthritis Rheum.* 1988;18:111–120.

[38]Buchwald D, Goldenberg DL, Sullivan JL, Komaroff AL. The "chronic, active Epstein-Barr virus infection" syndrome and primary fibromyalgia. *Arthritis Rheum.* 1987;30:1132–1136.

[39]Goldenberg DL. Fibromyalgia and its relation to chronic fatigue syndrome, viral illness and immune abnormalities. *J Rheumatol.* 1989;19[Suppl]:91–93.

[40]Berg AM, Naides SJ, Simms RW. Established fibromyalgia syndrome and parvovirus B19 infection. *J Rheumatol.* 1993;20:1941–1943.

[41]Wolfe F. The clinical syndrome of fibrositis. *Am J Med.* 1986;81:7–14.

[42]Greenfield S, Fitzcharles MA, Esdaile JM. Reactive fibromyalgia syndrome. *Arthritis Rheum.* 1992;35:678–681.

[43]Waylonis GW, Perkins RH. Post-traumatic fibromyalgia: A long-term follow-up. *Amer J Phys Med Rehabil.* 1994;73:403–412.

[44]Wolfe F. Post-traumatic fibromyalgia: A case report narrated by the patient. *Arthritis Care Res.* 1994;7:161–165.

[45]Bennett RM. Disabling fibromyalgia: Appearance versus reality (editorial). *J Rheumatol.* 1993;11:1821.

[46]Bruusgaard D, Evensen AR, Bjerkedal T. Fibromyalgia—a new cause for disability pension. *Scand J Soc Med.* 1993;21:116–119.

[47]Moldofsky H, Wong MTH, Lue FA. Litigation, sleep, symptoms and disabilities in postaccident pain (fibromyalgia). *J Rheumatol.* 1993;20:1935–1940.

[48]Reilly PA. Fibromyalgia in the workplace—a management problem. *Ann Rheum Dis.* 1993;52:249–251.

[49]Wolfe F. Disability and the dimensions of distress in fibromyalgia. *J Musc Pain.* 1993;1:65–88.

[50]Whorton D, Weisenberger BI, Milroy WC, *et al.* Does fibromyalgia qualify as a work-related illness or injury. *J Occup Med.* 1992;34:968.

[51]Littlejohn GO. Medicolegal aspects of fibrositis syndrome. *J Rheumatol.* 1989;19[Suppl]:169–173.

[52]Littlejohn GO. Fibrositis/fibromyalgia syndrome in the workplace. *Rheum Dis Clin North Am.* 1989;15:45–60.

[53]McCain GA, Cameron R, Kennedy JC. The problem of longterm disability payments and litigation in primary fibromyalgia: the Canadian perspective. *J Rheumatol.* 1989;19[Suppl]:174–176.

[54]Saskin P, Moldofsky H, Lue FA. Sleep and posttraumatic rheumatic pain modulation disorder (fibrositis syndrome). *Psychosom Med.* 1986;48:319–323.

[55]Dubner R. Neuronal plasticity and pain following peripheral tissue inflammation or nerve injury. In: Bond MR, Charlton JE, Woolf CJ, eds. *Proceedings of the Fifth World Congress on Pain.* New York: Elsevier Science, 1991;263–276.

[56]Coderre TJ, Katz J, Vaccarino AL, Melzack R. Contribution of central neuroplasticity to pathologic pain: Review of clinical and experimental evidence. *Pain.* 1993;52:259–285.

[57]Bennett GJ, Xie Y-K. Peripheral mononeuropathy in rat that produces disorders of pain sensation like those seen in man. *Pain.* 1988;33:87–107.

[58]Wolfe F, Vancouver Fibromyalgia Consensus Group. The fibromyalgia syndrome: A consensus report on fibromyalgia and disability. *J Rheumatol.* 1996;(in press).

[59]Holmes GP, Kaplan JE, Gantz NM, *et al.* Chronic fatigue syndrome: A working case definition. *Ann Intern Med.* 1988;108:387–389.

[60]Fuduka K, Straus SE, Hickie I, Sharpe MC, Dobbins JG, Komaroff A. The chronic fatigue syndrome: A comprehensive approach to its definition and study. *Ann Intern Med.* 1994;121:953–959.

[61]Schluederberg A, Strauss SE, Peterson P, *et al.* NIH conference chronic fatigue syndrome research. Definition and medical outcome assessment. *Ann Intern Med.* 1992;117:325–331.

[62]Hickey I, Lloyd A, Wakefield D, Parker G. The psychiatric status of patients with the CFS. *Br J Psychiatry.* 1990;156:534–540.

[63]Lane TJ, Manu P, Matthews DA. Depression and somatization in the CFS. *Am J Med.* 1991;91:335–344.

[64]Manu P, Matthews DA, Lane TJ. The mental health of patients with a chief complaint of chronic fatigue. *Arch Intern Med.* 1988;148:2213–2217.

[65]Manu P, Matthews DA, Lane TJ. Panic disorder among patients with chronic fatigue. *South Med J.* 1991;84:451–456.

[66]Goldenberg DL, Simms RW, Geiger A, Komaroff AL. High frequency of fibromyalgia in patients with chronic fatigue seen in a primary care practice. *Arthritis Rheum.* 1990;33:381–387.

[67]Wolfe F, Smythe HA, Yunus MB, *et al.* The American College of Rheumatology 1990 criteria for the classification of fibromyalgia: Report of the Multicenter Criteria Committee. *Arthritis Rheum.* 1990;33:60–72.

[68]Lewis G, Wessely S. The epidemiology of fatigue: More questions than answers. *J Epidem Comm Health.* 1992;46:92–97.

[69]Buchwald D, Umali P, Umali J, Kith P, Pearlman T, Komaroff A. Chronic fatigue and the chronic fatigue syndrome: Prevalence in a Pacific Northwest health care system. *Ann Intern Med.* 1995;123:81–88.

[70]Dale JK, Di Bisceglie AM, Hoofnagle JH, *et al.* Chronic fatigue syndrome: Lack of association with hepatitis C virus infection. *J Med Virol.* 1991;34:119–121.

[71]Bode L, Komaroff AL, Ludwig N. No serologic evidence of Borna disease virus in patients with CFS. *Clin Infect Dis.* 1992;15:1049–1012.

[72]Komaroff AL, Wang SP, Lee J, Grayston JT. No association of chronic chlamydia pneumoniae infection with CFS. *J Infect Dis.* 1992;165:184.

[73]Khan AS, Heneine WM, Chapman LE, *et al.* Assessment of a retrovirus sequence and other possible risk factors for the chronic fatigue syndrome in adults. *Ann Intern Med.* 1993;118:241–245.

[74]Helinger WC, Smith TF, Van Scoy RE, *et al.* Chronic fatigue syndrome and the diagnostic utility of antibody to Epstein-Barr virus early antigen. *JAMA.* 1988;260:971–973.

[75]Klimas NG, Salvato FR, Morgan R, Fletcher MA. Immunologic abnormalities in CFS. *J Clin Microbiol.* 1991;28:1403–1410.

[76]Salvaggio JE. Psychological aspects of "environmental illness," "multiple chemical sensitivity," and building-related illness. *J Allergy Clin Immunol.* 1994;94:366–370.

[77]Abbey SE, Garfinkel PE. Chronic fatigue syndrome and the psychiatrist. *Can J Psychiatry.* 1990;35:625–633.

[78]Abbey SE, Garfinkel PE. Chronic fatigue syndrome and depression: Cause, effect or covariate. *Rev Infect Dis.* 1991;13(Suppl 1):S73–S83.

[79]Pepper C, Krupp LB, Friedberg F, *et al.* Comparison of psychiatric characteristics in chronic fatigue syndrome, multiple sclerosis, and depression. *J Neuropsychiatry Clin Neurosci.* 1993;5:1–7.

[80]Krupp LB, Sliwinski M, Masur D, Friedberg F, Coyle PK. Cognitive functioning and depression in patients with chronic fatigue syndrome and multiple sclerosis. *Arch Neurol.* 1994;51:705–710.

[81]Black DW, Rathe A, Goldstein RB. Measures of distress in 26 "environmentally ill" subjects. *Psychosomatics.* 1993;34:131–138.

[82]Demitrack MA, Dale JK, Straus SE, *et al.* Evidence for impaired activation of the hypothalamic-pituitary-adrenal axis in patients with CFS. *J Clin Endocrinol Metab.* 1991;73:1224–1234.

[83]Demitrack MA. Chronic fatigue syndrome: A disease of the hypo-thalamic-pituitary-adrenal axis? *Ann Med.* 1994;26:1–5.

[84]Jefferies W. Mild adrenocortical deficiency, chronic allergies, autoimmune disorders and the chronic fatigue syndrome: A continuation of the cortisone story. *Med Hypoth.* 1992;42:183–189.

[85]Rutherford OM, White PD. Human quadriceps strength and fatigability in patients with post viral fatigue. *J Neurol Neurosurg Psychiatry.* 1991;54:961–964.

[86]Scheffers MK, Johnson R Jr, Grafman J, *et al.* Attention and short-term memory in CFS patients. *Neurology.* 1992;42:1667–1675.

[87]Stokes MJ, Cooper RG, Edwards RT. Normal muscle strength and fatigability in patients with effort syndromes. *Br Med J.* 1988;297:1014–1017.

[88]Bou-Holaigah I, Rowe PC, Kan J, Calkins H. The relationship between neurally mediated hypotension and the chronic fatigue syndrome. *JAMA.* 1995;274:961–967.

[89]Sisto SA, Tapp W, Drastal S, *et al.* Vagal tone is reduced during paced breathing in patients with the chronic fatigue syndrome. *Clin Autonom Res.* 1995;5:139–143.

[90]DeLuca J, Johnson SK, Beldowicz D, *et al.* Neuropsychological impairments in chronic fatigue syndrome, multiple sclerosis, and depression. *J Neurol Neurosurg Psychiatry.* 1995;58:38–43.

[91]Grafman J, Schwartz V, Dale JK, Scheffers M, Houser C, Straus SE. Analysis of neuropsychological functioning in patients with chronic fatigue syndrome. *J Neurol Neurosurg Psychiatry.* 1993;56:684–689.

[92]McDonald E, Cope H, David A. Cognitive impairment in patients with chronic fatigue: A preliminary study. *J Neurol Neurosurg Psychiatry.* 1993;56:812–815.

[93]Ray C, Phillips L, Weir W. Quality of attention in chronic fatigue syndrome: Subjective reports of everyday attention and cognitive difficulty, and performance on tasks of focused attention. *J Clin Psychol.* 1993;32:357–364.

[94]Schmaling KB, DiClementi JD, Cullum CM, *et al.* Cognitive functioning in chronic fatigue syndrome and depression: A preliminary comparison. *Psychosomat Med.* 1994;56:383–388.

15

The Multiple Chemical Sensitivity Syndrome

Mark R. Cullen

INTRODUCTION

During the 1980s an apparently new syndrome was described whose hallmark is clinical intolerance to low levels of man-made chemicals. Although there is not yet a widely accepted definition or designation, the disorder is easily recognized, especially when it occurs in patients following an episode of overexposure to chemicals such as solvents or pesticides. Instead of recovering, patients begin to complain that commonplace environmental contaminants in air, food or water elicit symptoms at doses far below those which usually induce toxic reactions. These symptoms typically include central nervous system complaints such as fatigue, dizziness or cognitive problems, and often have an associated musculoskeletal component. Characteristically the symptoms are not associated with objective impairment of the organs to which they are referable, but both the complaints and their pattern of occurrence may be impressive, with resulting dysfunction and disability.

Although this type of adverse response to chemicals and odors is probably not new, most clinicians who treat patients with occupational and environmental health problems have the impression that multiple chemical sensitivities (MCS) is occurring more frequently than in the past.[1] While little is known about its pattern of occurrence, it has become prevalent enough to have attracted clinicians specializing in its diagnosis and treatment—clinical ecologists or environmental physicians—and has created controversy among medical associations, specialty groups, insurance carriers and policy makers. Despite intense debate over who should treat patients suffering with the disorder and who should pay, research has not yet clarified the cause or pathogenesis of the disease, and strategies for treatment and prevention of MCS remain empiric.

Notwithstanding limited knowledge, MCS is probably distinctive enough as a clinical problem to merit separate consideration, especially in view of the morbidity of the disorder. It is the goal of this chapter to elucidate what is known about MCS, with particular attention to the rheumatologic features, and offer strategies for evaluation and management based on the best available information.

DEFINITION AND DIAGNOSIS

There is no consensus on the definition of MCS. Certain features allow differentiation from other clinical entities[2-3]:

1) Symptoms appear after the occurrence of an occupational or environmental illness such as a systemic chemical intoxication or an injury to upper or lower respiratory tract mucosa. This "initiating" event may be one episode, such as a smoke inhalation, or repeated insults, such as indoor air pollution or solvent overexposure. These episodes may be severe or very mild, but are typically significant enough in the experience of the patient to prompt medical attention.

2) Symptoms, often similar to those of the precipitating illness, begin to occur when the patient is exposed to various "triggering" odors or chemicals, often at low levels which are far below those usually associated with clinical effects.

3) Generalization of symptoms occurs such that multiple organ-system complaints are involved. Central nervous system symptoms (for example, fatigue, headache, dizziness, cognitive difficulties) are always prominent. Other systems symptomatically affected may include the respiratory tract (throat constriction, dyspnea, chest tightness), GI tract (abdominal pain, altered bowel habit, food intolerances), skin and cardiovascular system (palpitations, chest pain). Rheumatologic complaints are relatively common, and will be described in greater detail below. Importantly, these symptoms may occur only after chemical exposures perceived by the patient, or may be chronic and persistent, exacerbated by triggering exposures.

4) Evaluation reveals minimal or no objective impairment of organs which would explain the pattern or intensity of complaints.

5) Psychosis or organic disease which could explain the multiorgan symptoms is excluded.

While clinical patterns are variable, and not every patient displays each of these features, it is very important to consider all of the criteria before classifying a patient as having MCS. Each criterion serves to rule out other disorders with which MCS may be confused: somatization disorder, sensitization to environmental antigens (for example, occupational asthma), chronic sequelae of organ system damage (for example, bronchiolitis obliterans) or a masquerading systemic disease (for example, vasculitis or connective tissue disease). On the other hand, MCS is not a diagnosis of exclusion, and extensive tests, which often accentuate patient fears and illness perception, are unnecessary in most cases. While many variations are seen, MCS actually has an unmistakable character which usually allows prompt recognition.

In practice, the most difficult diagnostic problems with MCS fall into two categories. In the early stages of the disorder, it is often difficult to distinguish MCS from the occupational or environmental health problem which typically precedes it. For example, patients who have experienced organic solvent toxicity may find that their reactions continue after they have been removed from high-exposure areas or when these exposures have been controlled. Failing to appreciate that a complication has occurred, clinicians may assume that high exposures are still occurring and try to control them, an admirable but unhelpful approach. This is especially troublesome in the office setting, where MCS may be seen as a complication of the so-called sick building syndrome. Whereas most office workers will respond to efforts which improve indoor air quality, the patient who has acquired MCS will continue to have problems despite the modifications. Efforts to further improve the air quality will likely frustrate patient and employer alike.

Later, the MCS patient may become depressed or anxious, as do patients with other chronic diseases. Combined with other features of the disease which already suggest a possible nonorganic basis, clinicians may inappropriately focus primarily on psychiatric aspects.

RHEUMATOLOGIC MANIFESTATIONS OF MCS

Although musculoskeletal complaints are very common among MCS patients, there are no case series from which to derive an estimated prevalence. In as many as 10%, these complaints may dominate the clinical profile.

Neither complaints nor physical findings are specific. The most widely appreciated pattern closely overlaps fibromyalgia, with diffuse tenderness over major muscle groups of the upper torso and trunk; trigger points are often definable, and some patients will have overlapping findings for fibromyalgia. Pain and periarticular swelling, usually around large weight-bearing joints, are frequent complaints, but are not typically associated with physical signs of tenderness or edema at the sites in question. Complaints are often described as migratory, developing in association with other symptoms after triggering exposures. Arthritis or anatomically defined tenosynovial changes cannot be attributed to MCS *per se,* although the author has treated patients with inflammatory arthritis who attribute fluctuations in their arthritis to environmental exposures or avoidance. Objective abnormalities should prompt a search for an alternative or additional diagnosis to MCS.

LABORATORY TESTS

As with other organ systems in MCS, the laboratory is no more helpful in defining the musculoskeletal problems in these patients than the physical examination. Radiographs are normal, as is the erythrocyte sedimentation rate. Serologic tests for antinuclear antibodies and rheumatoid factor are negative.

Nevertheless, some reports suggest that various laboratory abnormalities in MCS patients support the diagnosis. Several authors have described high rates of nonspecific autoantibodies among these patients,[4] including low-titer antinuclear antibodies and antithyroid antibodies. Antibodies against myelin or ubiquitous low-molecular-weight compounds such as formaldehyde have been described,[5–7] but the reliability of laboratory techniques demonstrating such abnormalities have been challenged.

Tests of neurologic dysfunction have also been suggested as useful in evaluating patients with MCS. Anecdotal reports indicate abnormalities on SPECT and PET scanning of the central nervous system,[8–10] but adequate control data have not yet been presented. A growing literature has shown mild decrements on standardized neuropsychological testing protocols, though the most pervasive abnormalities have been in psychological function rather than actual cognitive performance.[11,12] There is no indication for the use of the nuclear scans in the evaluation of MCS patients outside well-defined research protocols. On the other hand, the neuropsychological testing may be of use not so much diagnostically, as for reassuring patients about their level of CNS function and/or defining functional limitations for treatment and rehabilitation (see below).

EPIDEMIOLOGY

In the absence of a uniform case definition, the prevalence of MCS is unknown. Nevertheless, some general demographic observations can be made. MCS appears most commonly in the fourth and fifth decades of life, though younger patients, including children, have been widely reported.[13–15]

Many patients come from higher socioeconomic classes, with the economically disadvantaged and nonwhites underrepresented in most reports[13-15]; this may be explained by differential access to care, differing perception of disease in different social strata or diagnostic bias. Women are more frequently affected than men.[13-15] Even after large outbreaks of occupational or environmental illnesses which might predispose to MCS, only isolated cases occur. However, clusters have been reported after some outbreaks,[16,17] and families with multiple cases have also been reported, suggesting higher risk associated with certain initiating chemical factors in these clusters.

In addition to these features, the settings in which the illness occurs have also been partially characterized. Both occupational and nonoccupational exposures have been implicated, and several classes of chemicals appear to account for the majority of initiating events: organic solvents, pesticides and respiratory irritants. A related condition, "sick building syndrome," typically affects most individuals sharing a specific ("sick") environment; clinical improvement of almost all affected people closely follows environmental modification. MCS, on the other hand, most commonly occurs in isolation and does not abruptly respond to modifications of the environment, such as better ventilation or substitution of troublesome materials.

It is uncertain whether MCS represents a new disorder. Those who suspect a primarily pathogenic role for toxic environmental agents argue that MCS is a twentieth-century disease with rapidly rising incidence due to increased chemical contamination of the environment.[18,19] Others, especially those who suspect that psychological mechanisms are central to MCS, have argued that only the societal context of the disease is new.[20,21]

PATHOGENESIS

The pathway which in certain individuals leads from an apparently self-limited episode or episodes of toxic effect from an environmental exposure to the development of potentially disabling symptomatic responses to very low levels of ubiquitous chemicals remains unknown. Several theories have been offered.

1) Immune dysfunction due to cumulative exposures to xenobiotic materials.

2) Limbic sensitization or limbic kindling.[22,23] Drawing from the growing body of scientific literature on the biology of drug dependence and habituation, symptoms are attributed to acquired alterations of limbic-thalamic and limbic-cortical pathways. Advocates point to the rich interconnection between olfactory nerves and the limbic system, coupled with the clinical observation of the importance of nasal odors and irritation to many MCS patients as evidence

supporting this view, which otherwise remains largely conjectural.

3) Classification of MCS as a somatoform illness.[20,24,25] It has been suggested that MCS is a variant of classic post-traumatic stress disorder,[26] a conditioned response to an unpleasant experience,[27] or a manifestation of early childhood trauma.[28] In these views, the initial illness plays a symbolic role in the pathogenesis of the disorder.

Unfortunately, despite considerable literature on this subject, little compelling clinical or experimental data has been published to confirm or refute any of these views. Therefore, most existing data must be characterized as anecdotal.

The psychiatric view of the disorder has been the most extensively explored. A growing body of evidence indicates that MCS subjects have both more extensive histories of psychiatric problems, and more significant psychopathology than patients with other chronic diseases.[21,24,25] Such data fail to explain the striking occurrence of MCS in many individuals without such features, however. As noted above, despite reports of laboratory abnormalities in selected groups of patients, evidence for the immunologic theory of MCS is very weak, because of problems with laboratory methods, interpretation of laboratory tests themselves and inadequacy of population comparisons. Controlled studies were unable to duplicate positive results.[12,29]

Most unfortunate of all, the debate over the etiologic basis of the disorder has been shrouded by dogmatism. Important financial decisions often hinge on how an individual case or cases of MCS is interpreted (for example, patient benefit entitlements, physician reimbursement acceptance and so on). Therefore, physicians and physician organizations have expressed strong views concerning diagnosis and management which have inhibited scientific progress as well as patient care.[30,31] Physicians with conflicting views may find it impossible to conduct research in this climate of controversy. In this way MCS differs markedly from other environmentally related questions such as the issue of scleroderma in coal miners, in which uncertainty about pathogenesis has not interfered with efforts to study the problem or treat its victims.

NATURAL HISTORY

MCS has yet to be subjected to sufficient clinical study to elucidate its course and outcome. Nevertheless, anecdotal experience with large numbers of patients has provided evidence for a general pattern of illness characterized by cyclical periods of improvements and exacerbations. While these cycles may be viewed by the patient as related to changes in his or her environment or responses to a therapy or other behavior, the pattern can rarely linked to a specific factor.

Two important observations follow from this. First, other than during the early stages during which the process evolves, there is little evidence to suggest that MCS is a progressive disorder. Patients do not deteriorate from year to year, nor have complications such as infections or organ system failure been observed. There is no evidence of mortality from MCS, although many patients become convinced that progression and death are inevitable, based on their experience of debilitating and frightening symptoms.

While this observation provides the basis for reassurance, it must be qualified by the recognition that complete remission of symptoms is infrequent. While good outcomes have been described, these are based on enhanced patient function and sense of well-being. The underlying tendency to react adversely to low-level chemical exposures persists, although symptoms may become sufficiently tolerable to permit resumption of a near-normal lifestyle.

Overall, MCS appears to be a disorder which is neither self-limited nor progressive. While neither has been confirmed by long-term follow-up study, it is not premature to include these assumptions in planning and evaluating treatments and assisting patients in vocational and personal rehabilitation efforts.

CLINICAL MANAGEMENT

There is no specific treatment for MCS. Although a vast array of modalities has been proposed and some extensively practiced, none has been subjected to controlled evaluation to determine efficacy. Theories of treatment have closely followed the theories of pathogenesis. Clinical ecologists, viewing MCS as an immune dysfunction syndrome caused by excessive burdens of xenobiotics, have directed therapy to reduction of burden by strict avoidance of chemicals. This approach is often accompanied by efforts to identify "specific" sensitivities with various forms of nontraditional skin and blood testing and by utilizing therapies based on the principles of desensitization with a goal of inducing "tolerance." Coupled with this may be strategies to bolster underlying immunity with dietary supplementation, eradication of "infections" such as candida, and provision of other nutritional supports. A more radical approach involves efforts to eliminate toxins from the body by chelation or accelerated turnover of fat (a putative source of causal substances such as organic hydrocarbons).

Clinicians inclined to a more psychological view of the disorder have explored alternative treatment approaches. Supportive individual or group therapies and behavioral modification have been described (personal observation). However, as with the more biological approaches, the efficacy of these modalities remains unproven for more than palliative purposes, except insofar as they are treating coexisting, underlying or complicating psychiatric manifestations of the disease (see below).

Although none of these modalities is dangerous, limitations in present knowledge suggest that they are best reserved for well-controlled trials. Certain treatment principles can be justified, based on present knowledge and experience. These include:

1) Taking steps to limit, to the extent possible, the search for the mysterious "cause" of the disease is an important first aspect of treatment. This will help to minimize extensive diagnostic testing which often perpetuates uncertainty.

2) Whatever the scientific belief of the clinician, it is crucial that the existing knowledge and uncertainty about MCS be explained to the patient, including specifically that the cause is unknown. The patient must be reassured that the possibility of a psychological basis does not mean that the illness is less real, less serious or less worthy of treatment. Conversely, neither would demonstration of a biologic cause make MCS more important, more honorable nor more treatable. Further reassurance that the condition will not progress or lead to death is valuable, coupled with caution that curative therapy is unavailable.

3) Steps to remove the patient from the most obviously offensive aspects of their environment are often necessary, especially if the patient still lives or works in the same environment where the initiating illness developed. While radical avoidance is counterproductive given the main goal of improving patient function, protection from daily misery is important in establishment of the therapeutic relationship which the patient deserves and needs. Most disturbingly, this sometimes means a vocational change, with assistance in obtaining workers' compensation or other disability benefits to make this possible.

4) Having established this foundation of support, the goal of all subsequent therapy should be symptomatic control with development of improved function. Musculoskeletal complaints should be controlled with symptomatic approaches, such as NSAIDs, sleep modification and so on. Psychological distress, as with adjustment difficulties, anxiety or depression must also be treated. Unfortunately, since MCS patients generally do not tolerate pharmacologic agents, nonpharmacologic approaches may be necessary. Special value may be garnered from judicious use of physical therapy or related modalities where rheumatologic symptoms dominate.

5) Beyond these measures, supportive counseling and reassurance initiate the task of adjusting to an illness without established treatment. To the extent consistent with tolerable symptoms, patients must be encouraged to expand the range of their activities and should be discouraged from passivity, dependence or resignation, which often appear during the course of treating MCS, however supportive the clinician.

6) Although it is appropriate to provide patients with all available factual information about MCS as well as representing the views of the treating clinician, many patients will try available alternative treatment modalities proposed by a friend, support group or lay literature. It is probably not reasonable to resist such efforts strongly or to undermine one's therapeutic relationship on this account. Rather, hold steadily

to a single coherent perspective, treating the "treatment" as yet another disturbing manifestation of a troublesome condition.

PREVENTION

Primary prevention of MCS cannot be seriously discussed given the incomplete knowledge of the pathogenesis of the disorder and the host factors which make certain individuals susceptible. At this time the most reasonable approach is reduction of the opportunities in the workplace and ambient environment for the kinds of acute exposures which appear to precipitate MCS in some people, especially solvents and pesticides. Elimination of poorly ventilated offices is also likely to help prevent cases because of the importance of sick building syndrome as a precipitant.

Secondary prevention, that is, intervening after a noxious exposure but before MCS begins, may offer greater control opportunities, although no intervention has been studied. Because psychological factors may play a role in victims of environmental mishaps, careful early management of all individuals is important, even if the prognosis from a strictly biologic perspective appears good. For example, patients seen in clinics or emergency rooms after acute illnesses should be queried about their reactions to the events and should receive close follow-up if exaggerated fears of long-term effects or recurrence are expressed. Equally important, efforts should be made to prevent recurrences of the exposures, since repeated insults may be an important pathway leading to MCS.

REFERENCES

[1]Mooser SB. The epidemiology of multiple chemical sensitivities. *Occupational Med State of the Art Reviews.* 1987;2:663–668.

[2]Cullen MR. The worker with multiple chemical sensitivities: An overview. *Occupational Med State of the Art Reviews.* 1987;2:655–661.

[3]Sparks PJ, Daniell W, Black DW, et al. Multiple chemical sensitivity syndrome: A clinical perspective. I. Case definition, theories of pathogenesis, and research needs. *JOM.* 1994;36:718–730.

[4]Thrasher JD, Broughton A, Micevich P. Antibodies and immune profiles of individuals occupationally exposed to formaldehyde: Six case reports. *Am J Ind Med.* 1988;14:479–488.

[5]Thrasher JD, Wojdani A, Cheung G, Heuser G. Evidence for formaldehyde antibodies and altered cellular immunity in subjects exposed to formaldehyde in mobile homes. *Arch Environ Health.* 1987;42:347–350.

[6]Broughton A, Thrasher JD, Gard Z. Immunological evaluation of four arc welders exposed to fumes from ignited polyurethane (isocyanate) foram: Antibodies and immune profiles. *Am J Ind Med.* 1988;13:463–472.

[7]Vojdani A, Ghoneum M, Brautbar N. Immune alteration associated with exposure to toxic chemicals. *Toxicol Indus Health.* 1992;8:239–253.

[8]Callender TJ, Morrow L, Subramanian K, Duhon D, Ristovv M. Three-dimensional brain metabolic imaging in patients with toxic encephalopathy. *Environ Res.* 1993;60:295–319.

[9]Heuser G, Mena I, Francisca A. Neurospect findings in patients exposed to neurotoxic chemicals. In: Mitchell FL. *Multiple Chemical Sensitivity: A Scientific Overview.* Princeton, NJ: Princeton Scientific Publishing, 1995;561–571.

[10]Simon T. *Single Photon Emission Computed Tomography of the Brain in Patients with Chemical Sensitivities.* Princeton, NJ: Princeton Scientific Publishing, 1995;573–577.

[11]Fiedler N, Kipen HM, DeLuca J, Kelly-McNeil K, Natelson B. A controlled comparison of multiple chemical sensitivity and chronic fatigue syndrome. *Psychosomatic Med.* 1996;58:38–49.

[12]Simon GE, Daniell W, Stockbridge H, Claypoole K, Rosenstock L. Immunologic, psychological and neuropsychological factors in multiple chemical sensitivity: A controlled study. *Ann Intern Med* 1993;19(2):97–103.

[13]Cullen MR, Pace PE, Redlich CA. The experience of the Yale occupational and environmental medicine clinics with multiple chemical sensitivities. *Toxicol Indus Health.* 1992;8:15–19.

[14]Buchwald D, Garrity D. Comparison of patients with chronic fatigue syndrome, fibromyalgia and multiple chemical sensitivities. *Arch Intern Med.* 1994;154:2049–2053.

[15]Miller CS, Mitzel HC. Chemical sensitivity attributed to pesticide exposure versus remodeling. *Arch Environ Health.* 1995;50(2):119–129.

[16]Welch LS, Sokas R. Development of multiple chemical sensitivity after an outbreak of sick-building syndrome. *Toxicol Indus Health.* 1992;8:47–50.

[17]Sparks PJ, Simon GE, Katon WJ, Altman IC, Ayars GH, Johnson RL. An outbreak of illness among aerospace workers. *West J Med.* 1990;153:28–33.

[18]Ashford NA, Miller CS. *Chemical Exposures: Low Levels and High Stakes.* New York: Van Norstrand Reinhold, 1991.

[19]Dickey LD. *Clinical Ecology.* Springfield, IL: Charles C. Thomas, 1976.

[20]Brodsky CM. Allergic to everything: A medical subculture. *Psychosomatics.* 1983;24:731–736.

[21]Stewart DE, Raskin J. Psychiatric assessment of patients with "20th century disease" ("total allergy syndrome"). *Can Med Assoc J.* 1985;133:1001–1006.

[22]Bell IR. White paper. Neuropsychiatric aspects of sensitivity to low-level chemicals: A neural sensitization model. *Toxicol Indus Health.* 1994;10:277–312.

[23]Bell IR, Miller CS, Schwartz GE. An olfactory-limbic model of multiple chemical sensitivity syndrome: Possible relationships to kindling and affective spectrum disorders. *Biol Psychiatry.* 1992;32:218–242.

[24]Simon GE, Katon WJ, Sparks PJ. Allergic to life: Psychological factors in environmental illness. *Am J Psychiatry.* 1990;147(7);901–906.

[25]Black DW, Rathe A, Goldstein R. Environmental illness—a controlled study of 26 subjects with "20th century disease." *JAMA.* 1990;264(24):3166–3170.

[26]Schottenfeld RS, Cullen MR. Recognition of occupational-induced post-traumatic stress disorders. *J Occup Med.* 1986;28:365–369.

[27]Shusterman D, Balmes J, Cone J. Behavioral sensitization to irritants/odorants after acute overexposure. *J Occup Med.* 1988;30: 565–567.

[28]Staudenmayer H, Selner ME, Selner JC. Adult sequelae of childhood abuse presenting as environmental illness. *Ann Allergy.* 1993a;71:538–546.

[29]Kipen H, Fiedler N, Maccia C, Yurkow E, Todaro J, Laskin D. Immunologic evaluation of chemically sensitive patients. *Toxicol Ind Health.* 1992;8(4):125–135.

[30]American College of Physicians. American College of Physicians position statement: clinical ecology. *Ann Intern Med.* 1989;111: 168–178.

[31]American Medical Association, Council of Scientific Affairs. Clinical ecology. *JAMA.* 1992;268:3465–3467.

V

Rheumatic Syndromes and the Workplace

16

Occupation-Associated Upper-Extremity Disorders

Louis Bessette and Jeffrey N. Katz

INTRODUCTION

Musculoskeletal disorders of the upper extremity have become the subject of growing interest in the past 15 years, especially because of the increased incidence and prevalence of cases related to work. Injuries due to repetitive trauma have increased eightfold over the last decade and are currently the largest source of workplace-related morbidity, accounting for more than 50% of all occupational illnesses in the United States.[1] Consequently, workers' compensation claims for these disorders have risen rapidly over the past 15 years in most industrialized countries.

The rise in the frequency of these disorders is thought to result from several factors. The most important is probably the increasing automation and specialization of work.[1] Although new technologies have generally reduced workload, the redesign of jobs in many industries requires that the worker perform a limited number of tasks faster and repeatedly.[2] Other factors are thought to be the improved accuracy of reporting, heightened awareness of the problem by employees and employers, and advances in diagnostic tests.[3]

The first part of this chapter will define the terminology used in this field and address ambiguities. Then existing information on epidemiology, occupational risk factors, clinical evaluation, medical management and prevention of musculoskeletal disorders of the upper extremity will be reviewed. Major emphasis is placed on carpal tunnel syndrome (CTS) because it is one of the most common upper-extremity disorders and its pathophysiology is reasonably well understood. The final section provides a brief review of work-associated shoulder disorders.

REVIEW OF TERMINOLOGY

The nomenclature describing upper-extremity disorders of occupational origin is confusing and inconsistent. Some terms refer to well-defined clinical entities (CTS, tendonitis or bursitis); others are vague or inclusive of a wide variety of less well-defined disorders (for example, cumulative trauma disorder, repetition strain injury and overuse syndrome).

Cumulative trauma disorders (CTD) have been defined as "those disorders of the muscles, tendons, nerves, and blood vessels that are caused, precipitated, or aggravated by repeated exertions or movements of the body."[4] The term CTD is by no means a diagnosis, but refers to a class of disorders with similar characteristics such as exposure, pathogenesis and symptoms. *Repetition strain injury* (RSI) is a term popularized in Australia about two decades ago during an apparent epidemic of diffuse arm pain in a variety of occupational groups. RSI was defined by the National Occupational Health and Safety Commission as "a collective term for a range of conditions characterized by discomfort or persistent pain in muscles, tendons, and other soft tissues, with or without physical manifestations. RSI is usually caused or aggravated by work, and is associated with repetitive movement, sustained or constrained postures and/or forceful movements."[5] As with CTD, some well-defined conditions fall within the group of RSI disorders, but the etiology and pathomechanism of many problems in the RSI categories are obscure. *Overuse syndrome* was characterized as "a musculoskeletal disorder characterized by pain, tenderness, and often functional loss in muscle groups and ligaments subjected to heavy or unaccustomed use."[6] Pain anywhere from the hand to the scapular and neck region was noted to be the predominant symptom.[7,8] On physical examination, the patient with overuse syndrome experiences tenderness on palpation of the affected muscles, joints, and ligaments.

These diverse terms refer to upper-extremity musculoskeletal disorders that have in common an apparent increase in prevalence under certain occupational conditions. This terminology is confusing and should be avoided. Well-defined nomenclature of known entities (for example, CTS or tendonitis) should be used in most cases. The term "musculoskeletal disorders of occupational origin" to regroup musculoskeletal disorders associated with occupational factors has been proposed.[9]

CARPAL TUNNEL SYNDROME

CTS is a frequent cause of disability of the upper extremity and is the most common peripheral neuropathy. In the last two decades, there has been increasing interest in CTS as an occupational disease.[10] Data from some industries, showing that an estimated 15% of workers are affected annually, raise concerns about the occupational causes of CTS, losses in productivity or work time, rising worker compensation costs, disabilities and disease management.[11–14] These concerns and the clinical manifestations of CTS are discussed in detail in this section.

Epidemiology

CTS in the General Population

The annual incidence of CTS has been estimated to be 0.1% for a defined general population in Rochester, Minnesota, using the record-linkage system based at the Mayo Clinic.[15] In that population, the peak age of incidence was between 45 and 54 years, with a rate three times higher in women than men. Diagnosis was based on a combination of clinical and electromyographic findings in the majority of cases.

In a Dutch population survey of 504 adults interviewed, 64 potential cases (defined as tingling, pain, and/or numbness in the fingers innervated by the median nerve, occurring twice a week or more, with nocturnal awakening in most cases) were found.[16] Upon neurophysiological examination, 5.6% (women: 5.8%; men: 0.6%) had CTS. Among 170 million U.S. adults who had "ever worked" according to the 1988 National Health Interview Survey data, a prevalence of 1.6% of self-reported CTS was found.[17] The prevalence was higher in women (1.9%) than in men (1.2%), and among whites was 1.8 times higher than among nonwhites.

CTS in the Workplace

The incidence and prevalence of CTS in the workplace is a subject of debate. A population-based incidence study of occupational CTS (OCTS) using the Washington State Workers' Compensation database found an industrywide incidence rate of 1.74 claims per 1,000 full-time-equivalent workers, much higher than in the general population.[18] The mean age was 37.4 years, with a female to male ratio of 1.2:1, in contrast to nonoccupational CTS (mean age, 51 years, female/ male ratio, 3:1). In the same study, the highest industry-spe-

cific OCTS rates were found in the food processing, carpentry, egg production, wood products and logging industries. In cross-sectional studies from different industries the prevalence of CTS was 1.1% to 2.1%.[19,20] However, in these studies the diagnosis was made on clinical grounds with no specific criteria and no electrophysiological measurements.

Occupational Risk Factors

The causal relationship between ergonomic factors and CTS is a subject of controversy.[21,22] Six major occupational risk factors have been associated with CTS and other musculoskeletal disorders of occupational origin (Table 16-1.) CTS, hand/wrist tendonitis, hand-arm vibration syndrome, and shoulder tendonitis are the musculoskeletal disorders of the upper extremity that have most convincingly been associated with occupational factors. Other upper-extremity disorders, such as cervical radiculopathy, tension neck (occupational cervicobrachial syndrome), epicondylitis and RSI, have been associated with work, but there is insufficient evidence to demonstrate a causal link.[23–27]

In a review of 54 studies relating occupational exposure to upper-extremity musculoskeletal disorders (excluding hand-arm vibration syndrome), it was concluded that there is a causal relationship between ergonomic risk factors and upper-extremity musculoskeletal disorders.[22]

Force and Repetitiveness

The median nerve and flexor tendons pass through the carpal tunnel, which is bounded by rigid bones on three sides and by the flexor retinaculum ligament on the palmar side.[28]

Table 16-1 Occupational risk factors associated with carpal tunnel syndrome

Occupational Risk Factor[+]	Strength of Association from Epidemiologic Studies[‡]
Repetitiveness	+++
Force	+++
Posture	++
Vibration	++
Mechanical stress concentration	+
Glove and exposure to cold	+

+++: Good epidemiologic studies that support a strong relationship between the ergonomic factor and CTS.

++: Epidemiologic studies that support the association between the ergonomic factor and CTS, but with important methodologic flaws.

+: No epidemiologic data that support the association between the ergonomic factor and CTS or poorly designed studies.

[+]All risk factors (repetitiveness, force, posture, etc) refer specifically to the hand and wrist.

[‡]See Stock[22] for criteria to measure methodologic quality of epidemiologic studies.

Finger movement with a flexed or extended wrist causes the tendons to move against the adjacent walls of the carpal tunnel. Repetitive movements in flexion and extension (without adequate recovery time) may cause irritation and inflammation of the synovial membrane of the tendons.[29-31] Surgical specimens in idiopathic CTS generally reveal a low-grade inflammatory infiltrate, increased vascularity, edema, and fibrosis of the flexor tendon sheaths.[32,33] Inflammatory thickening of the synovial membrane may in turn compress the median nerve inside the stiff boundary of the carpal tunnel. Forceful contraction of muscle also adds to the risk by stretching the tendons, which causes ischemia, inflammation, and eventually fibrillar tearing of the tendons.[34] Repetitive movements and force are the occupational risk factors for which there is the strongest epidemiologic support for a relationship with CTS. However, it has not been determined what constitutes a safe level of force and repetitive work.[19,35-37]

Force and Posture

Extreme wrist postures or movement (flexion and hyperextension), particularly in combination with pinch, are often described as risk factors for CTS. Carpal tunnel pressure in volunteers with 90° of wrist flexion or extension reached that of patients with CTS in a neutral position (31 mg Hg).[38] Pressure in the canals of patients with CTS reached 94 mg Hg with flexion and 110 mg Hg with hyperextension. Increased carpal canal pressure may cause an ischemic insult by compromising epineural and endoneural circulation.

It has been demonstrated that force exerted by the muscles on the tendons and fingers is related to the posture of the hand.[39-42] For example, four to five times more muscle force must be exerted to pinch objects with the fingertips than with a power grip.

Vibration

Vibration exposure is known to cause both a vasospastic disorder of the upper extremity and a diffuse distal neuropathy called *hand-arm vibration syndrome*.[43-45] This syndrome is characterized by episodic vasospasm, numbness and tingling of the fingers, and diffuse neuropathy on nerve conduction study.[44-49] A high prevalence of such symptoms has been reported among foundryman and grinders,[50-51] forestry workers,[52-55] railroad mechanics,[56] rock drillers,[57] and shipyard workers.[47]

Vibration has also been suggested as a possible risk factor for CTS.[10,58,59] However, the association observed between vibration and CTS might be explained by the effect of force, awkward posture, and repetitiveness when vibrating hand tools are used.[59,60,61] Although focal slowing of median nerve conduction velocity suggestive of CTS has been described in vibration-exposed workers, a diffuse neuropathy is more common. Pathological examination of nerves in finger biopsies in persons suffering from vibration-induced neuropathy revealed fibrosis, increased thickness of the epineurium or perineurium, extensive destruction of the myelin sheath and a reduction in the number of nerve fibers.[62]

Mechanical Stress Concentration

Direct pressure at the base of the palm can increase the pressure in the carpal tunnel, compressing the median nerve and the underlying tendons and vessels, with resultant ischemia.[30,63-65] Tasks that often produce pressure on the base of the palm include the use of screwdrivers, scrapers, paint brushes and buffers. No study to date has adequately separated direct compression from that of other risk factors.

Gloves and Exposure to Cold

Gloves may inhibit sensory feedback and attenuate worker strength,[65] thus increasing the strength required for a task.[66] Furthermore, a glove that is too tight at the wrist may apply external pressure that contributes to compression of the nerve. There is no evidence that low temperatures cause direct soft-tissue injury or CTS. However, cold temperature may cause loss of tactile sensitivity and decrease in motor function.[67,68] Reduction of manual dexterity may increase the force or awkwardness of posture needed to accomplish a task and thus accentuate the symptoms of nerve impairment.

In one study of 207 workers from two frozen food plants, the prevalence of CTS in subjects exposed to cold and repetitive movements was evaluated.[69] Workers were classified into three groups: 1) low exposure to cold and low rate of repetition; 2) low exposure to cold and high rate of repetition; 3) high exposure to cold and high rate of repetition. Group 3 had a significantly higher risk of CTS than groups 1 and 2, which suggests a combined effect of the two factors.

Nonoccupational Risk Factors

A variety of disorders considered to be risk factors for CTS are outlined in Table 16-2. The conditions most frequently documented in 1,016 residents of Rochester, Minnesota diagnosed with CTS were Colles' fracture, rheumatoid arthritis, hormonal agents, oophorectomy, diabetes mellitus and pregnancy.[70]

Clinical Manifestations and Diagnosis

Carpal tunnel syndrome results from compression of the median nerve. Typically, patients experience episodes of burning pain or tingling in the hand that may spread above

Table 16-2 Nonoccupation conditions associated with carpal tunnel syndrome

Condition
Space-Occupying Lesions
Ganglia[145]
Hemangioma[146]
Osteoid osteoma[147]
Lipoma[148]
Thickened transverse carpal ligament (familial)[149,150]
Nonspecific tenosynovitis[151]
Hematoma[152]
Trauma
Colles' fracture and other forearm fracture[153,154]
Old wrist fracture[155]
Carpal bone fracture[156]
Blunt trauma to wrist[157]
Operative procedure of the wrist[158]
Inflammatory Musculoskeletal Diseases
Rheumatoid arthritis[159]
Progressive systemic sclerosis[160]
Polymyalgia rheumatica[161]
Polymyositis[162]
Crystal-Induced Rheumatic Diseases
Gout[163]
Calcium pyrophosphate dihydrate disease[164]
Hydroxyapatite disease[165]
Degenerative Arthritis of the Wrist Metabolic and Endocrine Diseases
Diabetes[166]
Thyroid (myxedema)[167]
Acromegaly[168]
Mucoppolysaccharidosis[169]
Infection
Osteomyelitis of the carpal bones[170]
Mycobacterium tuberculosis[171]
Atypical mycobacteria[172,173]
Histoplasmosis[174]
Miscellaneous Conditions
Pregnancy[175]
Hormonal agent[176]
Oophorectomy[177]
Amyloidosis[178]
Dialysis[179]

the wrist and that often occur at night.[71] Numbness, affecting the index and middle fingers, the radial side of the ring finger and occasionally the thumb, is also a common complaint. Symptoms may be precipitated by activities such as driving or holding a newspaper or a book. Abnormalities on physical examination may or may not be present. Loss of sensation may be demonstrated in the index and middle fingers or radial side of the ring finger. The muscles of the thenar eminence may develop weakness and atrophy, especially in severe or chronic cases.[72] Bilateral involvement occurs in approximately 50% of cases.[37,73–75]

CTS lesions may exist in isolation or in various combinations, causing more diffuse and less typical symptoms. For example, the "double crush" syndrome is due to the combination of cervical radiculopathy with peripheral nerve entrapment. In addition, 30% to 40% of CTS patients have also been reputed to have lateral epicondylitis of the elbow or ulnar nerve entrapment.[76,77] Many workers with CTS complain of more diffuse symptoms of the cervicobrachial region.[78] Using a hand symptom diagram, recipients of workers' compensation had more numbness/tingling of the arm and shoulder region than nonrecipients (25% versus 9.5%).[79] This finding suggests that patients with work-related CTS have other lesions.

A diagnosis of CTS is generally made on the basis of a characteristic history and physical findings. In fact, the diagnostic impression of an experienced clinician based on a history and physical examination is more accurate than any other test.[80] Positive responses to provocative tests, such as Tinel's and Phalen's signs, are often absent, even in patients with classic symptoms.[80–83] Table 16-3 presents the results of a study evaluating the utility of the history and physical examination findings for the diagnosis of CTS.[80] A hand diagram, on which patients draw in the location of their symptoms, was a valuable adjunct in diagnosing CTS.

Electromyographic study of nerve conduction latency is considered to be the gold standard.[84,85] A slowed conduction velocity, along with prolongation of distal motor latency, lends support to the diagnosis of CTS. However, false-negative nerve conduction tests are well documented, occurring in 8% of the cases in one series.[86] The National Institute for Occupational Safety and Health (NIOSH) case definition[87] (Table 16-4) was found to have a sensitivity of 0.67 and a specificity of 0.58.[88] Its predictive positive value would be 0.22 in a hypothetical occupational setting with a 15% prevalence of CTS. Although the case definition may be adequate for surveillance in high-risk workplaces, it should not be used as a diagnostic tool in clinical practice.

Prevention, Treatment and Outcome

Despite treatment advances, prevention of CTS remains the highest priority. Prevention of work-related musculoskeletal disorders encompasses three main strategies.[59,78] *primary prevention*—eliminating or minimizing risks to workers' health before the development of symptoms; *secondary prevention*—alleviating and preventing the development of impairment; *tertiary prevention*—management and rehabilitation of those with disabilities, and prevention of recurrence. The effectiveness of a prevention program requires a multidisciplinary approach involving ergonomists, occupational therapists, physicians, epidemiologists, and administrators of the workplace.

For primary prevention, three strategies have been proposed[59]: 1) reduction of exposure to known risk factors; 2) a

Table 16-3   Utility of history and physical findings in the diagnosis of CTS

Findings	Sensitivity	Specificity	Sample with 40% Prevalence of CTS		Sample with 15% Prevalence of CTS	
			PPV[+]	NPV[‡]	PPV	NPV
Tinel's sign	0.6	0.67	0.55	0.72	0.25	0.91
Phalen's sign	0.75	0.47	0.48	0.74	0.2	0.91
Sensory loss	0.32	0.81	0.54	0.63	0.23	0.87
Hand diagram rating	0.61	0.71	0.59	0.73	0.27	0.91
Neurologist assessment	0.84	0.72	0.67	0.87	0.34	0.96
Age ≥ 40 years	0.8	0.42	0.48	0.76	0.2	0.92
Nocturnal symptoms	0.77	0.28	0.42	0.64	0.16	0.87
Bilateral symptoms	0.61	0.58	0.49	0.69	0.2	0.89
Tinel's sign plus hand diagram rating	0.39	0.89	0.71	0.69	0.39	0.89

Adapted from Katz, *et al.*[8]
[+]Positive predictive value
[‡]Negative predictive value

Table 16-4   NIOSH surveillance case definition of work-related carpal tunnel syndrome

Criteria A, B and C must be met:
A. Symptoms suggestive of carpal tunnel syndrome: Paresthesia, hypoesthesia, pain or numbness affecting at least part of the median nerve distribution of the hand.
B. Objective findings consistent with carpal tunnel syndrome: Either (1) One or more of the following physical findings: Tinel's sign, or decreased or absent sensation to pin prick in the median nerve distribution of the hand.
   or   (2) Electrodiagnostic findings of the median nerve dysfunction across the carpal tunnel.
C. Evidence of work-relatedness: One or more of the following: Frequent, repetitive or forceful hand work on the affected side; sustained awkward position; use of vibrating tools; prolonged pressure over wrist or base of palm; temporal relationship of symptoms to work or association with carpal tunnel syndrome noted in coworkers.

Adapted from Matte, *et al.*[87]

conditioning or training process that increases tolerance of workers; or 3) a preplacement process to identify those persons at high risk for developing CTS. A conditioning or training period for persons in repetitive or forceful jobs in which the workers can gradually adapt their muscles and tendons might be useful.[89–91] The identification of specific characteristics of the person's job to control exposure to occupational risk factors is the most valuable preventive strategy: ergonomically designed tools, workstations, work tasks, or work organization may prevent musculoskeletal disorders. However, there is no good study of outcomes of prospective primary prevention.[63,65,92–101]

At the level of secondary prevention, it is important to educate the worker and reduce obstacles that prevent the reporting of symptoms to a physician.[59,102] Once symptoms are reported, not only should appropriate medical treatment be considered, but a thorough work history should be obtained to identify risk factors that might be eliminated. It is important to follow these cases to ensure that medical treatment and job changes have been effective.

At the stage of tertiary prevention, workers with established CTS are usually treated conservatively with nonsteroidal anti-inflammatory drugs, local injection of steroids into the carpal tunnel, splinting of the wrist and occupational therapy.[103–105] Conservative treatment is successful in up to 50% of cases and may produce complete relief in 10% to 22%.[103] Surgical decompression is usually recommended to patients with persistent symptoms and disability despite conservative management, and is generally considered the first intervention in severe cases. Carpal tunnel release may be accomplished with a traditional incision allowing direct exposure, or by endoscopic techniques. Both are effective, with success rates ranging from 70% to greater than 90%.[32,75,105–112]

Despite the effectiveness of medical and surgical treatment, a substantial proportion of workers remain out of work or disabled for a long period. CTS has been reported to have the highest mean duration of work absence of all disorders in the workers' compensation population. More than 20% are out of work for longer than six months[13] and 8% remains out of work for more than one year.[113] In the non-workers'-compensation population, work disability has averaged about two to six months.[106,114]

Symptom relief and functional improvement appear to be the most important predictors of return to work.[113,114] In one retrospective study, patients who had greatest relief of symptoms were most likely to return to work, and workers in occupations that required intensive use of hands and wrists were least likely to return to work.[113] The limited data on work disability in CTS also suggest a biopsychosocial model that includes economic, workplace, psychological and social dimensions.[114,115]

A rehabilitation program after surgery should be considered to speed recovery and functional improvement. One study showed that the most important factor influencing return to work after carpal tunnel release was the number of hand therapy sessions per week.[116]

An important error at the stage of tertiary prevention is to focus on medical and surgical treatment to improve symptoms and functional status, without attempting to reduce the risk factors at work. The recurrence of CTS is frequent if a worker returns to a job involving multiple risk factors. Measures such as job changes, transitional workshops and graded retraining under the supervision of an experienced hand therapist may help to reduce the risk of recurrence.

SHOULDER DISORDERS

Shoulder complaints include a wide variety of conditions and diseases and may also originate from multiple sites and anatomic structures.[117,118] Studies addressing shoulder disorders use many different names for the same condition or nonspecific terms such as shoulder pain syndrome, shoulder-neck disorders and occupational cervicobrachial disorders.[119] This lack of generally accepted criteria and classification of shoulder complaints makes the interpretation of epidemiologic studies difficult.

Shoulder Disorders in the General Population and the Workplace

The prevalence of shoulder disorders in the general population is estimated at 7% to 15% for individuals less than 50 years old[120,121] and 15% to 25% for those over the age of 50.[120-126] Most studies have shown a slightly higher prevalence in women.[122,123,125,127] The prevalence of shoulder complaints in high-risk exposure groups in the workplace varies from 2.3%[20] to more than 50%,[128,129] depending on the definition of the condition and the job title or risk factors evaluated.

Occupational Risk Factors

The principal occupational risk factors that have been associated with shoulder complaints are repetitive arm movement, posture (including dynamic and static postures), force and vibration.[117] As in the case of CTS, most of the risk factors occur together in varying degrees of intensity, and it

is very difficult to isolate the role of one exposure from that of another. Workers whose jobs involve highly repetitive arm movements associated with shoulder symptoms include spray painters,[130] assembly line workers.[126,130] winders,[130] garment workers,[131] food packers[132] and fish processors.[133]

Tasks that require a worker to sustain a position in abduction or forward flexion (dynamic or static tasks) for a protracted period or to use the arm at shoulder level or above have been associated with shoulder tendonitis or diffuse symptoms in the shoulder region. Jobs described as requiring awkward postures include operation of a cash register,[134] electronic part assembly[135] or other assembly line works,[126] welding,[136] keyboarding[137-139] and use of a computer mouse.[140] The explanation for shoulder symptoms related to keyboarding and mouse use can be thought of as time spent in a static position with arms unsupported, which increases static muscle loading.[140] Exposure to vibration has been suggested to increase the risk of shoulder tendinitis.[141] However, most workers exposed to vibration have jobs that also require heavy lifting and awkward postures.

Rotator cuff syndromes (tendonitis and tendon rupture) are probably the most common shoulder disorders. The predisposing factors are degeneration caused by impairment of perfusion and nutrition and mechanical stress.[142] The tendons of the supraspinatus, the biceps brachii (long head) and the upper parts of the infraspinatus muscles have a zone of avascularity.[143] Factors such as direct compression of the tendons under the coracoacromial arch during elevation and muscle tension impair circulation.[142]

Management

The basic preventive approaches described for CTS also apply to shoulder problems. Another efficient treatment of acute shoulder tendonitis is a single subacromial injection of a corticosteroid with a local anesthetic and/or administration of an oral nonsteroidal anti-inflammatory agent.[144] In chronic severe cases, surgical removal of the lateral part of the acromion may relieve pain.[142]

REFERENCES

[1]*Bureau of Labor Statistics Report on Survey of Occupational Injuries and Illnesses in 1977–1989.* Washington, DC: Bureau of Labor Statistics, US Dept of Labor, 1990.

[2]Bammer G. How technological change can increase the risk of repetitive motion injuries. *Semin Occup Med.* 1987;2:25–30.

[3]Rempel DM, Harrison RJ, Barnhart S. Work-related cumulative trauma disorders of the upper extremity. *JAMA.* 1992;267:838–842.

[4]Armstrong TJ. Introduction to occupational disorders of the upper extremities. In: Ann Arbor MOHE, ed. *Occupational Disorders of the Upper Extremities.* MI: 1990.

[5]National Institute of Occupational Safety Commission (Australia). Repetition strain injury (RSI): A report and model code of practice. Canberra, Aust. Gov. Publ. Serv. 1986.

[6]Dennett X, Fry HJ. Overuse syndrome: A muscle biopsy study. *Lancet.* 1988;1:905–908.

[7]Fry HJ. Physical signs in the hand and wrist seen in the overuse injury syndrome of the upper limb. *Aust N Z J Surg.* 1986;56:47–49.

[8]Puffer JC, Zachazewski JE. Management of overuse injuries. *Am Fam Physician.* 1988;38:225–232.

[9]Gerr F, Letz R, Landrigan PJ. Upper-extremity musculoskeletal disorders of occupational origin. *Annu Rev Public Health.* 1991;12:543–566.

[10]Cannon LJ, Bernacki EJ, Walter SD. Personal and occupational factors associated with carpal tunnel syndrome. *J Occup Med.* 1981;23:255–258.

[11]Liss GM, Armstrong C, Kusiak RA, Gailitis MM. Use of provincial health insurance plan billing data to estimate carpal tunnel syndrome morbidity and surgery rates. *Am J Ind Med.* 1992;22:395–409.

[12]Kraut A. Estimates of the extent of morbidity and mortality due to occupational diseases in Canada. *Am J Ind Med.* 1994;25:267–278.

[13]Cheadle A, Franklin G, Wolfhagen C, et al. Factors influencing the duration of work-related disability: A population-based study of Washington State workers' compensation. *Am J Public Health.* 1994;84:190–196.

[14]Palmer DH, Hanrahan LP. Social and economic costs of carpal tunnel surgery. *Instr Course Lect.* 1995;44:167–172.

[15]Stevens JC, Sun S, Beard CM, O'Fallon WM, Kurland LT. Carpal tunnel syndrome in Rochester, Minnesota, 1961 to 1980. *Neurology.* 1988;38:134–138.

[16]de Krom MC, Knipschild PG, Kester AD, et al. Carpal tunnel syndrome: Prevalence in the general population. *J Clin Epidemiol.* 1992;45:373–376.

[17]Tanaka S, Wild DK, Seligman PJ, et al. The US prevalence of self-reported carpal tunnel syndrome: 1988 National Health Interview Survey data. *Am J Public Health.* 1994;84:1846–1848.

[18]Franklin GM, Haug J, Heyer N, Checkoway H, Peck N. Occupational carpal tunnel syndrome in Washington State, 1984–1988. *Am J Public Health.* 1991;81:741–746.

[19]Silverstein BA, Fine LJ, Armstrong TJ. Occupational factors and carpal tunnel syndrome. *Am J Ind Med.* 1987;11:343–358.

[20]McCormack RR Jr, Inman RD, Wells A, Berntsen C, Imbus HR. Prevalence of tendinitis and related disorders of the upper extremity in a manufacturing workforce. *J Rheumatol.* 1990;17:958–964.

[21]Hadler NM. Work-related disorders of the upper extremity. Part I: cumulative trauma disorders—a critical review. In: Hadler NM, Bunn, ed. *Occupational Problems in Medical Practice.* New York: Lawrence DellaCorte Publication, Inc, 1989;1–8.

[22]Stock SR. Workplace ergonomic factors and the development of musculoskeletal disorders of the neck and upper limbs: A meta-analysis. *Am J Ind Med.* 1991;19:87–107.

[23]Kurppa K, Waris P, Rokkanen P. Tennis elbow. Lateral elbow pain syndrome. *Scand J Work Environ Health.* 1979;5 Suppl 3:15–18.

[24]Maeda K, Horiguchi S, Hosokawa M. History of the studies on occupational cervicobrachial disorder in Japan and remaining problems. *J Hum Ergol.* 1982;11:17–29.

[25]Anderson JA. Shoulder pain and tension neck and their relation to work. *Scand J Work Environ Health.* 1984;10:435–442.

[26]Viikari-Juntura E. Tenosynovitis, peritendinitis and the tennis elbow syndrome. *Scand J Work Environ Health.* 1984;10:443–449.

[27]Bammer G, Martin B. The arguments about RSI: An examination. *Community Health Stud.* 1988;12:348–358.

[28]Robbins H. Anatomical study of the median nerve in the carpal tunnel and etiologies of the carpal tunnel syndrome. *J Bone Joint Surg Am.* 1963;45A:953–966.

[29]Armstrong TJ, Chaffin DB. Some biomechanical aspects of the carpal tunnel. *J Biomech.* 1979;12:567–570.

[30]Tichauer ER. Some aspects of stress on forearm and hand in industry. *J Occup Med.* 1966;8:63–71.

[31]Lamphier T, Crooker C, Crooker J. DeQuervain's disease. *Ind Med Surg.* 1965;34:847–856.

[32]Phalen GS. The carpal-tunnel syndrome. Seventeen years' experience in diagnosis and treatment of six hundred fifty-four hands. *J Bone Joint Surg Am.* 1966;48:211–228.

[33]Yamaguchi D, Lipscomb P, Soule E. Carpal tunnel syndrome. *Minn Med.* 1965;22:31.

[34]Perrott JW. Anatomical factors in occupational trauma. *Med J Aust.* 1961;1:73–81.

[35]Silverstein BA, Fine LJ, Armstrong TJ. Hand wrist cumulative trauma disorders in industry. *Br J Ind Med.* 1986;43:779–784.

[36]Nathan PA, Meadows KD, Doyle LS. Occupation as a risk factor for impaired sensory conduction of the median nerve at the carpal tunnel. *J Hand Surg Br.* 1988;13:167–170.

[37]Birkbeck MQ, Beer TC. Occupation in relation to the carpal tunnel syndrome. *Rheumatol Rehabil.* 1975;14:218–221.

[38]Gelberman RH, Hergenroeder PT, Hargens AR, Lundborg GN, Akeson WH. The carpal tunnel syndrome. A study of carpal canal pressures. *J Bone Joint Surg Am.* 1981;63:380–383.

[39]Chao EY, Opgrande JD, Axmear FE. Three-dimensional force analysis of finger joints in selected isometric hand functions. *J Biomech.* 1976;9:387–396.

[40]Swanson AB, Matev IB, de Groot G. The strength of the hand. *Bull Prosthet Res.* 1970;10:145–153.

[41]Smith EM, Sonstegard DA, Anderson WH Jr. Carpal tunnel syndrome: Contribution of flexor tendons. *Arch Phys Med Rehabil.* 1977;58:379–385.

[42]Armstrong TJ, Chaffin DB. Carpal tunnel syndrome and selected personal attributes. *J Occup Med.* 1979;21:481–486.

[43]Gupta A, McCabe SJ. Vibration white finger. *Hand Clin.* 1993;9:325–337.

[44]Brammer AJ, Taylor W, Piercy JE. Assessing the severity of the neurological component of the hand-arm vibration syndrome. *Scand J Work Environ Health.* 1986;12:428–431.

[45]Brammer AJ, Pyykko I. Vibration-induced neuropathy. Detection by nerve conduction measurements. *Scand J Work Environ Health.* 1987;13:317–322.

[46]Cherniack MG. Raynaud's phenomenon of occupational origin. *Arch Int Med.* 1990;150:519–522.

[47]Cherniack MG, Letz R, Gerr F, Brammer A, Pace P. Detailed clinical assessment of neurological function in symptomatic shipyard workers. *Br J Ind Med.* 1990;47:566–572.

[48]Brammer AJ, Taylor W, Lundborg G. Sensorineural stages of the hand-arm vibration syndrome. *Scand J Work Environ Health.* 1987;13:279–283.

[49]Gemne G, Pyykko I, Taylor W, Pelmear PL. The Stockholm Workshop scale for the classification of cold-induced Raynaud's phenomenon in the hand-arm vibration syndrome (revision of the Taylor-Pelmear scale). *Scand J Work Environ Health.* 1987;13: 275–278.

[50]National Institute of Occupational Safety and Health. Vibration white finger diseases in US workers using pneumatic chipping and grinding hand tools. I: Epidemiology. *DHHS.* 1982;81:118.

[51]Letz R, Cherniack MG, Gerr F, Hershman D, Pace P. A cross-sectional epidemiological survey of shipyard workers exposed to hand-arm vibration. *Br J Ind Med.* 1992;49:53–62.

[52]Farkkila M, Aatola S, Starck J, Pyykko I, Korhonen O. Vibration-induced neuropathy among forestry workers. *Acta Neurol Scand.* 1985;71:221–225.

[53]Pyykko I, Korhonen O, Farkkila M, Starck J, Aatola S, Jantti V. Vibration syndrome among Finnish forest workers, a follow-up from 1972 to 1983. *Scand J Work Environ Health.* 1986;12:307–312.

[54]Miyashita K, Shiomi S, Itoh N, Kasamatsu T, Iwata H. Epidemiological study of vibration syndrome in response to total hand-tool operating time. *Br J Ind Med.* 1983;40:92–98.

[55]Futatsuka M, Ueno T. Vibration exposure and vibration-induced white finger due to chain saw operation. *J Occup Med.* 1985;27: 257–264.

[56]Yu ZS, Chao H, Qiao L, Qian DS, Ye YH. Epidemiologic survey of vibration syndrome among riveters, chippers and grinders in the railroad system of the People's Republic of China. *Scand J Work Environ Health.* 1986;12:289–292.

[57]Chatterjee DS, Barwick DD, Petrie A. Exploratory electromyography in the study of vibration-induced white finger in rock drillers. *Br J Ind Med.* 1982;39:89–97.

[58]Farkkila M, Pyykko I, Jantti V, Aatola S, Starck J, Korhonen O. Forestry workers exposed to vibration: A neurological study. *Br J Ind Med.* 1988;45:188–192.

[59]Silverstein BA, Fine LJ, Armstrong TJ. Carpal tunnel syndrome: Causes and a preventive strategy. *Semin Occup Med.* 1986; 1:213–221.

[60]Armstrong TJ, Fine LJ, Radwin RG, Silverstein BS. Ergonomics and the effects of vibration in hand-intensive work. *Scand J Work Environ Health.* 1987;13:286–289.

[61]Carlsoo S. The effect of vibration on the skeleton, joints and muscles: A review of the literature. *Appl Ergono.* 1985;13:251–258.

[62]Takeuchi T, Futatsuka M, Imanishi H, Yamada S. Pathological changes observed in the finger biopsy of patients with vibration-induced white finger. *Scand J Work Environ Health.* 1986; 12:280–283.

[63]Armstrong TJ. Ergonomics and cumulative trauma disorders. *Hand Clin.* 1986;2:553–565.

[64]Kendall D. Aetiology, diagnostic, and treatment of paraesthesiae in the hands. *Br Med J.* 1960;2:1633–1640.

[65]Tichauer ER, Gage H. Ergonomic principles basic to hand tool design. *Am Ind Hyg Assoc J.* 1977;38:622–634.

[66]Hertzberg T. Some contributions of applied physical anthropometry to human engineering. *Ann NY Acad Sci.* 1955;63:616–629.

[67]Mackworth N. Finger numbness in very cold winds. *J Appl Phys.* 1950;5:533–543.

[68]Williamson D, Chrenko F, Hamley E. A study of exposure to cold in cold stores. *Appl Ergono.* 1984;15:25–30.

[69]Chiang HC, Chen SS, Yu HS, Ko YC. The occurrence of carpal tunnel syndrome in frozen food factory employees. *Kao-Hsiung i Hsueh Ko Hsueh Tsa Chih [Kaohsiung Journal of Medical Sciences.]* 1990;6:73–80.

[70]Stevens JC, Beard CM, O'Fallon WM, Kurland LT. Conditions associated with carpal tunnel syndrome. *Mayo Clin Proc.* 1992;67:541–548.

[71]Spinner RJ, Bachman JW, Amadio PC. The many faces of carpal tunnel syndrome. *Mayo Clin Proc.* 1989;64:829–836.

[72]Biundo JJ. Regional rheumatic pain syndromes. In: Schumacher HR, ed. *Primer on the Rheumatic Diseases.* Atlanta: Arthritis Foundation, 1993;277–287.

[73]Masear VR, Hayes JM, Hyde AG. An industrial cause of carpal tunnel syndrome. *J Hand Surg Am.* 1986;11:222–227.

[74]Tanzer RC. The carpal tunnel syndrome—A clinical and anatomical study. *J Bone Joint Surg Am.* 1959;41A:626–634.

[75]Cseuz KA, Thomas JE, Lambert EH, Love JG, Lipscomb PR. Long-term results of operation for carpal tunnel syndrome. *Mayo Clin Proc.* 1966;41:232–241.

[76]Murray-Leslie CF, Wright V. Carpal tunnel syndrome, humeral epicondylitis, and the cervical spine: A study of clinical and dimensional relations. *Br Med J.* 1976;1:1439–1442.

[77]Jones JG. Ulnar tunnel syndrome. *Am Fam Physician.* 1991; 44:497–502.

[78]Pfalzer LA, McPhee B: Carpal tunnel syndrome research. In: Isernhagen SJ, ed. *The Comprehensive Guide to Work Injury Management.* First edition. Gaithersburg, MD: An Aspen Publication Inc, 1995;127–192.

[79]Bessette L, Keller RB, Lew RA, *et al.* Prognostic value of a hand symptom diagram in surgery for carpal tunnel syndrome. *J Rheumatol.* (in press).

[80]Katz JN, Larson MG, Sabra A, *et al.* The carpal tunnel syndrome: diagnostic utility of the history and physical examination findings. *Ann Intern Med.* 1990;112:321–327.

[81]Gellman H, Gelberman RH, Tan AM, Botte MJ. Carpal tunnel syndrome. An evaluation of the provocative diagnostic tests. *J Bone Joint Surg Am.* 1986;68:735–737.

[82]Golding DN, Rose DM, Selvarajah K. Clinical tests for carpal tunnel syndrome: An evaluation. *Br J Rheumatol.* 1986;25:388–390.

[83]Seror P. Sensitivity of the various tests for the diagnosis of carpal tunnel syndrome. *J Hand Surg Br.* 1994;19:725–728.

[84]Stevens JC. AAEE minimonograph 26: The electrodiagnosis of carpal tunnel syndrome. *Muscle Nerve.* 1987;10:99–113.

[85]Dorwart BB. Carpal tunnel syndrome: A review. *Semin Arthritis Rheum.* 1984;14:134–140.

[86]Grundberg AB. Carpal tunnel decompression in spite of normal electromyography. *J Hand Surg Am.* 1983;8:348–349.

[87]Matte TD, Baker EL, Honchar PA. The selection and definition of targeted work-related conditions for surveillance under SENSOR. *Am J Public Health.* 1989;79suppl:21–25.

[88]Katz JN, Larson MG, Fossel AH, Liang MH. Validation of a surveillance case definition of carpal tunnel syndrome. *Am J Public Health.* 1991;81:189–193.

[89]Lutz G, Hansford T. Cumulative trauma disorder controls: the ergonomics program at Ethicon, Inc. *J Hand Surg Am.* 1987;12:863–866.

[90]Hansford T, Blood H, Kent B, Lutz G. Blood flow changes at the wrist in manual workers after preventive interventions. *J Hand Surg Am.* 1986;11:503–508.

[91]Silverstein BA, Armstrong TJ, Longmate A, Woody D. Can implant exercise control musculoskeletal symptoms? *J Occup Med.* 1988;30:922–927.

[92]Sunderland S. The nerve lesion in the carpal tunnel syndrome. *J Neurol Neurosurg Psychiatry.* 1976;39:615–626.

[93]Chatterjee DS. Workplace upper limb disorders: A prospective study with intervention. *Occup Med.* 1992;42:129–136.

[94]Isernhagen SJ. Principles of prevention for cumulative trauma. *Occup Med.* 1992;7:147–153.

[95]Carson R. Proper medical management can reduce cumulative trauma disorder incidence. *Occup Health Saf.* 1993;62:41–44.

[96]Fisher DL, Andres RO, Airth D, Smith SS. Repetitive motion disorders: The design of optimal rate-rest profiles. *Hum Factors.* 1993;35:283–304.

[97]Johnson SL. Ergonomic hand tool design. *Hand Clin.* 1993;9:299–311.

[98]Silverstein BA, Fine LJ. Cumulative trauma disorders of the upper extremity. A preventive strategy is needed. *J Occup Med.* 1991;33:642–644.

[99]Dortch HL, 3d, Trombly CA. The effects of education on hand use with industrial workers in repetitive jobs. *Am J Occup Ther.* 1990;44:777–782.

[100]McKenzie F, Storment J, Van Hook P, Armstrong TJ. A program for control of repetitive trauma disorders associated with hand tool operations in a telecommunications manufacturing facility. *Am Ind Hyg Assoc J.* 1985;46:674–678.

[101]McCasland LJ. Development of an ergonomic program—for the meatpacking industry. *AAOHN J.* 1992;40:138–142.

[102]Maizlish N, Rudolph L, Dervin K, Sankaranarayan M. Surveillance and prevention of work-related carpal tunnel syndrome: An application of the Sentinel Events Notification System for Occupational Risks. *Am J Ind Med.* 1995;27:715–729.

[103]Green DP. Diagnostic and therapeutic value of carpal tunnel injection. *J Hand Surg Am.* 1984;9:850–854.

[104]Gelberman RH, Aronson D, Weisman MH. Carpal-tunnel syndrome. Results of a prospective trial of steroid injection and splinting. *J Bone Joint Surg Am.* 1980;62:1181–1184.

[105]Muhlau G, Both R, Kunath H. Carpal tunnel syndrome—course and prognosis. *J Neurol.* 1984;231:83–86.

[106]Brown RA, Gelberman RH, Seiler JG III, et al. Carpal tunnel release. A prospective, randomized assessment of open and endoscopic methods. *J Bone Joint Surg Am.* 1993;75:1265–1275.

[107]Hybbinette CH, Mannerfelt L. The carpal tunnel syndrome. A retrospective study of 400 operated patients. *Acta Orthop Scand.* 1975;46:610–620.

[108]Harris CM, Tanner E, Goldstein MN, Pettee DS. The surgical treatment of the carpal-tunnel syndrome correlated with preoperative nerve-conduction studies. *J Bone Joint Surg Am.* 1979;61:93–98.

[109]Semple JC, Cargill AO. Carpal-tunnel syndrome. Results of surgical decompression. *Lancet.* 1969;1:918–919.

[110]Tountas CP, MacDonald CJ, Meyerhoff JD, Bihrle DM. Carpal tunnel syndrome. A review of 507 patients. *Minn Med.* 1983;66:479–482.

[111]Posch JL, Prpic I. Surgical treatment of the carpal tunnel syndrome. *Handchirurgie.* 1975;7:95–98.

[112]Kulick MI, Gordillo G, Javidi T, Kilgore ES Jr, Newmayer WL III. Long-term analysis of patients having surgical treatment for carpal tunnel syndrome. *J Hand Surg Am.* 1986;11:59–66.

[113]Adams ML, Franklin GM, Barnhart S. Outcome of carpal tunnel surgery in Washington State workers' compensation. *Am J Ind Med.* 1994;25:527–536.

[114]Katz JN, Fossel AH, Punnett L, Mooney N, Bessette L, Keller RB. Predictors of return to work following carpal tunnel release. *Am J Ind Med.* 1996 (in press).

[115]Bongers PM, de Winter CR, Kompier MA, Hildebrandt VH. Psychosocial factors at work and musculoskeletal disease. *Scand J Work Environ Health.* 1993;19:297–312.

[116]Nathan PA, Meadows KD, Keniston RC. Rehabilitation of carpal tunnel surgery patients using a short surgical incision and an early program of physical therapy. *J Hand Surg Am.* 1993;18:1044–1050.

[117]Sommerich CM, McGlothlin JD, Marras WS. Occupational risk factors associated with soft tissue disorders of the shoulder: A review of recent investigations in the literature. *Ergonomics.* 1993;36:697–717.

[118]Bjelle A. Epidemiology of shoulder problems. *Baillieres Clin Rheumatol.* 1989;3:437–451.

[119]Katz JN, Buchbinder R. Soft tissue syndromes. *Baillieres Clin Rheumatol.* 1995;9:585–598.

[120]Allander E. Prevalence, incidence, and remission rates of some common rheumatic diseases or syndromes. *Scand J Rheumatol.* 1974;3:145–153.

[121]Takala J, Sievers K, Klaukka T. Rheumatic symptoms in the middle-aged population in southwestern Finland. *Scand J Rheumatol.* 1982;47suppl.:15–29.

[122]Bergenudd H, Lindgarde F, Nilsson B, Petersson CJ. Shoulder pain in middle age. A study of prevalence and relation to occupational work load and psychosocial factors. *Clin Orthop.* 1988;234–238.

[123]Chard MD, Hazleman R, Hazleman BL, King RH, Reiss BB. Shoulder disorders in the elderly: A community survey. *Arthritis Rheum.* 1991;34:766–769.

[124]Cunningham LS, Kelsey JL. Epidemiology of musculoskeletal impairments and associated disability. *Am J Public Health.* 1984;74:574–579.

[125]Bergstrom G, Bjelle A, Sorensen LB, Sundh V, Svanborg A. Prevalence of symptoms and signs of joint impairment at age 79. *Scand J Rehabil Med.* 1985;17:173–182.

[126]Bjelle A, Hagberg M, Michaelson G. Occupational and individual factors in acute shoulder-neck disorders among industrial workers. *Br J Ind Med.* 1981;38:356–363.

[127]Manahan L, Caragay R, Muirden KD, et al. Rheumatic pain in a Philippine village. A WHO-ILAR COPCORD Study. *Rheumatol Int.* 1985;5:149–153.

[128]Tola S, Riihimaki H, Videman T, Viikari-Juntura E, Hanninen K. Neck and shoulder symptoms among men in machine operating, dynamic physical work and sedentary work. *Scand J Work Environ Health.* 1988;14:299–305.

[129]Ekberg K, Karlsson M, Axelson O, Malm P. Cross-sectional study of risk factors for symptoms in the neck and shoulder area. *Ergonomics.* 1995;38:971–980.

[130]Kvarnstrom S. Occurrence of musculoskeletal, disorders in a manufacturing industry with special attention to occupational shoulder disorders. *Scand J Rehabil Med Suppl.* 1983;8:1–114.

[131]Punnett L, Robins JM, Wegman DH, Keyserling WM. Soft tissue disorders in the upper limbs of female garment workers. *Scand J Work Environ Health.* 1985;11:417–425.

[132]Luopajarvi T, Kuorinka I, Virolainen M, Holmberg M. Prevalence of tenosynovitis and other injuries of the upper extremities in repetitive work. *Scand J Work Environ Health.* 1979;5Suppl 3:48–55.

[133]Chiang HC, Ko YC, Chen SS, Yu HS, Wu TN, Chang PY. Prevalence of shoulder and upper-limb disorders among workers in the fish-processing industry. *Scand J Work Environ Health.* 1993;19:126–131.

[134]Sallstrom J, Schmidt H. Cervicobrachial disorders in certain occupations, with special reference to compression in the thoracic outlet. *Am J Ind Med.* 1984;6:45–52.

[135]Kilbom A, Persson J. Work technique and its consequences for musculoskeletal disorders. *Ergonomics.* 1987;30:273–279.

[136]Herberts P, Kadefors R, Hogfors C, Sigholm G. Shoulder pain and heavy manual labor. *Clin Orthop.* 1984;166–178.

[137]Kamwendo K, Linton SJ, Moritz U. Neck and shoulder disorders in medical secretaries. Part I. Pain prevalence and risk factors. *Scand J Rehabil Med.* 1991;23:127–133.

[138]Knave BG, Wibom RI, Voss M, Hedstrom LD, Bergqvist UO. Work with video display terminals among office employees. I. Subjective symptoms and discomfort. *Scand J Work Environ Health.* 1985;11:457–466.

[139]Rossignol AM, Morse EP, Summers VM, Pagnotto LD. Video display terminal use and reported health symptoms among Massachusetts clerical workers. *J Occup Med.* 1987;29:112–118.

[140]Karlqvist L, Hagberg M, Selin K. Variation in upper limb posture and movement during word processing with and without mouse use. *Ergonomics.* 1994;37:1261–1267.

[141]Stenlund B, Goldie I, Hagberg M, Hogstedt C. Shoulder tendinitis and its relation to heavy manual work and exposure to vibration. *Scand J Work Environ Health.* 1993;19:43–49.

[142]Matsen III FA, Arntz CT. Subacromial impingement. In: Rockwood CA, F.A., ed. *The Shoulder.* Philadelphia: W.B. Saunders Company, 1990;623–646.

[143]Ling SC, Chen CF, Wan RX. A study on the vascular supply of the supraspinatus tendon. *Surg Radiol Anat.* 1990;12:161–165.

[144]Hollingworth GR, Ellis RM, Hattersley TS. Comparison of injection techniques for shoulder pain: Results of a double blind, randomised study. *Br Med J Clin Res.* 1983;287:1339–1341.

[145]Harvey FJ, Bosanquet JS. Carpal tunnel syndrome caused by a simple ganglion. *Hand.* 1981;13:164–166.

[146]Peled I, Iosipovich Z, Rousso M, Wexler MR. Hemangioma of the median nerve. *J Hand Surg Am.* 1980;5:363–365.

[147]Herndon JH, Eaton RG, Littler JW. Carpal-tunnel syndrome. An unusual presentation of osteoid-osteoma of the capitate. *J Bone Joint Surg Am.* 1974;56:1715–1718.

[148]Louis DS, Dick HM. Ossifying lipofibroma of the median nerve. *J Bone Joint Surg Am.* 1973;55:1082–1084.

[149]Poilvache P, Carlier A, Rombouts JJ, Partoune E, Lejeune G. Carpal tunnel syndrome in childhood: report of five new cases. *J Pediatr Orthop.* 1989;9:687–690.

[150]Leifer D, Cros D, Halperin JJ, Gallico GG III, Pierce DS, Shahani BT. Familial bilateral carpal tunnel syndrome: Report of two families. *Arch Phys Med Rehabil.* 1992;73:393–397.

[151]Rosenthal EA. Tenosynovitis: Tendon and nerve entrapment [published erratum appears in *Hand Clin* 1988;4(2):x]. *Hand Clin.* 1987;3:585–609.

[152]Hartwell SW Jr, Kurtay M. Carpal tunnel compression caused by hematoma associated with anticoagulant therapy. Report of a case. *Cleve Clin Q.* 1966;33:127–129.

[153]Lusthaus S, Matan Y, Finsterbush A, Chaimsky G, Mosheiff R, Ashur H. Traumatic section of the median nerve: An unusual complication of Colles' fracture. *Injury.* 1993;24:339–340.

[154]Paley D, McMurtry RY. Median nerve compression by volarly displaced fragments of the distal radius. *Clin Orthop.* 1987;139:147.

[155]Soccetti A, Carloni S, Giovagnoni M, Misericordia M. MR findings in post-traumatic carpal tunnel syndrome. *Chir Organi Mov.* 1993;78:233–239.

[156]Lee DJ, Fechter J, Schnall SB. Old displaced fracture of the scaphoid. An unusual cause of carpal tunnel syndrome. *Orthop Rev.* 1993;22:842–844.

[157]Mack GR, McPherson SA, Lutz RB. Acute median neuropathy after wrist trauma. The role of emergent carpal tunnel release. *Clin Orthop.* 1994;141–146.

[158]Leibovic SJ, Geissler WB. Treatment of complex intra-articular distal radius fractures. *Orthop Clin North Am.* 1994;25:685–706.

[159]Vemireddi NK, Redford JB, PombeJara CN. Serial nerve conduction studies in carpal tunnel syndrome secondary to rheumatoid arthritis: Preliminary study. *Arch Phys Med Rehabil.* 1979;60:393–396.

[160]Berth-Jones J, Coates PA, Graham-Brown RA, Burns DA. Neurological complications of systemic sclerosis—a report of three cases and review of the literature. *Clin Exp Dermatol.* 1990;15:91–94.

[161]O'Duffy JD, Hunder GG, Wahner HW. A follow-up study of polymyalgia rheumatica: Evidence of chronic axial synovitis. *J Rheumatol.* 1980;7:685–693.

[162]Quinones CA, Perry HO, Rushton JG. Carpal tunnel syndrome in dermatomyositis and scleroderma. *Arch Dermatol.* 1966;94:20–25.

[163]Pai CH, Tseng CH. Acute carpal tunnel syndrome caused by tophaceous gout. *J Hand Surg Am.* 1993;18:667–669.

[164]Gerster JC, Lagier R, Boivin G, Schneider C. Carpal tunnel syndrome in chondrocalcinosis of the wrist. Clinical and histologic study. *Arthritis Rheum.* 1980;23:926–931.

[165]Lagier R, Boivin G, Gerster JC. Carpal tunnel syndrome associated with mixed calcium pyrophosphate dihydrate and apatite crys-

tal deposition in tendon synovial sheath. *Arthritis Rheum.* 1984; 27:1190–1195.

[166]Chammas M, Bousquet P, Renard E, Poirier JL, Jaffiol C, Allieu Y. Dupuytren's disease, carpal tunnel syndrome, trigger finger, and diabetes mellitus. *J Hand Surg Am.* 1995;20:109–114.

[167]Frymoyer JW, Bland J. Carpal-tunnel syndrome in patients with myxedematous arthropathy. *J Bone Joint Surg Am.* 1973;55:78–82.

[168]Woo CC. Neurological features of acromegaly: A review and report of two cases. *J Manipulative Physiol Ther.* 1988;11:314–321.

[169]MacDougal B, Weeks PM, Wray RC Jr. Median nerve compression and trigger finger in the mucopolysaccharidoses and related diseases. *Plast Reconstr Surg.* 1977;59:260–263.

[170]Gerardi JA, Mack GR, Lutz RB. Acute carpal tunnel syndrome secondary to septic arthritis of the wrist. *J Am Osteopath Assoc.* 1989;89:933–934.

[171]Suso S, Peidro L, Ramon R. Tuberculous synovitis with "rice bodies" presenting as carpal tunnel syndrome. *J Hand Surg Am.* 1988;13:574–576.

[172]Prince H, Ispahani P, Baker M. A Mycobacterium malmoense infection of the hand presenting as carpal tunnel syndrome. *J Hand Surg Br.* 1988;13:328–330.

[173]Randall G, Smith PW, Korbitz B, Owen DR. Carpal tunnel syndrome caused by Mycobacterium fortuitum and Histoplasma capsulatum. Report of two cases. *J Neurosurg.* 1982;56:299–301.

[174]Strayer DS, Gutwein MB, Herbold D, Bresalier R. Histoplasmosis presenting as the carpal tunnel syndrome. *Am J Surg.* 1981;141:286–288.

[175]Heckman JD, Sassard R. Musculoskeletal considerations in pregnancy. *J Bone Joint Surg Am.* 1994;76:1720–1730.

[176]Vessey MP, Villard-Mackintosh L, Yeates D. Epidemiology of carpal tunnel syndrome in women of childbearing age. Findings in a large cohort study. *Int J Epidemiol.* 1990;19:655–659.

[177]Pascual E, Giner V, Arostegui A, Conill J, Ruiz MT, Pico A. Higher incidence of carpal tunnel syndrome in oophorectomized women. *Br J Rheumatol.* 1991;30:60–62.

[178]Gertz MA, Kyle RA. Primary systemic amyloidosis—a diagnostic primer. *Mayo Clin Proc.* 1989;64:1505–1519.

[179]Schwarz A, Keller F, Seyfert S, Poll W, Molzahn M, Distler A. Carpal tunnel syndrome: A major complication in long-term hemodialysis patients. *Clin Nephrol.* 1984;22:133–137.

17

Occupation-Related Physical Factors and Osteoarthritis

David T. Felson

Osteoarthritis (OA) is the most common form of arthritis. Symptomatic knee OA affects approximately 15% of elderly people and may affect up to 6% of all adults.[1] Hip OA and involvement of other joints are also exceedingly common. OA develops after many years of articular cartilage damage. This damage is brought on by both systemic and local factors.[1,2] Like other chronic, degenerative diseases of aging, such as heart disease, a multitude of factors combine to increase the risk of disease occurrence. Also like these other diseases, modifying some of these risk factors for disease may result in OA prevention.

There are several occupational groups with a high rate of OA. Appreciating whether and how occupation increases the risk of OA is important in understanding what causes this disease. Furthermore, since common jobs involve repetitive joint use, occupation-related disease may account for a large percentage of OA in the population and may be amenable to preventive intervention.

This chapter will review the effects of occupation-related physical factors on OA. It will focus on appendicular joints, where the correlation of symptoms and X-ray change is high. In addition, the relationship between occupation and radiographic changes of OA in the lumbar and cervical spines, including spinal osteophytosis, facet joint disease and disc disease, will be addressed. Some studies have defined OA by X ray, whereas in others only clinical evaluations have been performed. It is possible that factors causing clinical disease differ from those leading to radiographic changes. Also, since risk factors for OA are joint-specific,[1] this review will attempt to separate out the association of occupational physical factors and OA by joint.

Paralyzed limbs are rarely, if ever, affected by OA,[3] suggesting that joint use is required to induce OA. Also, amputations occurring below the knee protect against OA in that knee.[4] Lastly, some studies,[5,6] although not all,[7] report that people develop OA preferentially in the usually dominant right hand. Therefore, mechanical factors are necessary, although perhaps not sufficient by themselves, to cause OA.

DO OCCUPATIONAL PHYSICAL ACTIVITIES CAUSE OSTEOARTHRITIS?

Three types of studies have been utilized to evaluate the relationship between occupational activities and OA: First, studies comparing the rates of OA in geographic regions with contrasting types of occupations; second, studies of specific occupational groups to evaluate whether there are high rates of OA in overused joints. Lastly, studies that have explored particular physical activities in workers to identify activities correlated with high rates of OA.

Geographical Studies

Most studies comparing OA prevalence in different geographic regions have compared physical labor or farming areas with urban areas. For example, in one survey the frequency of self-reported OA in different regions of Sweden was highest in regions characterized by farming and forestry activities.[8] Stockholm, which had the lowest rate of farming, forestry, heavy industry and mining activities of all of the regions studied, had a particularly low rate of OA.

Farming communities report high rates of hip and knee OA.[9,10] Middle-aged men and women residents of the island of Gotland in the Baltic Sea, a predominantly agricultural community, had significantly higher rates of hip OA by pelvic X-ray than a comparable Swedish urban population. Similarly, a rural population in Japan experienced higher rates of OA than did a comparable urban population near Osaka;[11] however specific joint involvement was not reported.

Despite strong evidence that OA may arise more frequently than expected in agricultural communities, a comprehensive review of X rays from various studies around the world[12] did not reveal higher rates of hip OA in the farming communities of Wensleydale, England and Azmoos, Switzerland than in nonagricultural communities in Europe. Furthermore, a higher prevalence of radiographic knee OA was found in men and women on the industrialized western coast of Greenland than on the eastern coast, where the population consists of Eskimos who are hunters and fishermen.[13]

Studies of Specific Occupational Groups

Farming

The reports of high rates of OA in farming communities naturally led to focused studies of the disease in farmers. As shown in Table 17-1, these studies have all reported that male farmers have a higher prevalence of hip OA than non-farmers. Farming remains an independent risk factor for hip disease, even after adjusting for important confounding factors like age and weight. There is insufficient data on women, and little information on OA in other joints.

Specific occupational groups reported to have high rates of osteoarthritis are listed in Table 17-2. Case-control and cohort studies usually evaluate the association of exposures such as farming with incident or new cases of disease. Stud-

Table 17-1   Controlled studies of farming and osteoarthritis

Reference #	Authors/Yr	Design of Study	OA: Radiographic Versus Clinical Diagnosis	Sex of Subjects	Joint(s) Studied	Results
14	Louyot and Savin 1966	Survey of jobs of hip OA cases	Clinical	M & F	hip	Higher than expected rates in farmers (M&F)
49	Typpo 1985	Case control	X-ray	M & F	hip	Increased proportion of farmers among cases
19	Thelin et al. 1990	Case Control	Clinical	M & F	hip	Increased risk of hip OA in farmers (especially ≥ 10 years)
15	Vingard et al. 1991	Cohort	Clinical	M & F	hip & knee	High risk of hip OA in male farmers (RR = 3.8) but risk of knee OA only marginally increased (RR = 1.46, p < .05). No significant increase in hip or knee OA in females.
16	Croft et al. 1992	Case control	X-ray[+]	M	hip	Increased hip OA, especially if ≥10 years farming (OR = 9.3)
17	Croft et al. 1992	Cohort	X-ray[+]	M	hip	Marked increase in hip OA especially if ≥10 years farming
50	Axmacher and Lindberg 1993	Cohort	X-ray	M & F	hip	Increased hip OA (RR = 12.0) in male farmers

[+]OA based on joint space narrowing but subjects also designated as OA if underwent total hip replacement.
Modified from Felson DT.[53]
M = male; F = female.

Table 17-2   Specific occupational groups reported to have high rates of osteoarthritis

Occupational Group(s)	Joint(s) Affected	Controlled Study	Reference
Pneumatic Drill Operators	Shoulders, wrists, elbows, MCPs	No	See text; multiple studies
Farmers	Hips, knees	Yes	See text; multiple studies
Cotton Mill Workers	DIPs, PIPs	Yes	Lawrence 1961[30]
Miners	Knees, lumbar spine	Yes	Kellgren and Lawrence 1952[31]
Shipyard Laborers	Knees	Yes	Lindberg and Montgomery 1987[35]
Dockers	DIPs, elbows knees	Yes	Partridge and Duthie 1968[51]
Foundry Workers	Lumbar spine	Yes	Lawrence et al. 1966[52]
Ballet Dancers	Ankle, subtalar & MTP	Yes	Brodelius 1961[33]; van Dijk et al. 1995[34]
Soccer Players	Talar joints, knees, hips	Yes	See text; multiple studies

Modified from Felson DT.[53]
MCP = metacarpophalangeal joints.
DIP = distal interphalangeal joints.
PIP = proximal interphalangeal joints.
MTP = metatarsophalangeal joints.

ies have, without exception, evaluated prevalent disease, raising concerns that the strength of the relationship may be underestimated (could those with hip OA have discontinued farming?), and about a biased selection of cases (prevalent cases are usually those with the most long-standing disease). The choice of hospital cases[14,15] or cases selected because they were undergoing total hip arthroplasty[16,17] suggests that farming may predispose to severe OA.

What is the explanation for the higher-than-expected rate of hip OA among farmers? Hip OA may be in part due to developmental abnormalities in the hip joint,[1] although this has not been proven.[16] Many individuals who grow up on the farm begin work during childhood when the hip is not fully developed, and there may be a high rate of slipped capital femoral epiphysis, a developmental abnormality that often leads to subsequent OA.[1,19] However, one study[14] reported that farmers with hip OA actually have a lower rate of abnormal morphologies than nonfarmers with this disease, suggesting no preexisting developmental problem.

Given the long-term intensive heavy physical labor associated with farming,[14] it seems more reasonable to postulate that some particular aspect of this labor is associated with mechanical damage of the hip and perhaps of other joints, including the knee. Physical activities that might be implicated include: long periods of standing, excessive bending and kneeling, walking long distances, climbing, lifting or moving heavy objects and driving, especially on tractors or trucks for long periods which may expose the hips to repeated vibration. In an effort to isolate these different activities, it has been demonstrated that standing, bending, walking long distances over rough ground, tractor driving and lifting or moving heavy weights were associated with particularly high rates of hip OA in farmers.[17-19] Of these various activities, standing is unlikely to be implicated as it does not especially increase force across the hip joint.[15]

Jackhammer Operators

The jackhammer is a heavy pneumatic tool generally held by both hands and used to drill concrete or stone. Other pneumatic drills that are smaller and hand-held generally vibrate faster than large pneumatic drills but impart less force with each vibration. Pneumatic drill workers are at high risk of developing Raynaud phenomenon, especially after they have been working with pneumatic tools for many years.[20,21] The rate of Raynaud among various types of pneumatic tool operators rises above 30% in those using these tools for at least 10 years, especially in those working on hard material. Also, the frequency of vibration appears to correlate with the risk of Raynaud, in that tools which vibrate 2,000 to 3,000 times per minute are more likely to induce white fingers than tools which vibrate less frequently. Working in the cold may also increase this risk.

Osteoarthritis was first described in pneumatic tool operators before World War II.[20,22] The joints involved are other-wise not usually affected by OA, and include the shoulder, metacarpophalangeal (MCP) joint and even the wrist.[23]

Initial reports suggested that up to one-third of jackhammer operators developed elbow OA,[20] but subsequent studies reported lower rates of disease in the elbow and wrist.[23,24] Although pathologic changes in the capitellum are commonly found at autopsy, clinical OA of the elbow and wrist are extremely rare in middle-aged men. The presence of clinical elbow disease in 5% to 10% of subjects strongly suggests an association.

Recent case reports document unusually severe MCP joint arthritis in a jackhammer operator[25] and severe wrist OA in a worker who had been a jackhammer operator for 30 years.[26] On the other hand, while acromioclavicular (AC) joint OA is increased in frequency among Swedish rock blasters[27] compared to their foremen, bricklayers, who are unexposed to vibratory tools, experience the same high rate of AC joint OA, suggesting it is heavy manual lifting which causes OA in the AC joint, rather than exposure to vibratory tools.

In summary, given the severity of unusual upper-extremity OA found in pneumatic drill workers, it seems extremely likely that pneumatic drill use is associated with higher-than-expected rates of OA in the wrist, elbow and MCP joints.

Why are jackhammer operators prone to develop OA in these upper-extremity joints? First, workers who use heavy tools experience tremendous impact loads across non-weight-bearing joints, which are ill-designed to sustain these loads. In general, impact loads are born by two major shock absorbers, muscles and tendons on the one hand and sub-chondral bone on the other.[28,29] Vibratory tools could subvert the effectiveness of these major shock absorbers in several ways and therefore lead to the transmission of excess force across joints. Muscles and tendons operate by assuming the correct tension and position to withstand anticipated force. Input to muscles and tendons arises from muscle spindles, which could be overwhelmed by the repetitive stimulus of vibration. This could immobilize or impair the tendons' ability to assume proper tension to deflect load from the cartilage of the joint. The commonly experienced sensation of numbness which occurs after the use of pneumatic tools could be a signal that neurologic input is temporarily dysfunctional after prolonged tool use. Furthermore, pneumatic tools could simply lead to the fatigue of protective muscles. Lastly, with impact loads transmitted to joints, the subchondral bone could sustain microfractures which could alter the deformability of the subchondral bone, leading to increased force transmitted to the cartilage.

Other Occupational Groups with High Risks of Osteoarthritis

In addition to pneumatic drill operators and farmers, other occupational groups have been reported to have high rates of OA in overused joints. For example, cotton mill workers[30] had high rates of radiographic and clinical disease in their distal interphalangeal (DIP) and proximal interphalangeal (PIP) joints, but not in the cervical or lumbar spines compared to coal mining males and female homemakers. Miners, however, had an increased prevalence of radiographic and symptomatic OA of the knee and lumbar spine compared to office workers and manual workers who never worked in mines.[31] Miners did not have higher rates of hand OA than manual workers, although office workers appeared to have slightly less hand OA than either manual workers or miners. A study of lumbar spine OA in miners reported that longer duration of heavy work was associated with an increased rate of osteophytosis but not necessarily higher rates of disc narrowing.[32]

In other studies, ballet dancers were found to have more OA in the ankle, subtalar and first metatarsophalangeal (MTP) joints than age-matched female controls,[33,34] and long-time manual laborers in a Swedish shipyard had higher rates of knee OA (3.9%) than controls (1.5%, p < 0.05).[35]

Controlled studies of OA in current and former soccer players have yielded conflicting results.[1] One study found no higher rate of hip OA than in controls but reported that 28% of soccer players' knees had patellofemoral OA, a much higher rate than controls.[36] Many of these subjects had sustained identifiable knee injuries which may have accounted for some of their disease. Another study, however, found that 28 out of 57 subjects had hip osteophytes (without joint space narrowing) versus only 15 controls, a significant difference, whereas there was no difference in the rate of knee OA.[37]

While most studies of specific occupational groups have reported higher-than-expected rates of OA, others have been negative. For example, female physical education teachers had no more knee or hip OA than aged-matched controls.[38] In addition, experience with runners and other sports enthusiasts suggests that increased rates of OA are not consistently found.

Insight into how occupational activities induce OA may be gleaned from reports of unusual OA in certain workers. For example, seven manual laborers, of whom three were farmers, had painful and palpably enlarged MCP joints.[39] Radiographic changes included not only joint space loss but also large osteophytes and cystic changes, especially in the second and third metacarpal heads. For all these subjects, heavy work had demanded prolonged gripping motions in both hands over at least 30 years. In the MCPs, the prolonged gripping may have led to fatigue of the protective muscles across the joint, transmitting excess force to the joint cartilage. Also, foundry workers may develop severe elbow OA if they have long-term jobs that require daily use of tongs for lifting and twisting hot metal rods.[40]

Almost all studies of specific occupational groups have been cross-sectional. Failure to assess OA in (usually former) workers who quit or switch to less demanding work may cause underestimates of the association of occupation with OA. However, case-control studies in which OA cases are drawn from those with severe disease (such as total joint replacement patients, or hospitalized patients) may introduce several biases. First, these studies may be best conceptualized as studies of severe OA and its causes. Second, in these studies, occupational physical activity may act as a disease promoter, especially if the physical demands from the occupation continue after OA has begun. In this case, occupational activities are not causing OA but contributing to worsening symptoms or disease progression.

Notwithstanding these methodologic caveats, specific occupational groups are at high risk for OA in repetitively used joints. The question remains as to which particular activities induce the joint damage.

Which Activities Cause Osteoarthritis?

Studies of Specific Occupation Groups

Several intensive investigations of specific occupational groups at high risk for OA have attempted to determine particular activities that lead to disease. The first of these was a study of coal miners, a group found to have an unexpectedly high rate of knee OA and radiographic lumbar disc degeneration.[31] In an exhaustive investigation of occupational factors thought to increase the risk of back and knee problems, several different groups of miners, including those who worked in wet versus dry environments, those who worked at different heights, and those who worked on the mine face versus the roadway, were compared with dockers who also performed heavy manual labor and with sedentary workers.[41] For lumbar disc disease, the severity of radiologic change was similar in miners and heavy manual laborers, but miners more often had multiple discs affected. The single factor best identified with a higher risk of severe disc disease was the duration of time the miner had been performing heavy lifting. Radiographic changes in the spine were unrelated to whether the miner worked in a wet or a dry environment (although back symptoms were more frequent in those from wet mines), and were unaffected by the height at which the miner worked or history of previous back injury. Radiographic knee OA was more common in the miners than in laborers or sedentary workers. The prevalence of knee OA was unrelated to the distance walked, kneeling, heavy lifting or the duration of work in wet mines. Indeed, the only factor clearly associated with knee OA in this group of miners was a history of knee injury, a risk factor identified in many other studies.[1]

In another study, repetitive hand motion was examined in three groups of women mill workers, burlers, spinners and winders who had performed their jobs for at least 20 years.[42] Importantly, winding involves using a power grip with a preponderance of load across the wrist and little load across finger joints. On the other hand, burling and spinning both use the second and third fingers in a precision or pincer grip which puts large forces across the DIP and PIP joints. Burlers and spinners had unusually high rates of (OA) in the DIP joints. Furthermore, they had malalignment of the PIP joint of the second finger. Winders, on the other hand, had few, if any, of these radiographic changes. This study provided strong evidence that repetitive use with increased force across a joint can induce OA.

In one of the few longitudinal studies of occupational physical activity, the physical workload of 502 Finnish metal industry workers was examined.[43] Physical work was characterized by its physical load demand, which was based primarily on how much carrying and lifting was required, static phase, which summarized static muscle work, stereotypy, which summarized whether the job activities contained stereotypic or repeated movements of a given joint, and lastly, physical strain, which graded other quantitative measures. Musculoskeletal disease, evaluated both at the baseline assessment and five years later, was defined by self-report and by a physical examination done by physiotherapists. Among men and women at baseline, blue-collar workers had higher rates of musculoskeletal findings on physical examination and more chronic musculoskeletal disease by self-report. Baseline physical load and static load were correlated strongly with the presence of musculoskeletal findings and self-reported disease, although neither stereotypy nor overall physical strain had an association with musculoskeletal morbidity. At the five-year follow-up, none of the aspects of physical labor, except for the physical load (men only)—a measure of carrying during the job—was associated with higher-than-expected rates of musculoskeletal findings. To explain the negative longitudinal findings, it was postulated that there was loss to follow-up, and that a selection of workers were able to remain in physically demanding jobs. It was also noted that some workers would never enter physically demanding jobs because of preexisting musculoskeletal conditions. Physical load and strain may be global summaries of physical work, which may contain particular activities that are damaging to joints. This study points out the complexity of defining ergonomic tasks in a multioccupational work environment.

A POPULATION PERSPECTIVE

Studies of Multiple Occupational Groups

While specific and unusual occupational activities, including pneumatic drill operation, may increase the risk of OA, the importance of occupation-induced OA in the population at large is not clear from the studies so far reviewed. Do occupational physical activities play an important role as a cause of knee or other joint OA?

In a nationwide study of hospital admissions for OA in Sweden, workers with high levels of exposures to dynamic (impact loading) and static compression forces were compared to those with low exposures to these forces.[44] Occupational groups at high risk of hip OA included farmers, firefighters, mill workers, butchers, dockers and, to a lesser degree, unskilled manual workers, fisherman and miners. Those at high risk of knee OA hospitalization included firefighters, farmers and construction workers. Women mailcarriers had a very high rate of hip OA, and women employed in house or hotel cleaning had a high rate of knee OA compared to low-exposure controls. This study suggests that there are many occupational groups who are at a high risk of OA in overused joints.

To evaluate the association of occupational status and concurrent knee OA by radiograph, data was evaluated[45] from the National Health and Nutrition Examination Survey (NHANES) I, a U.S. federal survey that included nonweight-bearing knee X rays. In general, workers who were craftsmen, laborers or service workers had the highest prevalence of radiographic knee OA. Each person was characterized by whether his or her occupation required bending, kneeling and/or carrying or lifting. After adjusting for age, race, body mass index and education level, the authors found that strength demand of job and knee-bending were powerful correlates of knee OA. For persons in the 55-to-64-year age-group, the proportion of radiographic knee OA attributable to job-related knee-bending was greater (32%) than for obesity (24%), a major risk factor for knee OA. This strongly suggests that occupation-related overuse has an important role in OA.

In a longitudinal evaluation of occupational activity and knee OA, job activity was correlated with the prevalence of subsequent knee OA.[46] Among men, those with jobs that required both knee-bending and at least moderate carrying (frequent lifting of at least 25 lbs) were at a higher than expected risk of subsequent radiographic OA (OR = 2.22 [95% CI 1.38, 3.58 p < .01]). For men, as in the NHANES I study, the proportion of OA attributable to jobs in which there were both knee-bending and physical demands was slightly higher than the proportion of OA attributable to obesity.

In a case-control study of women with symptomatic knee OA, previous jobs which entailed either squatting, kneeling or climbing more than 10 flights per day were more frequent than expected in cases.[47] Furthermore, the risk of OA seemed especially high when the subject's previous job combined kneeling or squatting with heavy lifting.

Activities that increase force across the hip joint involve walking, lifting a heavy package and, especially, kneeling or running. In a case-control study of hip OA, the prevalence of disease was increased in men if more than one-half of the working day entailed activities such as kneeling, walking, heavy work standing or a combination of these three activities.[48] Other work activities, including light standing and sitting, were unassociated with a risk for hip OA.

In summary, multiple studies of individual occupations and of populations have suggested that occupation-related joint overuse is an important cause of knee, hip and other joint OA. Much of the burden of OA in our society may, in fact, be attributable to occupational overuse.

Occupational overuse is not an easy target for prevention, since occupational physical activities are complex, and identifying the particular activity which may induce OA in a given joint may be difficult. Well-defined ergonomic evaluations such as that in the Virginia textile mill[42] are difficult in most environments where workers often change their jobs or particular physical activities evolve over time. Recent studies from Finland are representative of the complexity of defining specific ergonomic activities and the difficulty of isolating the effect of carrying or bending activities on disease.[43] Studies of farmers, in whom there is an increased risk of hip OA, have failed to identify a specific activity associated with disease. An additional problem in establishing a relationship between a particular activity and its effect on joints is the time required for OA to develop. Furthermore, since the causation of OA is multifactorial, risk factors other than occupation may play a role and should be controlled for in these studies. Notwithstanding these difficulties, the impact of occupation on OA is so clear and has such a substantial impact on the burden of disease that future studies are clearly warranted. Such investigations should include better definitions of ergonomic activities and a more focused attempt to isolate the specific activities which predispose to the development of OA.

Supported by NIH Grants AR20613 and AG09300

REFERENCES

[1]Felson DT. Epidemiology of hip and knee osteoarthritis. *Epidemiol Rev.* 1988;10;1–28.

[2]Dieppe P. The Classification and Diagnosis of Osteoarthritis. In: *Osteoarthritic Disorders.* Kuettner, Goldberg, eds. Rosemont, IL: Am Acad Ortho Surg. 1995;5–12.

[3]Glyn JH, Sutherland I, Walker GF, *et al.* Low incidence of osteoarthrosis in hip and knee after anterior poliomyelitis: A late review. *Br Med J.* 1966;2:739–742.

[4]Peyron JG. Review of the main epidemiologic-etiologic evidence that implies mechanical forces as factors in osteoarthritis. *Engineering Med.* 1986;15:77–79.

[5]Hadler NM. Industrial rheumatology. Clinical investigations into the influence of the pattern of usage on the pattern of regional musculoskeletal disease. *Arthritis Rheum.* 1977;20:1019–1025.

[6]Acheson RM. New Haven survey of joint disease XII: Distribution and symptoms of osteoarthrosis in the hands with reference to handedness. *Ann Rheum Dis.* 1970;29:275–285.

[7]Lane NE, Block DA, Jones HH, *et al.* Osteoarthritis in the hand: A comparison of handedness and hand use. *J Rheumatol.* 1989;16:637–642.

[8]Bjelle A, Allander E, Lundquist B. Geographic distribution of rheumatic disorders and working conditions in Sweden. *Scand J Soc Med.* 1981;9:119–126.

[9]Zinn WM. Reflections on degenerative hip disease. *Ann Phys Med.* 1970;X:209–217.

[10]Jordan JM, Linder GF, Renner JB, *et al.* The impact of arthritis in rural populations. *Arthritis Canc Res.* 1995;8:242–250.

[11]Shichikawa K, Mayeda A, Komatsubara Y, *et al.* Rheumatic complaints in urban and rural populations in Osaka. *Ann Rheum Dis.* 1966;25:25–31.

[12]Lawrence JS, Sebo M. The geography of osteoarthrosis. In: *The Aetiopathogenesis of Osteoarthrosis.* Baltimore: University Park Press 1980;155–183.

[13]Andersen S. The epidemiology of primary osteoarthrosis of the knee in Greenland. *Scand J Rheum.* 1978;7:109–112.

[14]Louyot P, Savin R. La coxarthrose chez l'argriculteur. *Revue du Rhumatisme.* 1966;33:625–632.

[15]Vingard E, Alfredsson L, Goldie I, *et al.* Occupation and osteoarthrosis of the hip and knee: A register-based cohort study. *Int J Epidemiol.* 1991;20:1025–1031.

[16]Croft P, Cooper C, Wickham C, *et al.* Osteoarthritis of the hip and occupational activity. *Scand J Work Environ Health.* 1992;18:59–63.

[17]Croft P, Coggon D, Cruddas M. Osteoarthritis of the hip: An occupational disease in farmers. *Br Med J.* 1992;304:1269–1272.

[18]Jacobsson B, Dalen N, Tjornstrand B. Coxarthrosis and labour. *Int Orthop.* 1987;11:311–313.

[19]Thelin A. Hip joint arthrosis: An occupational disorder among farmers. *Am J Indus Med.* 1990;18:339–343.

[20]Hunter D, McLaughlin AIG, Perry KM. Clinical effects of the use of pneumatic tools. *Br J Indus Med.* 1945;2:10–16.

[21]Miyashita K, Shiomi S, Itoh N, *et al.* Epidemiological study of vibration syndrome in response to total hand-tool operating time. *Br J Indus Med.* 1983;40:92–98.

[22]Copeman WSC. The arthritic sequelae of pneumatic drilling. *Ann Rheum Dis.* 1940;2:141–146.

[23]Gemne G, Saraste H. Bone and joint pathology in workers using hand-held vibrating tools: An overview. *Scand J Work Environ Health.* 1987;13:296–300.

[24]Burke MJ, Fear EC, Wright V. Bone and joint changes in pneumatic drillers. *Ann Rheum Dis.* 1977;36:276–279.

[25]Fam AG, Kolin A. Unusual metacarpophalangeal osteoarthritis in a jackhammer operator. *Arthritis Rheum.* 1986;29:1284–1289.

[26]Schumacher HR, Agudelo C, Labowitz R. Jackhammer arthropathy. *JOM.* 1972;14(7):563–564.

[27]Stenlund B, Goldie I, Hagberg M. Radiographic osteoarthrosis in the acromioclavicular joint resulting from manual work or exposure to vibration. *Br J Indus Med.* 1992;49:588–593.

[28]Brandt KD, Flusser D. Osteoarthritis. In: N Bellamy, ed. *Prognosis of the Rheumatic Diseases.* Kluwer Academic Publishers, 1991;11–35.

[29]Radin EL. The relationship between biological and mechanical factors in the etiology of osteoarthritis. *J Rheumatol.* 1983;10(suppl 9):20–21.

[30]Lawrence JS. Rheumatism in cotton operatives. *Br J Indus Med.* 1961;18:270–276.

[31]Kellgren JH, Lawrence JS. Rheumatism in miners; Part II: X-ray study. *Br J Indus Med.* 1952;9:197–207.

[32]Caplan PS, Freedman LMJ, Connelly TP. Degenerative joint disease of the lumbar spine in coal miners—a clinical and x-ray study. *Arthritis Rheum.* 1966;9:693–702.

[33]Brodelius A. Osteoarthrosis of the talar joints in footballers and ballet dancers. *Acta Orthop Scand.* 1961;30:9–314.

[34]Van Dijk CN, Lim LS, Poortman A, Strubbe EH, Marti RK. Degenerative joint disease in female ballet dancers. *Am J Sports Med.* 1995;23(3):295–300.

[35]Lindberg H, Montgomery F. Heavy labor and the occurrence of gonarthrosis. *Clin Orthop.* 1987;214:235–236.

[36]Solonen KA. The joints of the lower extremities of football players. *Ann Chir et Gynaecol Fenniae.* 1966;55:176–180.

[37]Klunder K. Osteoarthritis of the hip and knee joint in retired football players. *Acta Orthop Scand.* 1980;51:925–927.

[38]Eastmond CJ, Hudson A, Wright V. A radiological survey of the hips and knees in female specialist teachers of physical education. *Scand J Rheum.* 1979;8:264–268.

[39]Williams WV, Cope R, Gaunt WD. Metacarpophalangeal arthropathy associated with manual labor (Missouri metacarpal syndrome). *Arthritis Rheum.* 1987;30:1362–1371.

[40]Mintz G, Fraga A. Severe osteoarthritis of the elbow in foundry workers: An occupational hazard. *Arch Environ Health.* 1973;27:78–80.

[41]Lawrence JS. Rheumatism in coal miners: Part III. Occupational factors. *Br J Indus Med.* 1955;12:249–261.

[42]Hadler NM, Gillings DB, Imbus HR, *et al.* Hand structure and function in an industrial setting. *Arthritis Rheum.* 1978;21(2):210–220.

[43]Leino P, Hasan J, Karpppi S. Occupational class, physical workload, and musculoskeletal morbidity in the engineering industry. *Br J Indus Med.* 1988;45:672–681.

[44]Vingard E, Hogstedt C, Alfredsson L. Coxarthrosis and physical work load. *Scand J Work Environ Health.* 1991;17:104–109.

[45]Anderson J, Felson DT. Factors associated with osteoarthritis of the knee in the first national health and nutrition examination survey (HANES I). *Am J Epidemiol.* 1988;128:179–189.

[46]Felson DT, Hannan MT, Naimark A, *et al.* Occupational physical demands, knee bending, and knee osteoarthritis: Results from the Framingham Study. *J Rheumatol.* 1991;18:1587–1592.

[47]Cooper C, McAlindon T, Coggon D, Egger P, Dieppe P. Occupational activity and osteoarthritis of the knee. *Ann Rheum Dis.* 1994;53(2):90–93.

[48]Roach KE, Persky V, Miles T, Budiman-Mak, E. Biomechanical aspects of occupation and osteoarthritis of the hip: A case-control study. *J Rheumatol.* 1994;21:2334–2340.

[49]Typpo Osteoarthritis of the hip: Radiologic findings and etiology. *Ann Chir et Gynaecol.* 1985;74(suppl 201):5–38.

[50]Axmacher B, Lindberg H. Coxarthrosis in farmers. *Clin Orthop Rel Res.* 1993;287:82–86.

[51]Partridge REH, Duthie JJR. Rheumatism in dockers and civil servants: A comparison of heavy manual and sedentary workers. *Ann Rheum Dis.* 1968;27:559–568.

[52]Lawrence JS, Molyneux MK, Dingwall-Fordyce I. Rheumatism in foundry workers. *Br J Indus Med.* 1966;23:42–52.

[53]Felson DT. Do occupation-related physical factors contribute to arthritis? *Bailliere's Clin Rheumatol.* 1994;8:63–77.

18

Low Back Pain and the Workplace

David G. Borenstein

Low back pain is second only to the common cold as the most common affliction of mankind. Approximately 10% to 20% of the population of the United States has back pain each year,[1] and over 80% of the population will experience at least one significant episode of low back pain during their adult lives.[2] Epidemiologic studies in other industrial countries have shown that 35% to 90% of the adult population reports at least one episode of low back pain.[3-6] Low back pain is the fifth most common complaint resulting in a visit to a physician, according to a U.S. national ambulatory care survey.[7]

Low back pain is associated with a wide variety of mechanical and medical disorders.[8] Mechanical disorders of the lumbar spine are caused by overuse of a normal anatomic structure (muscle strain), or trauma or physical deformity of an anatomic structure (apophyseal joint osteophyte). Medical disorders affecting the spine are associated with constitutional symptoms, inflammatory or infiltrative disease of the vertebral structures or dysfunction in nonmusculoskeletal organ systems. Mechanical disorders are the cause of 90% of the pain in low back patients. However, a definitive anatomic cause is established in only 10% of individuals with low back pain.[9] The natural history of low back pain shows that over 50% of all patients improve within one week of the onset of pain, and more than 90% are pain-free at eight weeks.[10]

A subgroup of individuals develop low back pain associated with work activities. Injury of the lumbosacral spine related to occupational activities has a number of implications for workers, health professionals and employers. The injured individual is not only a patient but may also be a claimant in a workers' compensation process. Although the goal for all the participants in this process is restoration of the worker to preinjury status, several occupational, social and financial factors may undermine attainment of that goal. A number of questions may be asked to understand better the complexity and importance of this issue: Is work-related back pain a common problem for industry? What are the financial consequences of work-related back pain for industry and for the worker? Which worker is at greatest risk for developing this symptom? Can industry find effective means of identifying individuals prior to employment who may be at risk of developing back pain? How is work-related low back pain diagnosed and treated? What is the prognosis of work-related back injuries? Can work-related back injuries be prevented? The purpose of this chapter is to answer these questions concerning work-related low back pain.

EPIDEMIOLOGY AND ECONOMIC IMPACT OF WORK-RELATED BACK PAIN

Epidemiology

The frequency of low back pain in the general population can be more easily determined than the frequency of this disorder in workers. The difficulty in determining the occupational frequency of this disorder relates to the component of occupational back pain that is being measured. Low back pain may be defined as any uncomfortable sensation located between the first lumbar vertebra and the inferior border of the buttock. This pain may be acute (less than three months in duration) or chronic (more than three months in duration) and may be associated with sciatica (pain radiating down the leg below the knee). Occupational low back pain may be measured by the presence of *pain, impairment* or *disability.* Frequency determined by only *pain* will detect a large cohort of individuals with discomfort unassociated with occupational injury. Low back *impairment* is a decrease or loss of function in movement or physical activities of the lumbosacral spine. Low back *disability* is related to the inability to complete tasks required of a specific job. Low back compensation is the reimbursement for lost wages and medical expenses associated with work-related injuries. The frequency of occupational low back pain will differ with the measurement of pain, impairment, disability or those who file compensation claims.

The physical demands of employment have little effect on the incidence of low back pain compared to the general population but have a significant effect on the frequency of work-related low back disability and compensation. In one study, the prevalence of back pain was similar in nurses and teachers. However, back pain in nurses was related to occupational factors, whereas the occurrence of back pain in teachers was not.[11] In another study, light-duty laborers and heavy-duty laborers had similar frequencies of low back pain (53% and 64%, respectively). However, disability was twice as common in heavy-duty laborers compared to those workers engaged in light-duty work.[12] The duration of disabling back pain is longer in manual laborers compared to sedentary workers.[13] Sedentary workers are able to perform with a degree of physical impairment that is disabling to heavy duty laborers.[9]

The annual prevalence of industrially related back injuries in the United States was 2% in 1971.[14] Of 237 retiring employees at Eastman Kodak Company, 56% had severe low back pain requiring medical evaluation during their careers.[15] A similar frequency was noted in the steel industry.[16] Low back disorders have been reported to be the most common chronic condition resulting in decreased work capacity and reduced leisure-time activities for people below 45 years of age.[17] In Sweden during a period from 1960 to 1971, back pain was responsible for 12.5% of all sickness absences. An average of 2.5 days for each working person was lost per year.[18] In a more recent study of musculoskeletal symptoms in 1773 Swedish construction workers, low back symptoms were most common, experienced by 72% of those surveyed. The prevalence of low back pain was 54% when defined to include only those episodes that lasted one to seven days.[19]

The frequency of musculoskeletal symptoms among 308 apprentice and journeymen electricians was examined by Hunting and coworkers.[21] The median age was 26 years with a median of five years of experience. When a back disorder was defined as symptoms occurring three times or lasting greater than one week, back pain was reported in 51% of the respondents. Inexperience was associated with more frequent back symptoms. Back pain was more prevalent in electricians who were not currently working. When assessing visits to a health care provider, missed work or requirement for restricted work duties, low back pain was the most frequent cause in 34% of electricians.[20]

Cost of Low Back Pain

The cost of work-related low back pain is difficult to quantify. In the United States, the costs for work-related injuries are derived from a number of potential sources, including workers' compensation insurance (federal, state and private insurers), health insurance plans and social security benefits. Direct costs include wage loss, wage replacement, medical care, disability payments for temporary and permanent impairments, rehabilitation expenses and death benefits. The payment may be made as a lump sum or an annuity, or in payment for retraining. The generosity of the award may also be affected by labor contracts, the possibility of downsizing and the general state of the economy. Indirect costs of disability include the personal suffering of the workers, production losses, training of new employees, and administration and legal costs. Most data is taken from workers' compensation commission reports. These data underestimate the full extent of the expenses associated with low back pain. Not all workers are covered by compensation benefits, and not all back injuries are reported or qualify for compensation payments.[21] For example, only 2% to 5% of injured workers with back pain file compensation claims.[22]

The economic cost of low back pain to industry and society has increased over time. It was estimated that $14 billion were spent on the treatment and compensation of low back injuries in 1976. This amount exceeded all other industrial injury payments combined.[23] The impact of low back pain on the 1986 workmans' compensation claims for the state of Tennessee was calculated. Of 29,421 claims costing $160 million, 8000 cases (27%) were for back injuries, the largest category, of which 90% were nonspecific with regard to diagnosis. Compensatory payments for back injuries amounted to $55.8 million. Less than 25% of the total amount of dollars spent was for persons who returned to work within 90 days. More than 43% of the total payments was for persons who returned to work more than 90 days after injury. Ten percent of cases with the highest total benefits payments accounted for 57% of the total expenditures.[24] Workers' compensation data from 45 states during 1989 revealed that low back pain claims represented 16% of all compensation claims but 33% of the costs. Medical costs were 32.4% of the total costs, while days lost from work were the most expensive component of claims costs (65.8%).[25]

The median and mean costs per case of low back pain reflect the expense of a small number of compensable injuries. A number of studies have confirmed this finding, demonstrating that 10% of workers were responsible for 75% of direct costs,[26] and that 10% of back injuries were responsible for 90% of costs.[22]

The indirect costs associated with work-related low back pain are more difficult to quantify. A British report estimated that back pain costs the community more than $300 million a year in lost productivity. This is equivalent to the output from a British town of 120,000 people.[27] Other indirect costs to the community include decreased tax revenue and costs to the legal system.

RISK FACTORS

Industry has hoped that health professionals could reduce the problem of industrial back injuries by identifying individuals at increased risk. Specific risk factors for low back pain have been identified in the medical literature. Personal and job-related risk factors must be considered.

Individual Risk Factors

Women represent 40% of the working population in the United States, but account for only 20% of occupational low back problems. This may be due to employment in less physically demanding work. In a review of 31,000 employees, women who performed physically demanding jobs had a higher incidence of low back pain and file more expensive claims than men in similar work.[28] However, up to 80% of compensation claims are filed by men.

Age may be a risk factor for low back pain. Low back pain occurs in early life, reaches a maximum between 35 to 55 years of age, and recurs more often as the individual ages. Operations for herniated intervertebral discs are performed commonly on individuals between 35 and 45 years of age.[29,30] These data suggest that all age groups are at risk of back pain in the workplace. Younger workers may be at risk for herniated discs, while older workers have recurring episodes of pain.

Anthropomorphic data suggest that there is no strong correlation between height, weight, body build and low back pain.[31] Some studies have reported a correlation between height and the risk of back pain and sciatica.[31–33] Obesity is associated with increased risk of low back pain but may not cause an increased frequency of sciatica.[31,34]

The physical strength of individuals may play a role in increasing the risk of low back pain. Both extensor and flexor muscle weakness have been implicated among individuals with low back pain.[35,36] In one study the risk for back injury was increased threefold when the job requirement exceeded the strength capability of the worker when tested in preemployment strength testing.[37] In contrast, isometric trunk strength has been reported to have no predictive value for the identification of workers who will develop work-related back pain.[38] Therefore, assessment of trunk flexor and extensor strength is apparently of little value in determining risk for low back pain.

The association between radiographic abnormalities and the occurrence of back pain has been the subject of extensive investigation. Structural defects, such as scoliosis, kyphosis, leg length discrepancy, hyperlordosis, partial sacralization, spina bifida occulta, spondylolisthesis and spondylosis, are not always associated with low back pain.[9] In a cohort of 321 men, there was no correlation between back pain and transitional vertebra, Schmorl's nodes, or vacuum disc sign.[39] However, with traction spurs or disc space narrowing between the fourth and fifth lumbar vertebrae, an increased incidence of severe low back pain was evident.

Preemployment radiographic screening remains controversial because the ability to detect patients at risk for back pain has not been well established.[40] Furthermore, good workers might be excluded because of an anatomic abnormality that does not affect job performance (for example, spina bifida occulta). In the absence of data demonstrating the value of preplacement radiographic screening, these tests are not indicated on a cost- or risk-benefit basis.[41]

Restriction of lumbar spine mobility is not associated *per se* with low back pain. Adequate motion of the spine for normal activities can occur with unimpaired mobility of the thoracic spine and hips. Decreased flexion of the spine does not influence the duration of a low back pain event or affect the risk of recurrences.[13,42]

The role of cigarette smoking as a risk factor for back pain is controversial. Studies have reported an association between smoking and low back pain.[5,30] The association may be a result of increased intradiscal pressure from chronic coughing and straining or the adverse effects of nicotine on the biochemistry of the intervertebral disc. Other investigators have found no such association.[43]

Psychologic factors may play a role in work-related back pain. In workers who were not satisfied with their present occupation, place of employment or social situation, there was a high incidence of low back pain.[44] A correlation between back injuries and poor employee appraisal ratings by a supervisor has also been reported.[45] In a study of 3000 Boeing employees followed over a four-year period, 279 workers filed back injury reports. In this study, a strong association between back injury claims and dissatisfaction with work was noted.[46] In contrast, physical factors usually considered risk factors for back pain were unassociated with back pain claims.[47–50] Monotonous work, low job-related control, lack of social support and time pressures have been reported to increase the risk of musculoskeletal pain.[51] Additional studies are needed to determine whether psychological factors play a primary role in the development of low back pain or represent a secondary response to illness.

Low back pain occurs more commonly in individuals who have had previous episodes of back pain.[15,52] However, in a study of 154 postal workers, a history of prior back pain on screening examination was not associated with subsequent occupational injury.[53]

Job Risk Factors

In addition to individual worker characteristics, job factors influence the risk for low back pain. Heavy physical work that places increased stress on the lumbosacral spine has been associated with more frequent low back injuries.[13,54] Other studies have reported no significant differences between light and heavy physical jobs in the frequency of back pain.[55–57]

Contrary to conventional thinking, sedentary workers are also at risk for occupational low back pain. Several studies have shown that workers in jobs involving continuous sitting or standing have a greater point prevalence of back pain than jobs involving constant movement.[58–60] Sustained sedentary work in a forced nonneutral posture is a risk factor for low back pain.[61]

The combination of lifting, bending and twisting is a frequent cause of acute low back injuries. In one study, manual tasks including lifting, pushing, pulling or carrying were implicated as the cause of back pain in 70% of back injury workers.[62] Asymmetric lifting (with one or both hands at the side, with thoracic torsion or with lateral bending) results in significantly lower maximum voluntary muscle strength, higher compressive force, greater intradiscal pressure, increased myoelectric activity and antagonistic activity of trunk muscles. Lifting from this position places potentially hazardous stresses on the lumbar spine.[63] The weight of an object is also related to risk of back pain. Individuals lifting greater than 25 pounds more than 25 times per day have a threefold risk of developing a herniated intervertebral disc, compared to individuals lifting less than 25 pounds.[64] The moment (the product of the weight of the load and the distance from the spinal axis), rather than the weight of the load or lifting technique, has been implicated as the most important stress to the spine that causes low back pain.[9]

Frequent lifting can cause muscle fatigue, resulting in uncoordinated muscular effort associated with excessive utilization of energy. In this circumstance, endurance rather than maximal strength predicts development of back pain.[65] A sustained bent posture may also cause muscle fatigue and back pain. The maintenance of a slightly flexed trunk posture (by a housekeeper making beds, for example, or a draftsman working over a board) is a risk factor.

Vibration, or cyclic loading, has detrimental effects upon the spine. Repeated small stresses over time may lead to failure or degeneration of anatomic structures. Vibration at certain frequencies results in hastening of mechanical failure.

The resonant frequency in the lumbar region of the vertically vibrated, seated operator is 4.5 Hz.[66] Movement of a vehicle that resonates with a vibration of 4.5 Hz places an oscillating force on the lumbar spine, including the intervertebral axial disc and supporting tissues.[67] In addition to the skeleton, whole-body vibration produces adverse effects on the genitourinary and gastrointestinal systems.[68] Studies have reported the increased incidence of low back pain in a variety of vehicular drivers. Bus, truck, tractor, earth-moving equipment and crane drivers are all at similar risk.[68–73] These workers highlight the difficulty of identifying individual risk factors for work-related back pain. Truck drivers sit for prolonged periods of time in vehicles that vibrate and unload cargo that requires heavy lifting. Any one of these factors, singly or in combination, promotes low back pain.

DIAGNOSIS AND TREATMENT

The most frequently utilized classification system for work-related low back pain was reported by the Quebec Task Force on Spinal Disorders,[74] a multidisciplinary group established to formulate guidelines for the diagnosis and treatment of painful spinal conditions. The task force concentrated on occupation-related low back injury and disability. The data sources for their classification scheme included the Quebec Workers' Compensation Board and review of 469 publications. In an effort to simplify diagnoses, the task force classified activity-related spinal disorders into the 11 categories listed in Table 18-1. The categories were qualified further by duration of symptoms and work status.

These categorizations have major implications for prognosis. The duration of symptoms is divided into acute—less

Table 18-1   Quebec task force classification system

Classification	Symptoms	Duration of Symptoms from Onset	Working Status at Time of Evaluation
1	Pain without radiation	a (<7 days)	W (working)
2	Pain + radiation to extremity, proximally	b (7 days–7 weeks)	I (idle)
3	Pain + radiation to extremity, distally*	c (>7 weeks)	
4	Pain + radiation to upper/lower limb neurologic signs		
5	Presumptive compression of a spinal nerve root on a simple roentgenogram (i.e., spinal instability or fracture)		
6	Compression of a spinal nerve root confirmed by Specific imaging techniques (i.e., computerized axial tomography, myelography, or magnetic resonance imaging) Other diagnostic techniques (e.g., electromyography, venography)		
7	Spinal stenosis		
8	Postsurgical status, 1–6 months after intervention		
9	Postsurgical status, >6 months after intervention 9.1 Asymptomatic 9.2 Symptomatic		
10	Chronic pain syndrome		W (working)
11	Other diagnoses		I (idle)

*Not applicable to the thoracic segment.

than one month; subacute—one to three months; and chronic—greater than three months. The longer an individual with chronic back pain is out of work, the less opportunity there is to return to work. Similarly, the classifications "working" or "idle" have prognostic value for pain resolution. Idle workers are more likely to remain disabled compared to workers who return to work.

The task force also included a diagnostic and therapeutic algorithm in its monograph (Figure 18-1). The algorithm allows for the evaluation of individuals who have atypical characteristics. Individuals who are under 20 or over 50 years of age and have a history of neoplasm, trauma, fever, neurologic deficit or recurrent episodes are investigated by specific diagnostic techniques during the initial evaluation. Most work-related back pain patients can be treated conservatively without sophisticated diagnostic tests. Most individuals' symptoms will improve within seven weeks. For the 16% with persistent pain, consultation with a spine specialist is appropriate. By using this approach, workers are exposed to fewer invasive diagnostic and therapeutic interventions, and there are significant cost savings. The Quebec Task Force algorithm concentrates on the evaluation of mechanical disorders; however, other diagnostic and therapeutic algorithms are available that give equal emphasis to mechanical and nonmechanical low back disorders.[8]

Diagnostic Evaluation

The evaluation of an individual with low back pain begins with a history and physical examination. Inquiries concerning occupation are essential. The description should include estimates of the amount of time spent sitting, standing, bending, pushing, pulling and reaching. Other questions concern the approximate amount of weight lifted, the frequency of lifting tasks, the duration of overhead work, abnormal postures and exposure to whole-body vibration. Other normal daily activities, including sports and recreation, should be determined. A discussion of prior injuries, results of diagnostic tests, effective treatment and duration of disability should be included. A description of the injury is important to document if the event was related to an accident or defective equipment.

Physical examination concentrates on the lumbosacral spine and lower extremities. The patient is observed standing, sitting, lying supine, lying on one side and lying prone. Range of motion of the lumbosacral spine and lower extremities is determined. The pattern of motion as well as the extent is important. Muscle strength can be tested by asking the individual to walk on heels and on toes and to squat. These tasks require the function of L2, L3, and L4 for quadriceps power and L5 and S1 for foot strength. In the seated position, nerve tension signs are easily obtained by extending the legs. Positive findings can be confirmed by reproducing the same findings in the supine position. In the supine position, nerve tension signs and hip motion can be assessed.

Measurement of muscle bulk can suggest the duration of symptoms. Abductor muscle strength can be tested with the patient lying on his or her side. Palpation of the spine and sciatic notch is facilitated when the patient is prone. Neurologic examination for upper lumbar roots (femoral stretch test) and lower sacral roots (perineal sensation) is completed in the prone position. During the course of the examination, tests to determine consistency of patient responses should be included.[75] These tests include nonspecific tenderness, simulation tests of axial loading and rotation, distraction tests, nonanatomic regional disturbances and overreaction. Individuals with three or more of these findings may be exaggerating their symptoms and should be evaluated for malingering or a psychologic disorder.[80]

Radiographic and laboratory tests are not required during the initial evaluation of low back pain. In the majority of individuals, these studies are normal or do not provide diagnostic information. Radiographic evaluation is often associated with anatomic abnormalities that are not related to clinical symptoms.[76] Therefore laboratory or radiographic tests should be obtained only in individuals who do not respond to therapy, have recurrent episodes of back pain, demonstrate neurological abnormalities or develop constitutional symptoms and signs.

Treatment

The goals for treatment of work-related back pain include reduction of pain, improvement in physical function to facilitate return to work, and avoidance of recurrence or persistent pain. The number of workers who develop back pain from an obvious spinal injury is small. Most workers develop pain without a precipitating event, usually in the setting of frequent lifting or overexertion. There is a paucity of data validating the efficacy of low back pain therapies.[2] Interventions that are not costly, have little toxicity and improve patient function should be considered.

Patients should be encouraged to remain active and limit bed rest.[77] Individuals who remain active have less pain during the course of recovery. Individuals with severe pain may benefit from controlled physical activity, including periods of bed rest for the first two days.[78] Analgesics or nonsteroidal anti-inflammatory medications are helpful in decreasing pain and maintaining activity. Narcotic analgesics should be avoided. Muscle relaxants are useful as adjunctive therapy in patients with paraspinal muscle spasm.[79] Medications should be continued while daily physical activities are increased. Most individuals do not require physical therapy in the acute stage. Formal exercise programs, including back programs, are not helpful in hastening improvement in acute back pain patients. A physical therapy program may be helpful later in the course to promote mobility.

Individuals who have sciatica require more aggressive therapy and a longer period of controlled physical activity, and have a slower recovery. If sciatica persists despite max-

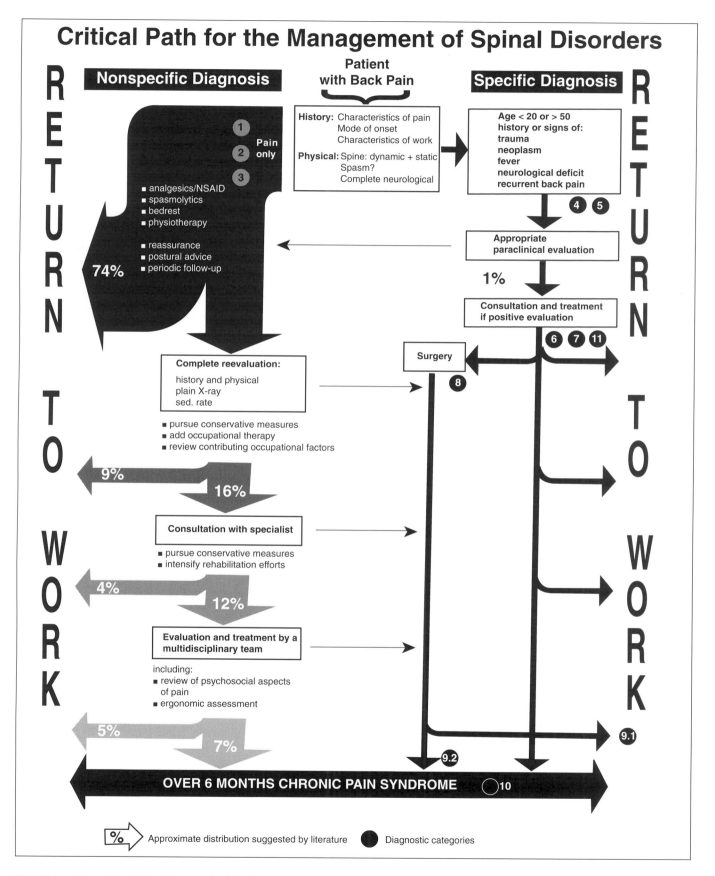

Fig. 18-1   Quebec Task Force Diagnostic Algorithm.

imal medical therapy, epidural corticosteroid injections may be helpful. Surgical decompression is indicated in patients who have persistent radicular pain, neurological signs and abnormalities on radiographic examination. With proper selection, discectomy can provide good to excellent results in 90% to 95% of cases. Unfortunately, the long-term success rate decreases to 70% over the subsequent decade due to recurrence or scarring.[80] Individuals who undergo discectomy are unable to return to heavy manual labor.

Work-hardening is a rehabilitation approach to patients with chronic occupational low back pain. Work-hardening recreates the work tasks of the injured worker in a protected environment. In a work-hardening program, the patient is involved on a daily basis in a combination of tasks that provide physical conditioning and simulate the demands of the patient's work. As the program progresses, additional tasks are added and activities are prolonged until a goal of eight hours is reached. The objective is to increase the worker's confidence in his or her ability to do work in a safe and effective manner. The program also identifies those patients who require a permanent adjustment of their work duties. These programs are effective in returning low back patients to work.[81]

PROGNOSIS

Several factors have been shown to affect the duration of work disability and absenteeism due to back pain. The importance of early return to work cannot be overemphasized. A decreased probability of returning to work is associated with prolonged pain beyond a six-week period. Workers with back pain who are absent from work for over six months have only a 50% likelihood of ever returning to productive employment.[82] If they are off work over one year, this decreases to 25%, and if more than two years, it is almost nil (see Figure 18-2).

The type and severity of the injury affects absenteeism. The injury may be difficult to evaluate because the history provided by the patient may be biased. Individuals who may benefit from compensation may identify the onset of a problem as acute rather than chronic. Since most low back injuries produce few objective findings, the physical examination is not helpful in identifying factors that will predict outcome.[89] In addition, low educational level and low income are strongly correlated with work absence.[83]

The role of secondary gain from workers' compensation payments and the prognosis of low back pain injuries is unresolved. One study found that patients injured on duty had a significantly longer period of disability than those injured off work.[84] The compensation patient may amplify the severity of the injury and the subsequent physical limitations. The financial considerations of the injured worker may make the "injured state" rewarding. In some circumstances, compensation payments amount to 100% of the worker's salary. High levels of benefits prolong the duration of work-related absenteeism.[85] However, not all studies find compensation payments to be predictors of work absence. In that regard, one study reported that six months after discharge from a hospital-based, interdisciplinary, occupational rehabilitation program, the numbers of compensation and noncompensation patients back at work were similar.[86] If injured workers are able to remain at work, their degree of disability is no different from other workers.

The duration of the initial episode of back pain may have a predictive value on the probability of a recurrent episode.

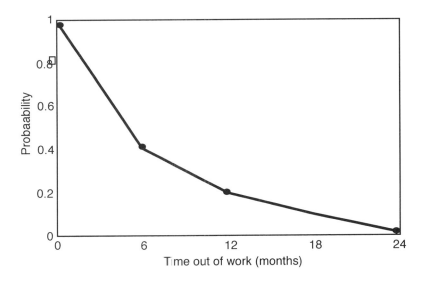

Fig. 18-2   The probability of return to work as a function of time out of work. Individuals absent from work for a 12 month or longer period have less than a 25% chance of returning to gainful employment.

In a group of 2342 workers who received compensation for a work absence secondary to back pain, 36.3% had at least one recurrence and had longer durations of absence compared to those with initial episodes of back pain.[87] A positive relationship was found between the duration of the initial episode of absence from work and the subsequent history of absence from work, both in terms of risk of recurrence and duration of absence. The risk for a recurrence of back pain was 19.9% if the initial episode was one day 639 in duration in the year following the injury versus 26.7% if the first episode was six months in duration. The chronicity of job absenteeism does not depend entirely on the worker. Characteristically, employers will not take workers back to their jobs until they are completely well, pain-free and capable of lifting heavy loads during an eight-hour day.[88] Physicians may wish to encourage the injured laborer to return to work, but find employers resistant to the notion of light-duty work. Until the cost-efficacy of early return to some form of work is impressed upon the employers, certain employees will become labeled as chronically disabled with a decreased opportunity to return to the workforce.

PREVENTION

Prevention of work-related back pain can be divided into three categories.[89] *Primary prevention* tries to prevent the onset of the illness in those at risk. *Secondary prevention* attempts to modify the progression of a disorder when the problem first becomes symptomatic. *Tertiary prevention* minimizes the consequences or complications of an injury in chronic stages once it is clinically manifest.

Primary prevention might be achieved through the use of preemployment screening, improvement in work habits and modifications of the workplace. Many prescreening tests are ineffective at identifying workers at risk for back injuries. Radiologic screening is neither cost- nor risk-benefit effective.[41] Strength testing that does not relate to the physical demands of the employees job is not successful in reducing injury claims.[48,90] However, workers who are physically fit may be the least likely to suffer disabling low back pain.[91]

Education regarding correct work habits may be helpful as employees start their jobs. Ergonomic modification of the workplace can help to design work that is within the physical capability of employees. Ergonomic tools to evaluate a job include analysis of energy expenditure, perceived stress on the musculoskeletal system and compressive force on the skeleton, among other factors. Ergonomic principles can be applied to the design of chairs to improve posture and decrease muscle fatigue.[92] Materials handling can be made safer by the design of appropriate vehicles to transport heavy weights. Containers can be made of the appropriate size and gripping surface to allow for ease of lifting and to improve line of sight to decrease falls. Although ideal conditions may be determined for a specific job, a reduction in the incidence of low back pain does not necessarily follow if recommendations are not followed by employees.

Secondary prevention of back injuries is approached through appropriate treatment and rehabilitation. An example of an effective system utilized for secondary prevention is a quality-based protocol with a standardized diagnostic and treatment algorithm devised for a large public utility company. A total of 5300 employees were evaluated and followed with an algorithm over a 10-year study.[93] The goal of the program was to reduce unjustified lost time from work and compensation costs by early functional return to work and avoidance of unnecessary surgery. Over a 10-year period, days lost from work fell by 55% and number of new injuries by 51%. The number of surgeries performed decreased by 67% and the operative success rate increased dramatically. Over the 10-year period, more than $4.1 million were saved in reduction of expenditures for lost time and replacement wages. The success of the program was based on close monitoring of treating physicians. Any variation from the usual protocol of diagnosis or treatment was questioned and reevaluated. By following a standard approach, extraneous tests and treatments were eliminated and more rapid recovery attained.

Tertiary prevention is needed for the injured worker with pain of three months duration or longer. These individuals have psychological, social and financial disruptions in their lives, as well as concerns involving their work. Work-hardening programs offer an aggressive approach to rehabilitation of the low back pain worker with a goal of return to gainful employment. In one such program consisting of five hours of treatment per week for three weeks, 82% of the graduates were reconditioned and returned to work. The control group had a 40% return-to-work rate.[94] Many of the patients had been disabled for 12 to 19 months. The return-to-work rate of these chronically disabled patients is an encouraging sign that tertiary prevention is effective.

DISABILITY AND IMPAIRMENT RATING

Some workers are unable to return to their preinjury level of function despite appropriate therapy. A determination of this loss of function is not exact and has few accepted guidelines. Physical impairment is an objective anatomic or pathologic dysfunction leading to loss of normal body ability. Permanent impairment is an objective assessment of functional abnormality or loss after the acute injury phase and after maximal medical rehabilitation. Physical disability is a measure of reduced capacity to engage in gainful activity as a result of some impairment.

Assessment of impairment is solely a medical responsibility. Disability ratings are best determined by administrative specialists based on the physician's impairment ratings. Determination of percentage impairment for specific back injuries is an inexact process. Assessment of motion of the spine as the sole criterion of impairment overlooks the contribution of pain to decreased function. Impairment ratings based on the "whole person" concept are the most current system. The length of time for complete healing is difficult to determine for some low back disorders. The usual three-month natural course of healing does not always apply to the impaired worker. In these individuals, healing is completed when there is no further reasonable progress toward resolution.

The physician has four responsibilities to the injured worker under workers' compensation law.[95] The first responsibility is to establish a causal relationship between the injury and the impairment. The second responsibility is to determine when maximal medical improvement has been attained. The third responsibility is to establish the presence and degree of permanent impairment when maximal healing has been reached. The fourth responsibility is to estimate work capacity and restrictions. Ideally, these determinations are made on an objective basis; however, the process is inexact. The physician should inform the patient about the nature of the process. The worker should understand both the role of the physician in measuring impairment and the administrative process as the final arbiter of disability. With a better understanding of this process, the patient's optimistic expectations concerning benefits can be tempered with reality.

REFERENCES

[1]Frymoyer JW, Pope MH, Costanza MC. et al. Epidemiologic studies of low-back pain. *Spine*. 1980;5:419–423.

[2]Deyo RA. Conservative therapy for low back pain. *JAMA*. 1983;250:1057–1062.

[3]Andersson GBJ. Epidemiologic aspects on low back pain in industry. *Spine*. 1981;6:53–60.

[4]Biering-Sorensen F. A prospective study of low back pain in a general population. *Scand J Rehabil Med*. 1983;15:71–96.

[5]Frymoyer JW, Pope MH, Clements JH, et al. Risk factor in low-back pain. An epidemiological survey. *J Bone Joint Surg*. 1983;65A:213–218.

[6]Riihimaki H. Low-back pain and occupation. A cross-sectional questionnaire study of men in machine operating, dynamic physical work, and sedentary work. *Spine*. 1989;14:204–209.

[7]Hart LG, Deyo RA, Cherkin DC. Physician office visits for low back pain: Frequency, clinical evaluation, and treatment patterns from a U.S. national survey. *Spine*. 1995;20:11–19.

[8]Borenstein DG, Wiesel SW, Boden SD. *Low Back Pain: Medical Diagnosis and Comprehensive Management*. 2nd ed. Philadelphia: W.B. Saunders, 1995;183–589.

[9]Garg A, Moore JS. Epidemiology of low-back pain in industry. *Occup Med St Art Rev*. 1992;7:593–608.

[10]Dillane JB, Fry J, Kaiton G. Acute back syndrome: A study from general practice. *Br Med J*. 1966;II:(1)82–84.

[11]Cust G, Pearson JCG, Mair A. The prevalence of low back pain in nurses. *Int Nurse Rev*. 1972;19:169–178.

[12]Hult L. Cervical, dorsal, and lumbar spine syndrome. *Acta Orthop Scand*. 1954;15(suppl):1–102.

[13]Bergquist-Ullman M, Larson U. Acute low back pain in industry. *Acta Orthop Scand*. 1977;170(suppl):1–117.

[14]Leavitt S, Johnston T, Beyer R. The process of recovery: Patterns in industrial back injury. Part 1. Cost and other quantitative measures of effort. *Indust Med*. 1971;40:7–14.

[15]Rowe ML. Low back disability in industry: Updated position. *J Occup Med*. 1971;13:476–478.

[16]Masset D. Low back pain: Epidemiologic aspects and work-related factors in the steel industry. *Spine*. 1994;19:143–146.

[17]Kelsey JL, Godlen AL. Occupational and workplace factors associated with low back pain. In: Deyo RA, ed. *Occupational Medicine St Art Rev*. 1988;3:7–16.

[18]Hansson T, Bigos S, Beecher P, Wortley M. The lumbar lordosis in acute and chronic low-back pain. *Spine*. 1985;10:154–155.

[19]Holmstrom EB, Lindell J, Moritz U. Low back and neck/shoulder pain in construction workers; occupational workload and psychological risk factors. Part 1: Relationship to low back pain. *Spine*. 1992;17:663–671.

[20]Hunting KL, Welch LS, Cuccherini BA, Seiger LA. Musculoskeletal symptoms among electricians. *Am J Indus Med*. 1994;25:149–163.

[21]Andersson GBJ, Pope MH, Frymoyer JW, Snook S. Epidemiology and cost. In: Pope MH, Andersson GBJ, Frymoyer JW, Chaffin DB, eds. *Occupational Low Back Pain: Assessment, Treatment, and Prevention*. St. Louis: Mosby Yearbook, 1991;95–113.

[22]Spengler DM, Bigos SJ, Martin NA, et al. Back injuries in industry: A retrospective study. I: Overview and cost analysis. *Spine*. 1986;11:241–245.

[23]Akeson WH, Murphy RW. Low back pain (editorial). *Clin Orthop*. 1977;129:2–3.

[24]Federspiel CF, Guy D, Kane D, Spengler D. Expenditures for nonspecific back injuries in the workplace. *J Occup Med*. 1989;31:919–924.

[25]Webster BS, Snook SH. The cost of 1989 workers' compensation low back pain claims. *Spine*. 1994;19:1111–1116.

[26]Abenhaim LL, Suissa S. Importance and economic burden of occupational back pain: A study of 2500 cases representative of Quebec. *J Occup Med*. 1987;29:670–674.

[27]Snook SH. The costs of back pain in industry. *Spine St Art Rev*. 1987;2:1–5.

[28]Bigos SJ, Spengler DM, Martin NA, et al. Back injuries in industry: A retrospective study. II. Injury factors. *Spine*. 1986;11:246–251.

[29]Spangfort EV. The lumbar disc herniation. *Acta Orthop Scand*. 1972;142(suppl):1–95.

[30]Svensson HO, Andersson GBJ. Low back pain in 40- to 47-year-old men: Work history and work environment factors. *Spine*. 1983;8:272–276.

[31]Battie MC, Bigos SJ. Industrial back pain complaints. A broader perspective. *Orthop Clin North Am*. 1991;22:273–282.

[32]Lawrence JS, Molyreaux MK, Dingwall-Fordyce I. Rheumatism in foundry workers. *Br J Indus Med*. 1966;23:42–52.

[33]Merriam WF, Burwell RG, Mulholland FC, *et al.* A study revealing a tall pelvis in subjects with low back pain. *J Bone Joint Surg.* 1983;65:153–156.

[34]Deyo RA, Bass JE. Lifestyle and low-back pain: The influence of smoking and obesity. *Spine.* 1989;14:501–506.

[35]Schultz A, Andersson G, Ortengren R, *et al.* Loads on the lumbar spine, validation and biochemical analysis by measurements of intradiscal pressures and myoelectric signals. *J Bone Joint Surg.* 1982;64:713–720.

[36]Nummi J, Jarvinen T, Stambej U, *et al.* Diminished dynamic performance capacity of back and abdominal muscles in concrete reinforcement workers. *Scand J Work Environ Health.* 1978;4(suppl 1):39–46.

[37]Chaffin DB, Herrin GD, Keyerling WM. Preemployment strength testing. An updated position. *J Occup Med.* 1978;20:403–408.

[38]Andersson GBJ, Pope MH. The patient. In: Pope MH, Andersson GBJ, Frymoyer JW, Chaffin DB, eds. *Occupational Low Back Pain: Assessment, Treatment, and Prevention.* St. Louis: Mosby Yearbook, 1991;132–147.

[39]Frymoyer JW, Cats-Baril W. Predictors of low back pain disability. *Clin Orthop.* 1987;221:89–98.

[40]Gibson ES. The value of preplacement screening radiography of the low back. *Spine St Art Rev.* 1987;2:91–107.

[41]Rowe ML. Are routine spine films on workers in industry cost- or risk-benefit effective? *J Occup Med.* 1982;24:41–43.

[42]Horal J. The clinical appearance of low back disorders in the city of Gothenburg, Sweden. *Acta Orthop Scand.* 1969;118(suppl):9–109.

[43]Astrand NE. Medical, psychological, and social factors associated with back abnormalities and self reported back pain: A cross sectional study of male employees in a Swedish pulp and paper industry. *Br J Indus Med.* 1987;44:327–336.

[44]Magora A. Investigation of the relation between low back pain and occupation. I. Age, sex, community, education, and other factors. *Indus Med Surg.* 1970;39:465–471.

[45]Bigos SJ, Spengler DM, Martin NA, *et al.* Back injuries in industry: A retrospective study. II. Injury factors. *Spine.* 1986;11:246–251.

[46]Bigos SJ, Battie MC, Fisher LD, *et al.* A prospective study of work perceptions and psychological factors affecting the report of back injury. *Spine.* 1990;16:1–6.

[47]Battie MC, Bigos SJ, Fisher LD, *et al.* A prospective study of the role of cardiovascular risk factors and fitness in industrial back pain complaints. *Spine.* 1989;14:141–147.

[48]Battie MC, Bigos SJ, Fisher LD, *et al.* Isometric lifting strength as a predictor of industrial back pain. *Spine.* 1989;14:851–856.

[49]Battie MC, Bigos SJ, Fisher LD, *et al.* The role of spinal flexibility in back pain complaints within industry: A prospective study. *Spine.* 1990;15:768–773.

[50]Battie MC, Bigos SJ, Fisher LD, *et al.* Anthropometric and clinical measurements as predictors of industrial back pain complaints: A prospective study. *J Spinal Disorders.* 1990;3:195–204.

[51]Bongers PM, de Winter CR, Kompier MA, Hildebrandt VH. Psychological factors at work and musculoskeletal disease. *Scand J Work Environ Health.* 1993;19:297–312.

[52]Buckle P, Kember P, Wood A, *et al.* Factors influencing occupational back pain in Bedfordshire. *Spine.* 1980;5:245–248.

[53]Zwerling C, Ryan J, Schootman M. A case-control study of risk factors for industrial low back injury. The utility of preplacement screening in defining high-risk groups. *Spine.* 1993;18:1242–1247.

[54]Dehlin O, Berg S, Andersson GBJ, *et al.* Effect of physical training and ergonomic counselling on the psychological perception of work and on the subjective assessment of low back insufficiency. *Scand J Rehabil Med.* 1981;13:1–9.

[55]Damkot DK, Pope MH, Lord J, Frymoyer JW. The relationship between work history, work environment and low-back pain in men. *Spine.* 1984;9:395–399.

[56]Partridge RE, Duthie JJR. Rheumatism in dockers and civil servants. A comparison of heavy manual and sedentary workers. *Ann Rheum Dis.* 1968;27:559–568.

[57]Sairanen E, Brushaber L, Kaskinen M. Felling work, low-back pain and osteoarthritis. *Scand J Work Environ Health.* 1981;7:18–30.

[58]Magora A. Investigation of the relation between low back pain and occupation: III. Physical requirements: Sitting, standing and weight lifting. *Indus Med Surg.* 1972;41:5–9.

[59]Nachemson AL, Elfstrom E. Intravital dynamic pressure measurements in lumbar discs: A study of common movements, maneuvers and exercises. *Scand J Rehabil Med.* 1970;1(suppl):1–40.

[60]Lawrence JS. Rheumatism in coal miners. Part III: Occupational factors. *Br J Ind Med.* 1955;12:249–261.

[61]Burdorf A, Naaktgeboren B, deGroot HCWM. Occupational risk factors for low back pain among sedentary workers. *J Occup Med.* 1993;35:1213–1220.

[62]Snook SH, Campanelli RA, Hart JW. A study of three preventive approaches to low-back injury. *J Occup Med.* 1978;20:478–481.

[63]Garg A. Occupational biomechanics and low-back pain. *Occup Med St Art Rev.* 1992;7:609–628.

[64]Kelsey JL, Githens PB, O'Connor T, *et al.* Acute prolapsed lumbar intervertebral disc: An epidemiologic study with special reference to driving automobiles and cigarette smoking. *Spine.* 1984;9:608–613.

[65]Parnianpour M, Nordin MA, Kahanovitz N, Frankel V. The triaxial coupling of torque generation of trunk muscles during isometric exertions and effect of fatiguing isoinertial movements on the motor output and movement. *Spine.* 1988;13:982–991.

[66]Pope MH, Wilder DG, Jorneus L, *et al.* The response of the seated human to sinusoidal vibration and impact. *J Biomech Eng.* 1987;109:279–284.

[67]Wilder DG. The biomechanics of vibration and low back pain. *Am J Indus Med.* 1993;23:577–588.

[68]Seidel H. Selected health risks caused by long-term, whole-body vibration. *Am J Indus Med.* 1993;23:589–604.

[69]Bovenzi M, Zadini A. Self-reported low back symptoms in urban bus drivers exposed to whole-body vibration. *Spine.* 1992;17:1048–1059.

[70]Bongers PM, Boshuizen HC, Hulshof CTJ, Koemeester AC. Back disorders in crane operators. *Int Arch Occup Environ Health.* 1988;60:129–137.

[71]Boshuizen HC, Bongers PM, Hulshof CTJ. Self-reported back pain in tractor drivers exposed to whole-body vibration. *Int Arch Occup Environ Health*. 1990;62:109–115.

[72]Brendstrup T, Biering-Sorensen F. Effect of fork-lift truck driving on low-back trouble. *Scand J Work Environ Health*. 1987;13: 442–452.

[73]Dupuis H, Zerlett G. Whole body vibration and disorders of the spine. *Int Arch Occup Environ Health*. 1987;59:323–336.

[74]Spitzer WO, LeBlanc FE, Dupuis M, *et al*. Scientific approach to the assessment and management of activity-related spinal disorders: Report of the Quebec Task Force on spinal disorders. *Spine*. 1987;12:S1–57.

[75]Waddell G, McCulloch JA, Kummel E, *et al*. Nonorganic physical signs in low back pain. *Spine*. 1980;5:117–125.

[76]Jensen MC, Brant-Zawadzki MN, Obuchowski N, Modic MT, Malkasian D, Ross JS. Magnetic resonance imaging of the lumbar spine in people without back pain. *N Engl J Med*. 1994;331:69–73.

[77]Malmivaara A, Hakkinen U, Aro T, *et al*. The treatment of acute low back pain—bed rest, exercises, or ordinary activity? *N Eng J Med*. 1995;332:351–355.

[78]Deyo RA, Diehl AK, Rosenthal M. How many days of bed rest for acute low back pain? A randomized trial. *N Engl J Med*. 1986;315: 1064–1070.

[79]Borenstein DG, Lacks S, Wiesel SW. Cyclobenzaprine and naproxen versus naproxen alone in the treatment of acute low back pain and muscle spasm. *Clin Ther*. 1990;12:125–131.

[80]Frymoyer JW. Back pain and sciatica. *N Engl J Med*. 1988;318: 291–300.

[81]Sachs BL, David JF, Olimpio D, *et al*. Spinal rehabilitation by work tolerance based on objective physical capacity assessment of dysfunction: A prospective study with control subjects and twelve month review. *Spine*. 1990;15:1325–1332.

[82]McGill CM. Industrial back problems—a control program. *J Occup Med*. 1968;10:174–178.

[83]Deyo RA, Tsio-Wu YJ. Functional disability due to back pain—a population-based study indicating the importance of socioeconomic factors. *Arthritis Rheum*. 1987;30:1247–1253.

[84]Sander RA, Meyers JE. The relationship of disability to compensation status in railroad workers. *Spine*. 1986;11:141–143.

[85]Walsh NE, Dumitru D. The influence of compensation on recovery from low back pain. In: Deyo RA, ed. *Occup Med St Art Rev*. 1988;3:109–121.

[86]Tollison CD. Compensation status as a predictor of outcome in nonsurgically treated low back injury. *South Med J*. 1993;86: 1206–1209.

[87]Rossignol M, Suissa S, Abenhaim L. The evaluation of compensated occupational spinal injuries: A three-year follow-up study. *Spine*. 1992;17:1043–1047.

[88]Spitzer WO. Low back pain in the workplace: Attainable benefits not attained. *Br J Indus Med*. 1993;50:385–388.

[89]Andersson GBJ. Concepts in prevention. In: Pope MH, Andersson GBJ, Frymoyer JW, Chaffin DB, eds. *Occupational Low Back Pain: Assessment, Treatment and Prevention*. St. Louis: Mosby Yearbook, 1991;211–216.

[90]Dueker JA, Ritchie SM, Knox TJ, Rose SJ. Isokinetic trunk testing employment. *J Occup Med*. 1994;36:42–48.

[91]Cady LD, Bischoff DP, O'Connell ER, *et al*. Strength and fitness and subsequent back injuries in fire fighters. *J Occup Med*. 1979;21:269–272.

[92]Chaffin DB, Pope MH, Andersson GBJ. Workplace design. In: Pope MH, Andersson GBJ, Frymoyer JW, Chaffin DB, eds. *Occupational Low Back Pain: Assessment, Treatment and Prevention*. St. Louis: Mosby Yearbook, 1991;251–265.

[93]Wiesel SW, Boden SD, Feffer HL. A quality-based protocol for management of musculoskeletal injuries: A ten-year prospective outcome study. *Clin Orthop*. 1994;301:164–176.

[94]Mayer TG, Gatchel RJ, Kishino N, *et al*. Objective assessment of spine function following industrial injury. A prospective study with comparison group and one-year follow-up. *Spine*. 1985; 10:482–493.

[95]Frymoyer JW, Haldeman S, Andersson GBJ. Impairment rating—The United States perspective. In: Pope MH, Andersson GBJ, Frymoyer JW, Chaffin DB, eds. *Occupational Low Back Pain: Assessment, Treatment and Prevention*. St. Louis: Mosby Yearbook, 1991;279–295.

VI

Surveillance, Regulatory, and Legal Approaches to Environmental Exposure-Associated Rheumatic Disease

19

Safety Surveillance of Food and Drugs

Patricia J. Rohan

Safety surveillance of products subject to regulation by the Food and Drug Administration (FDA) begins with preclinical investigations and continues through clinical trials and into the postmarketing period. This process is useful only if it is able to effect change when a significant public health risk is identified. Campaigns directly to inform the public of a health hazard cannot be guaranteed to reach those individuals most at risk, let alone change the behaviors and use patterns associated with an increased chance of injury or illness. In some cases, the pattern of serious illness or injury associated with the use, misuse or abuse of a product may necessitate removal of the product from the market.

At times, education and labeling changes, including warning statements, may be useful to consumers and health care providers. This is especially true when health care providers serve as an interface between the consumer and the product. Health care professionals are involved in the education and monitoring of patients to ensure that products are used properly according to a risk-benefit assessment. These professionals are motivated to adhere to current standards of care by personal, professional, legal and financial guidelines.

A different situation arises when the consumer bears direct responsibility for decisions on product use. A consumer usually assumes that any product on the market in the United States has been proven safe and possibly effective. Product information may be gleaned from advertisements or publications which may have a particular bias. Anecdotal testimony may replace standard of proof. Such testimony may be especially convincing when espoused by an authority figure (who is not required to have any relevant training or expertise) or by a personal acquaintance.[1] FDA experience with consumer focus groups shows that warning labels on products may be perceived as an irrelevant governmental requirement or as a laundry list used by the manufacturer to avoid product liability lawsuits. Consumers may not see any need to read a lengthy and often technical warning statement on a product, especially if the product is considered natural and/or safe.[2,3]

Thus, the totality of evidence is not always available to consumers or health care providers in a readily accessible format.

Furthermore, consumers are unlikely to know the types of illness or injuries most likely to occur with the use of a particular product or how to monitor themselves for the earliest signs of problems. Rather, consumers rely on symptoms, which don't always provide adequate warning before serious injury occurs. Consumers (and health care professionals) may neglect to consider the role of foods, dietary supplements and over-the-counter (OTC) products in evaluating health problems.

Finally, the prevailing attitude among the public is that OTC drugs and natural products are inherently safe and can affect the body positively. Consumers may not realize that these products exert pharmacologic effects.[4,5,6] There is insufficient awareness of the fact that up to 90% of the most widely used drugs in the United States are plant-derived or plant-based[7]; that some dietary supplements touted as being "natural" are in fact synthesized; or that as many as one in three consumers are using or have used alternative therapies.[8] These issues make safety surveillance a challenging undertaking.

In order better to appreciate the need for safety surveillance, one must understand what can be reasonably known about products at the time they are first introduced for widespread use. The role of the FDA has evolved through bills passed by Congress as well as by case law (Table 19-1). The terms "food," "drug," "device" and "biologic" have been defined by the Food, Drug and Cosmetic Act and through the courts. While consumers and health care providers may not think of or use such products according to these definitions, the FDA's authority is defined and limited by them.

Each center within the FDA has its own terms of authority for ensuring the safety of the products the centers regulate. Thus, while new drugs, biologics and food additives generally require premarket approval, some devices and infant

      Patricia J. Rohan

Table 19-1   Selected major events in the evolution of the Food and Drug Administration

Date	Act/Amendment, Regulation, Action	Summary	Comments
1938	Federal Food, Drug and Cosmetic Act	FDA established. Required proof of drug safety prior to approval (drugs marketed prior to 1938 were "grandfathered" and not affected by this requirement).	1937—elixir of sulfanilamide, containing diethylene glycol, results 107 deaths.[11]
1961	Spontaneous Reporting System	First systematic attempt to collect and evaluate adverse events related to use of drug products. Modeled after the AMA Committee on Blood Dyscrasias.	1952—chloramphenicol-associated aplastic anemia was brought to the attention of the FDA by a physician whose own 10-year-old son had died. This physician traveled cross-country and contacted local physicians. By the time he arrived in Washington DC, he had identified dozens of cases of aplastic anemia associated with the use of chloramphenicol. FDA's nationwide investigation immediately uncovered several hundred additional reports.[12]
1962	Kefauver-Harris Amendment	Requires: 1) proof of efficacy prior to marketing; 2) mandatory manufacturer reporting of adverse events to the FDA	Thalidomide use in the 1950s and 1960s resulted in 10,000 birth defects worldwide but only 11 in the U.S. because the drug had not yet been approved.[13]
1980	Infant Formula Act	Authorized establishment of minimum (and some maximum) nutrient specification requirements; quality factors, quality control procedures and record-keeping; and notification to the FDA of each new formula or change in formulation or processing (certain exemptions for special formulas used by infants with inborn errors of metabolism, low birth weight or unusual medical or dietary problems).	1979—infant formula manufactured with inadequate amounts of chloride resulted in at least 141 reports of hypochloremic metabolic alkalosis.[14] Affected infants displayed deceleration of growth, delayed neurologic development and other abnormalities. The addition of chloride alone to the diet resulted in a correction of the electrolyte abnormalities and the alkalosis.[15]
1992	Nutrition Labeling and Education Act (NDEA)	Required authorization of health claims used on food products relating a nutrient to a health benefit, based upon significant scientific agreement.	Kellogg's use of dietary guidelines for reducing cancer risk published by the National Cancer Institute (NCI) of the National Institutes of Health on the label of All-Bran cereal in 1984. The marketplace witnessed an unprecedented proliferation of nutrition-related claims.[16,17]
1993	MedWatch	Established by FDA as an education/promotional program to increase health care professionals awareness of product-associated illness and injury and to facilitate voluntary reporting of serious adverse events and product problems associated with the use of FDA-regulated products.[18]	Call 1–800–FDA–1088 to: 1) report serious adverse events/product problems; 2) obtain more information; 3) request the FDA Desk Guide for reporting.
1994	Dietary Supplement Health and Education Act (DSHEA)	Dietary supplements, including vitamins, minerals, amino acids, botanicals and other substances used to increase total dietary intake, are not subject to drug or food additive provisions of the Act and are not subject to FDA review for proof of safety or efficacy prior to marketing.[19–21]	Consumers and industry urge Congress to exempt dietary supplements from FDA review with a grassroots campaign promoted in health food stores.

formulas require only premarket notification submitted to the FDA. Most conventional food products, including dietary supplements, can be sold at the manufacturer's discretion.

PREMARKET APPROVAL

Premarket approval requires developing specifications for the product's identification and purity, manufacture and quality control, and testing, first in animals and then in humans. Testing in humans evaluates the efficacy of the product for one or more indications, defining an effective dosage or method of use in some cases, and monitoring for adverse events related to use of the product. Although a product may be tested in humans for up to 10 years, any one individual is usually exposed to the product for less than one year. Even in large premarket clinical trials on thousands of consumers, infrequent adverse events may escape detection. For example, to identify with 95% confidence *one* event occurring at a rate of one in 1000, approximately 3000 people would need to be exposed to a product for the appropriate length of time. This is for events that do not occur spontaneously in the control population. For conditions that do occur spontaneously in the control population (for example, cardiovascular events), an even larger study group would be needed. Therefore, premarket clinical studies are best at identifying relatively common adverse events or events anticipated on the basis of theoretical considerations or experience with similar agents already in use.

In contrast, dietary supplements and their ingredients are not required to undergo premarket review. In some cases there are no existing methods to analyze the product, whereas in others the active ingredient has not been identified. Manufacturers may list ingredients with obscure names, and requests by consumers for specific ingredient identification or source may be refused on the grounds that such information is a trade secret.[4] In the case of melatonin (a synthetic version of a naturally occurring hormone), four of six different products chemically analyzed were found to contain "impurities" which could not be characterized.[9] A dietary supplement marketed as melatonin would not have to show evidence of purity or that it actually contained melatonin.[4]

Postmarketing Surveillance

Safety cannot be thoroughly established until the product is widely marketed. It is only at this stage that it is possible to identify adverse events that are rare and/or unpredictable. With widely used products, this could affect hundreds of consumers, particularly if the product is used in a novel fashion not anticipated by the manufacturer. Such novel uses of approved products and devices are termed "off-label." Off-label product use is considered to be the practice of medicine and therefore is not regulated by the FDA. However, adverse events related to FDA-regulated products are collected regardless of the manner of product use, including off-label use, and consumer misuse or abuse. The FDA works with other federal agencies such as the Centers for Disease Control and Prevention, the United States Department of Agriculture and scientific and clinical organizations. In addition, the FDA monitors the medical and scientific literature for evolving knowledge relevant to specific substances and products.

Examples of safety concerns and safety surveillance are shown in Tables 19-2 and 19-3.

MANDATORY REPORTING—MANUFACTURERS

Manufacturers are required to submit to the FDA reports of all adverse events associated with the use of prescription drugs, some OTC drugs, biologics, devices and certain food additives. Dietary supplement manufacturers are not required to report adverse events. Serious, unexpected adverse events are generally required to be reported in an expedited manner. In the case of drugs, adverse events should be reported within 15 days of their receipt by the manufacturer. Other adverse events are reported on a regular basis. For drugs, this follows a quarterly schedule for the first three years of product life and annually thereafter. Regulations may vary from one class of product to another.

MEDWATCH

The MedWatch Program, initiated in 1993, is a system for voluntary reporting by health care professionals and indirectly by consumers of serious adverse events. The program focuses on events associated with the use of FDA-regulated products, including drugs, biologics, blood products, medical devices, infant formulas and dietary supplements. The FDA does not require that the reporter of adverse events be certain that the product caused a condition but merely that the product is suspect or, at the very least, that the affected individual was using the product.

The four goals of the program are: 1) to increase awareness of the possibility of product-induced illness or injury; 2) to focus on serious adverse events; 3) to make it easier for health professionals to report events directly to the FDA; and 4) to provide feedback to health care professionals (and indirectly to consumers) on the safety of health-care-related products.[9,10] MedWatch has developed partnerships with professional health care organizations to increase awareness and improve the reporting of serious adverse events. This passive surveillance system is uniquely suited to detecting previously unknown or unexpected adverse events under general conditions of use by a wide variety of consumers and in new product applications. Following individual reports of adverse outcomes, additional studies would be required to determine risk and potential causality.

Table 19-2   First identification of safety concerns at various points of product
development and use

Product Associated with Adverse Event	Premarket Testing		Postmarketing Surveillance		
	Preclinical Testing	Clinical Studies	Mandatory Reporting	Spontaneous Reporting	Medical/Scientific Literature
many products	x				
Fialuridine		x			
Terfenidine			x	x	
L-tryptophan				x	
Vitamin A					x

Table 19-3   Examples of safety surveillance

L-tryptophan (1989) Physicians in New Mexico noted three patients with marked eosinophilia and severe myalgia and also noted that in each case the patient had been using L-tryptophan. The state Health Department reviewed clinical laboratories for elevated eosinophil counts and identified a total of 30 cases of what came to be known as eosinophilia myalgia syndrome (EMS). The CDC, in cooperation with state health departments nationwide, developed a national surveillance program aided by extensive media coverage. More than 1500 cases and 38 deaths were reported. The FDA ordered a recall of all single-entity products containing L-tryptophan. Review linked most cases to one company that had changed manufacturing processes, and product analysis revealed several impurities in this particular product. No single impurity was conclusively identified as the causative agent. Reports in the United States and abroad have also linked EMS to L-5-hydroxytryptophan exposure.[22]

Terfenidine (1989–1990) After its introduction on the market, clinicians at Bethesda Naval Hospital in Maryland suspected a near-fatal arrhythmia in a healthy young woman was related to the concomitant use of terfenidine and ketoconazole. Blood analysis revealed high terfenidine blood levels. (Terfenidine is not normally detected in blood because of rapid metabolism.) A review of the FDA spontaneous reporting system revealed additional reports of torsades de pointes associated with the use of terfenidine, some in patients concomitantly receiving ketoconazole. Further study revealed high blood levels of terfenidine could lead to cardiac arrhythmias, which were seen in patients taking products that inhibit cytochrome P-450 3A4. Product labelling revisions contraindicate the use of terfenidine in patients receiving the antifungals ketoconazole and itraconazole, macrolide antibiotics erythromycin and troleandomycin, quinine, and those with hepatic dysfunction.[23–25]

Fialuridine (FIAU) (1995) This antiviral nucleoside analogue was under study in a group of 15 patients with chronic hepatitis B. During the thirteenth week of the study, one patient abruptly developed lactic acidosis and hepatic failure. The study was terminated at that point. Subsequently, seven patients developed severe, progressive hepatotoxicity despite the discontinuation of fialuridine. Of those, five died and two required liver transplantation. Several other patients also developed pancreatitis, neuropathy or myopathy.[26] Further investigation has shown that short-term studies were unable to predict tissue distributions and accumulation which occur with long-term exposure to FIAU.[27]

Vitamin A supplements (1995) A study reported that the use of high doses of preformed vitamin A supplements (retinol > 10,000 IU/d) in women before the seventh week of gestation was associated with an increased incidence of cranial neural crest birth defects. A weaker relationship was seen between birth defects and retinol from food (including dairy products, liver and fortified foods). Synthetic retinoids such as isotretinoin are known to cause birth defects in humans, and natural forms of preformed vitamin A are teratogenic in animals. B-carotene (a vitamin A precursor synthesized in plants) was not specifically studied, but animal studies of high intakes of B-carotene show neither toxicity nor teratogenicity.[28]

SIGNAL GENERATION

In order to generate a signal in safety surveillance, four things must occur: 1) the consumers or their health care providers must become aware of a problem or a change in body function; 2) all possible product exposures must be considered; 3) an association must be made between the event and the use of a product; and 4) the individual must know how to report the concerns directly or via a health care professional. The system does not function to determine causality in any one particular case. Rather, monitoring systems serve to identify patterns of complaints that then require further evaluation to establish an association with the use of a specific product.

Publicity about potential adverse effects may influence the rate of reporting. This can increase recognition and reporting of public health concerns or promote anxious overreporting of vague unverifiable complaints. Responsible media coverage can produce an accurate profile of the extent of the problem, an appreciation of the different presentations of affected consumers, confounders and risk factors, and geographic distribution.

ESSENTIAL ELEMENTS OF AN ADVERSE EVENT REPORT

To be useful, an adverse event report must contain specific information. Ideally, this includes 1) the *product* name and manufacturer (and the list of ingredients and directions for use if a dietary supplement); 2) the *problem* (adverse event or product problem); 3) the *use pattern* (amount, frequency, route of administration and stop and start dates); 4) *dechallenge and rechallenge* information (response to discontinuation and/or restarting the product); 5) consumer *demographics* (age, gender, geographic location); 6) relevant *medical records;* 7) *confounders* (other products in use, individual patient risk factors); and 8) the *outcome* of affected individuals.

THE FUTURE

The FDA is currently involved in a number of collaborative efforts to promote international harmony of disease classifications and medical terminology. Such efforts are expected to promote more rapid and effective identification of product-associated safety concerns.

Use of the Internet for exchanging information has improved access for reporting adverse events to the FDA and for obtaining specific FDA information. The various FDA centers are developing home pages to provide timely updates on safety concerns and to disseminate summary information on reported adverse events.

The views expressed herein are soley the professional opinions of the author and do not necessarily reflect those of the Food and Drug Administration.

REFERENCES

[1]Napier K. Unproven medical treatments lure elderly. *FDA Consumer Magazine.* Vol. 28 No. 2. 1994:publication no.(FDA):94–1218.

[2]Nies AS. Principles of therapeutics. In: Goodman and Gilman, eds. *The Pharmacological Basis of Therapeutics.* 8th edition New York: McGraw-Hill, Inc. 1990:62–83.

[3]Levy A. FDA, Center for Food Safety and Applied Nutrition, personal communication.

[4]Cetaruk EW, Aaron CK. Hazards of nonprescription medications. Concepts and controversies in toxicology. *Emerg Med Clin North Am.* 1994:12(2):483–510.

[5]Marwick C. Medical news and perspectives: Growing use of medicinal botanicals forces assessment by drug regulators. *JAMA.* 1995;273:607–609.

[6]D'Arcy PR. Adverse reactions and interactions with herbal medicines. Adverse drug reaction. *Toxicol Rev.* 1993;12(2):189–208.

[7]Fanning O. New survey shows majority of drugs originate in nature as well as in laboratory. *Intern Med World Rep.* 1995;31:16.

[8]Eisenberg DM, Kessler RC, Foster C, *et al.* Unconventional medicine in the United States: Prevalence, costs and patterns of use. *N Engl J Med.* 1993;328(4):246–252.

[9]Anonymous, Melatonin. *Med Lett Drugs Ther.* 1995;37(962): 111–112.

[10]Kessler DA. Introducing MedWatch: A new approach to reporting medication and device adverse effects and product problems. *JAMA.* 1993;269:2765–2768.

[11]Sulfanilamide—a warning (editorial). *JAMA.* 1937;109:1128.

[12]Maeder T. *Adverse Reactions.* New York: William Morrow, 1994.

[13]Schardein JL, ed. *Chemically Induced Birth Defects.* New York: Marcel Decker, 1985;215–259.

[14]Roy SD, Arrant BS Jr. Hypokalemic metabolic alkalosis in normotensive infants with elevated plasma renin activity and hyperaldosteronism: Role of dietary chloride deficiency. *Pediatrics.* 1981;67(3):423–429.

[15]Malloy MH, Graybeard B, Moss H, *et al.* Hypochloremic metabolic alkalosis from ingestion of a chloride-deficient infant formula: Outcome 9 and 10 years later. *Pediatrics.* 1991;87(6):811–822.

[16]Freimuth VS, Hammond SL, Stein JA. Health advertising: Prevention for profit. *Am J Pub Health.* 1988;78(5):557–561.

[17]Levy AS, Stokes RC. Effects of a health promotion advertising campaign on sales of ready-to-eat cereals. *Public Health Rep.* 1987;102(4):398–403.

[18]Clinical Therapeutics and the Recognition of Drug-Induced Disease. A MedWatch Continuing Education Article. Goldman SA, Kennedy DL, Lieberman R, eds. Rockville, MD: Food and Drug Administration. June 1995.

[19]The Dietary Supplement Health and Education Act of 1994. U.S. Food and Drug Administration Center for Food Safety and Applied Nutrition. *Consumer Information.* December 1, 1995.

[20]Silverglade BA. Dietary supplement safety under the dietary supplement Health and Education Act: Brave new world or pyrrhic victory? *Food Drug Law J.* 1996;51:319–322.

[21]McNamara SH. Dietary supplements of botanicals and other substances: A new era of regulation. *Food Drug Law J.* 1996;50: 341–348.

[22]Michelson D, Page SW, Casey R, *et al.* An eosinophilia-myalgia syndrome related disorder associated with exposure to L-5-hydroxytryptophan. *J Rheumatol.* 1994;21(12):2261–2265.

[23]Monahan BP, Ferguson CL, Killeavy ES, *et al.* Torsades de pointes occurring in association with terfenidine use. *JAMA.* 1990;264:2788–2790.

[24]Honig PK, Wortham DC, Zamani K, *et al.* Terfenadine-ketoconazole interaction: Pharmacokinetic and electrocardiographic consequences. *JAMA.* 1993;269:1513–1518.

[25]Janssen Pharmaceutica Inc. Letter to healthcare professionals. March 25, 1996

[26]McKenzie R, Fried MW, Sallie R, *et al.* Hepatic failure and lactic acidosis due to fialuridine (FIAU), an investigational nucleoside

analogue for chronic hepatitis B. *N Engl J Med.* 1995;333(17):1099–1105.

[27]Richardson FC, Engelhardt JA, Bowsher RR. Fialuridine accumulates in DNA of dogs, monkeys, and rats following long-term oral administration. *PNAS USA.* 1994;91(25):12003–12007.

[28]Rothman KJ, Moore LL, Singer MR, *et al.* Teratogenicity of high vitamin A intake. *N Engl J Med.* 1995;333(21):1369–1373.

20

Contrasting Views of Causation in Law, Science, and Medicine

Jack W. Snyder and Allan Gibofsky

Law, science and medicine increasingly confront the role of the environment in disease and injury processes. The ascent of environmentalism has led to recognition of "vectors," "etiologies" or "causes" of "injury" beyond those attributable to physicomechanical forces. Chemical, microbial and even psychological factors are currently viewed as significant causal agents of injury to a biologic matrix.

In parallel with developments in science and medicine expanding the concepts of injury and causes of those injuries, developments in workers' compensation and tort law were expanding concepts of compensable injury to include events associated with environmental agents. This expansion has been attributed, in part, to increasing acceptance by courts of the proposition that civil damage judgments provide an effective public policy instrument for internalizing costs to the parties that generate them. In environmental cases, courts have reasoned that by making a party compensate victims injured by its activities, the party will enhance its efforts to minimize injuries. However, the transfer of wealth from one party to another is not automatic. To obtain compensation in this arena, an individual must prove not only that he or she suffered legally cognizable damage or harm, but also that a particular agent (within the control or responsibility of the defendant) *caused* the damage or harm. In modern environmental, toxic tort and occupational disease litigation, the proof of causation as well as the proof of harm increasingly challenges judges and juries who must evaluate truly complex medical and scientific information.

This chapter compares and contrasts medical, scientific and legal approaches to the concepts of injury, risk, disability and causation. In reviewing these value-laden terms, a unifying theme is offered. We suggest that divergent views regarding causation can be largely attributed to equally divergent views of what represents "injury." That is, the definition of injury ultimately determines the nature and strength of evidence that may be required to prove the cause(s) of that injury. Importantly, a seemingly inexorable expansion of the definition of injury has become a critical driving force at the interface of law, science and medicine.[1] At this interface, injury or harm, however defined, becomes the basis for transfer of wealth from one party to another. Thus, in this chapter the only kind of injury that really matters is that which is compensable. Indeed, it is primarily in the context of compensable injury that those who seek further expansion of injury concepts are now pitted against those who would put the brakes on this process. The possibility of a causal connection between exposure to environmental agents and the development of rheumatic disorders may be viewed as one of the more highly publicized battlegrounds for these efforts.

INJURY IN SCIENCE AND MEDICINE

A conceptual road map for the analysis of the interaction between environmental agents and biological matrices (for example, cells, tissues, human beings) is presented in Figure 20-1. Western biomedical thought views human beings (or cells or tissues within) as targets that may be confronted by the *presence* of a foreign substance (agent). Presence, of course, is premised on the ability of the agent to gain access to the organelle, cell, tissue or intact animal of interest. In the presence of an agent, one of two things can happen. The agent either has an impact on the biomatrix or it does not. If the effect is adverse, the host (cell, tissue or organism) repairs, eliminates, or adapts to the adverse effect, or it does not. Failure to adapt or repair can be viewed as a form of permanent injury.

Most scientists and physicians characterize irreversible injury at more than one level. At least two levels of damage are distinguished by the concept of functionality. Some adverse effects that are not repaired represent a type of damage that is not accompanied by functional deficit. For exam-

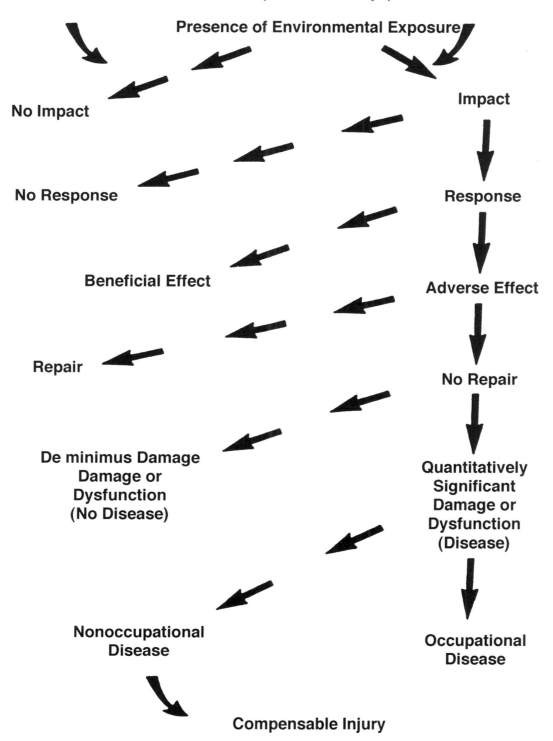

Fig. 20-1 A conceptual road map for analysis of interactions between environmental agents and biological matrices. Reprinted with permission from Snyder JW.[79]

Medical, legal and scientific professionals often use terms such as "presence," "impact," "response," "adverse effect," "repair," "de minimis damage," "disease" and "injury" to describe the consequences of environmental agents interacting with organelles, cells, tissues, organisms, animals and/or human beings. In medicolegal cases, one or more of these words may be employed as a synonym for the term "injury." Plaintiffs may contend that compensable injury has occurred because a benzene molecule was "present" in the bone marrow or had an "impact" on marrow progenitor cells, whereas defendants may deny that compensable injury has occurred even in a person with leukemia (a "disease") because the medical literature indicates that the cause of most leukemias remains unknown.

ple, some types of permanent changes in liver, kidney or other tissues may not be associated with perceivable or measurable loss of function. This level of injury is often called *de minimis* injury because it does not influence quality of life or lifestyle in ways that can be objectively verified or measured. By contrast, the nature and extent of adverse effects may be sufficient to cause dysfunction or disease, which is pragmatically defined as quantitatively verifiable or measurable biologically significant change that results in a negative change in lifestyle or quality of life. Examples of functional deficit include permanent changes in the motor cortex that decrease the ability to walk, or alterations of bone marrow that lead to aplastic anemia.

INJURY AND THE LAW

Most individuals generally do not employ the precepts of Western biomedicine to conceptualize or analyze injury. Thus, they may not distinguish impact, response, adverse effect, quantity of damage, disease and injury. These terms, which identify separate, scientifically verifiable events, are frequently used indiscriminately and interchangeably by claimants, insurers, lawyers, judges and legislators. Attempts have been made to equate each of these terms with compensable injury. In fact, even in the absence of measurable disease or adverse effect, proof of mere presence, access or impact—creating the *potential* or *risk* of disease—may be enough to award compensation.[2]

Evolution of the Principles of Compensation

The pressure to expand the concept of compensable harm in American culture reflects, at least in part, an inexorable evolution of the basic principles of compensation in the United States legal system. Three essential concepts that influence current rules and practices for awarding or denying compensation have been noted.[3] These are the *fault* principle, the *strict accountability* principle, and the *welfare* or *entitlement* principle.

The principle of fault, or blameworthiness, may be applied to either intended or unintended harm. For example, unless other interests served outweigh intended harms and are treated as justification (for example, defense of a person, defense of property or public necessity), conduct causing intended harm is socially undesirable, blameworthy and therefore compensable. Similarly, unintended harms are also blameworthy and compensable if they are caused by conduct that involves undue risks that, along with other costs, outweigh the benefits of the conduct causing the harm. If, however, the benefits of the conduct (or lack of conduct) are deemed to outweigh the costs, there is no fault and no compensable injury. Importantly, the outcome of the cost-benefit comparison in a *fault* analysis depends heavily on the values assigned to the various interests at stake. In some cases,

regardless of benefit, evolving societal concerns may assign the highest priority to the legal recognition of a "new" type of harm.[3] It is this context that innovative attempts to broaden the meaning of damage or harm have proliferated at the interface of law, science and medicine.

Despite legal recognition of new types of compensable injury, there may be significant social benefits from the conduct leading to those injuries. These benefits may be highly valued and therefore encouraged. If the benefits of the conduct outweigh the harms, fault cannot be found. Nevertheless, the conduct did cause injury. Should the harm be compensated in the absence of fault? By whom? To address these questions, U.S. law has embraced the principle of *strict accountability,* or liability without fault. That is, an actor, even though not at fault, should be liable for harms and risks within the scope of that actor's conduct. The actor, in turn, passes the liability and other costs of its conduct onto those who benefit from that conduct. If the added costs price the products of the conduct out of the market, this indicates that the conduct was not socially useful. Thus far, strict accountability has been primarily applied in no-fault statutes and in the law of nuisance, strict products liability, and strict liability for abnormally dangerous activities.[3]

To further address the problem of harm in the absence of fault, U.S. law has developed a third principle of compensation. The *welfare* or *entitlement* principle holds that compensation should not be paid by private enterprise or by the actor whose socially beneficial conduct caused the harm. Instead, through its government, society should pay. Furthermore, the government should compensate people not only because they are victims of accident, illness or misfortune, but also because they are needy, whatever the cause of the need may be. Of course, the exact nature of a government channel of accountability depends on how many segments of society will provide the governmental entity with the revenues to be used for purposes of compensation. If the sources of revenue are limited, the government could serve merely as a conduit for the application of strict accountability to private enterprise.

Each of these independent principles of compensation may influence both the definition of compensable harm and the quantum of proof needed to establish that harm. Thus, a willingness to define a particular outcome as compensable may depend on one's psychological preference for one principle over another. A willingness to recognize the validity of compensation for risk or fear or outrage may be guided, at least in part, by one's characterization of the transfer of wealth from one party to another. For example, those who prefer fault principles may argue that it is fundamentally unfair or unjust to award compensation for harms that many reasonable people would tolerate, especially if the benefits of an activity outweigh the costs. An advocate of fault would also contend that compensation via strict accountability or welfare/entitlement represents an enforced subsidy from persons whose activities are socially beneficial.

By contrast, an advocate of welfare principles may view negligence law or strict liability as a lottery; that is, the awards to victims under fault or strict accountability principles depend on factors other than need, and the obligations to pay depend on factors other than economic welfare. However, the pure entitlement perspective recognizes only that harm has occurred and a need for compensation has arisen. The source of the harm is largely irrelevant. Thus, at this end of the spectrum of principles of compensation, little or no proof of a causal connection between an action and an outcome is required.[3]

Who Can Be Injured?

Attempts to expand the scope of *who* can seek compensation for injury continue, especially at the extremes of life. For example, should the rights and privileges of "persons" attach to fetuses and young children? Increasingly, those fundamental common-law and constitutional rights that uniformly extend to both competent and incompetent adults have also been extended to children at the time of birth. By contrast, the law has struggled to determine which rights, if any, attach to a fetus. In most states now, a tort action for wrongful death can be filed by the estate of a stillborn child.[4]

The scope of who can seek compensation for injury has also been influenced by attempts to broaden the concept of *duty.* Using the "zone of danger" and other tests, courts have extended the general duty to prevent harm to protect wider nets of foreseeably injured plaintiffs. Thus, American jurisdictions have recognized: 1) the duty of confidentiality; 2) the duty of informed consent; 3) the duty to warn and control; 4) the duty to protect third parties; 5) the duty to report; and 6) the duty to disclose conflicts of interest.[5]

Where Can Injury Occur?

The setting in which harm occurs can further define "injury" and the nature of the proof required to establish that injury as compensable. What constitutes injury at work is not necessarily what constitutes injury elsewhere. As a result, what is required to prove causation in work-related cases may be quite different from what is required to prove causation elsewhere.

Historically, injury and disease have been conceptually distinct terms in law, science and medicine. The concept of injury has been used since antiquity for disorders that become apparent very shortly after the first interaction of an environmental agent with the host. The best known examples are disorders resulting from application of physical force or mechanical energy (trauma). By contrast, the term disease has been applied to disorders that first become manifest only after much longer periods following initial exposure. These disorders can result from application of chemical, biological or physical forces.

Compensation for work-related injury originally extended only to accidental, traumatic, relatively immediate, physical harm.[6] With recognition that the workplace could harbor agents of disease, the concept of compensable injury expanded. Coverage for occupational disease (OD) is now provided in all jurisdictions, but coverage methods vary considerably. Well-known schemes include: 1) use of a general definition of OD in a workers' compensation act; 2) use of an expanded definition of injury or personal injury to include OD; 3) use of a scheduled list of ODs coupled with a general disease catchall definition; 4) use of an unrestricted disease coverage provision; and 5) use of a separate OD act.

Not all languages and societies clearly distinguish between "injury" and "disease." In medicine, however, disease is viewed as one form of injury. In workers' compensation law, proof of disease is one method of proof of compensable injury. Thus, in law and medicine, injury is a broader concept than disease.

Compensable work injuries are not confined to those resulting in damage to the physical structure of the worker. Physical or mental dysfunction, including new-onset or unstable angina pectoris, cardiac arrhythmia or hypertension (in the absence of demonstrable physical changes) can serve as the basis of compensable harm. Furthermore, emotional distress originating in the workplace has become a recognized and accepted precipitant of various injuries and dysfunctions.[7]

When Can Injury Occur?

To further distinguish injury that is compensable from that which is not, courts must occasionally interpret the word "injury" as it appears in various statutes of limitations. The issue here is *when* did the harm occur? As in the medical malpractice, in the toxic tort context there are at least three possible interpretations of the timing of "injury." First, the injury can arise at the time of the alleged negligent act or omission.[8] One variation on this theme states that injury occurs on the date of last exposure to the offending substance.[9] Second, the injury can occur when the harm manifests itself in a physically objective and ascertainable manner.[10] Third, the injury can arise when the claimant discovers or gains knowledge of facts that would put a reasonable person on notice of the nature and extent of the harm, and that the injury was caused by the wrongful conduct of another.[11]

Most states have now adopted a version of the "discovery" rule to define when compensable harm occurs. However, the modern discovery rule creates problems. For example, does the statute of limitations begin to run when the initial harm surfaces or when the injury matures or worsens? Must the harm have reached its fullest manifestation before the statute begins to run? In addition, although created to be fair to claimants who suffer latent injuries, the discovery rule makes it difficult to predict losses because it creates a long period of time after an event during which a claim can be discovered.

NEWER FORMS OF COMPENSABLE INJURY

The evidentiary hurdles to be overcome in proving causation have also been influenced by newer legal concepts of *what* constitutes compensable injury. For example, a few courts have awarded compensation for the negligent or intentional infliction of emotional distress in the absence of physical, objectively demonstrable injury.[12] Others have compensated for loss of consortium.[13] Still others have recognized the loss of a chance for recovery or the loss of a chance to survive as an independent base for compensable injury.[14]

Perhaps the most controversial and challenging extension of the concept of what constitutes compensable harm is the recognition of an independent right to recover for the *risk* of future harm and/or for the *fear* that such a risk will materialize. Of interest here is the potential for at least three types of awards—namely, compensatory, punitive and medical surveillance damages. To appreciate how risk may be perceived as compensable injury, a brief review of the concept of risk may be helpful.

The Concept of Risk Control

The concept of risk has evolved substantially in recent decades. The older idea, that risk is essentially a wager that individuals make in the hope of gaining something significant, has almost disappeared from common parlance. Today risk is perceived as danger—to health, to property, to lifestyle—which must be controlled.[15]

Several factors have influenced both societal and individual perceptions of risk and the need to control it. First, instantaneous coverage by the media of spectacular environmental mishaps creates the impression that people can be "guinea pig" victims of involuntary and/or unknown exposures to physical, chemical or microbial agents. Second, the increasing ability to detect low amounts or concentrations of measurable entities encourages the use (or misuse) of numbers to influence positively or negatively the perception of risk. Third, the ability to control some aspects of risk, the recognized shortcomings of risk assessment and the general erosion of public trust in "experts" have created an atmosphere of doubt, apprehension and occasional outrage. These developments have, in turn, led to attempts to define risk as a distinct form of harm or injury that may be compensable in some circumstances.

The development of *risk control* as a central function of civil law has been most prominent in fields involving personal injury.[16] For example, the explosive growth of the field of products liability is largely the result of the law's increasing emphasis on risk control. The major issue is whether a manufacturer has appropriately minimized the risk of product injury.

Prior to 1960, actions subject to legal liability were those for which there was a dramatically greater chance than normal that loss would result. The law categorized acts as either qualifying as sufficiently abnormal to justify liability, or not. Typically, liability followed harms caused intentionally or recklessly. Modern law, however, has adopted a more expansive view of sources of loss. Today, some losses are viewed only as the outcome of some probabilistic process. Actions can be said to generate loss if they increase the probability of occurrence of a loss. All actions can be arrayed upon a continuum of contribution toward loss, from losses the probability of which is 100% (intentionally caused harms) to losses the probability of which is 0%.

Risk, Fear and Outrage as Compensable Injury

At least three new types of compensable injury may be evolving in U.S. tort law. The first tort transfers wealth for increased risk of future harm, the second compensates for fear of present or future harm, and the third transfers wealth on the basis of outrage.

Most courts have rejected claims seeking recovery for increased risk of contracting disease in the future where the plaintiff cannot establish the existence of present physical injury.[17] However, where the harm for which the claimant is allegedly at increased risk constitutes a separate and distinct ailment from the present harm, questions arise as to: 1) whether plaintiff may proceed now to seek recovery for both the present injury and the risk of prospective harm; 2) if plaintiff is permitted to seek recovery now only for the present injury, will he or she be barred from bringing a claim in the future for the separate and distinct injury; and 3) when does plaintiff's cause of action for a later-occurring injury accrue for purposes of the statute of limitations. Currently, most courts require reasonable medical probability or reasonable medical certainty that the anticipated harm will result in order to recover for a risk of future injury.[18]

Regarding *fear* as injury, a majority of courts require demonstrable present physical harm in order to recover for mental distress or fear associated with the possibility of future harm.[19] However, a few courts now recognize emotional distress or fear of future harm (including cancerophobia) as compensable injury even in the absence of present physical impact or harm.[20,21]

Jury awards on the basis of *outrage* remain a poorly defined and poorly understood aspect of toxic tort and product liability cases. The *Restatement (Second) of Torts* recognizes the tort of outrageous conduct, or negligent infliction of emotional distress. As with risk of injury and fear of injury claims, proof of physical injury, or at least contact, has traditionally been required. A few courts have recently applied the tort of outrage to deliberate or reckless infliction of mental suffering on another, even in the absence of physical injury.[22] To prove outrage, a plaintiff must show that: 1) the defendant either intended to cause emotional distress, or knew or should have known that his or her actions would cause emotional distress; 2) the conduct is outrageous, intolerable and offends generally accepted standards of decency and morality; 3) the defendant's conduct actually caused the emotional distress; and 4) the emotional distress must be severe.[23]

Some of the plaintiffs' counsel in the silicone breast implant litigation have suggested that verdicts for their clients are most likely based on the jury's collective outrage at what they perceive to be the conduct of the manufacturers in going to market before their products were adequately evaluated. By contrast, juror perceptions of the current state of medical and scientific knowledge may not factor prominently in their decisions. Whatever the critical factors influencing jury awards in silicone implant cases turn out to be, a major point for continuing debate is the propriety of imposing a 1996 standard of care with regard to premarket toxicology testing on a product that was marketed in the 1950s, 1960s and 1970s.

THE MEDICAL DETERMINATION OF IMPAIRMENT AND THE LEGAL DETERMINATION OF DISABILITY

Most physicians and attorneys who deal with rheumatologic disorders are familiar with the concept of *disability*.[24] Appropriate disposition of disability issues requires practitioners to make two fundamental medicolegal distinctions. First, they must realize that disability under the antidiscrimination laws is not always the same as disability for purposes of unemployment compensation. Second, they must appreciate the operational (procedural) difference between "impairment" and "disability."[25]

Disability and the Americans with Disabilities Act

Under the Americans with Disabilities Act of 1990,[26] the definition of disability is specifically designed to eliminate specific types of discrimination experienced by people with disabilities.[27] Thus, the ADA defines disability as 1) a physical or mental impairment that substantially limits one or more major life activities[28]; or 2) a record of such an impairment; or 3) being regarded as having such an impairment.[29] Physical impairment is defined as any "physiological disorder, or condition, cosmetic disfigurement, or anatomical loss affecting one or more of the following body systems: neurological, musculoskeletal, special sense organs, respiratory (including speech organs), cardiovascular, reproductive, digestive, genito-urinary, hemic and lymphatic, skin and endocrine"[30]; mental impairment is defined as any "mental or psychological disorder, such as mental retardation,

organic brain syndrome, emotional or mental illness, and specific learning disabilities."[31] The conclusion that an impairment substantially limits a major life activity must be reached only with reference to a specific individual and the effect of the impairment on that individual's life activities. An individualized approach, focusing on the nature, severity, expected duration and permanency or long-term impact of the impairment, is necessary because the same types of impairments often vary in severity and may restrict different people to different degrees.[32]

Disability in Compensation Systems

In the United States, three major compensation systems provide financial support to those who can no longer work because of illness or injury. These are workers' compensation, private disability insurance plans, and Social Security Disability Insurance (SSDI) plus Supplemental Security Income (SSI).[33] These programs differ in their definitions of disability, their legal and medical eligibility criteria and their schedules of benefits. In these systems, the disability evaluation process may require a physician to assume any one or more of three very different and potentially conflicting roles. He or she may function as a patient advocate and counselor, as a source of information for the compensating agency or as an adjudicator and certifier of impairment and/or disability.[34] In any of these situations, physicians may have at least an ethical obligation to tell patients which role(s) they are assuming and the potential conflicts that may arise.[35]

Disability in Social Security systems is typically defined as "the inability to engage in any substantial gainful activity by reason of any medically determinable physical or mental impairment which can be expected to result in death or which has lasted or can be expected to last for a continuous period of not less than 12 months."[36] To establish disability, the answers to five questions are typically sought.[37] First, is the applicant involved in substantial gainful activity? People who earn more than a threshold income (as defined by statute) are not considered disabled even though they are earning less money than before the onset of disability and can work only part-time at their previous occupation. Second, is there a severe impairment present? One of the most important requirements of any disability determination is that the individual have a medically determinable *impairment,* which has been defined as the presence of a specific disease that is of sufficient severity to justify the conclusion that a substantial reduction in functional ability has resulted. Whenever possible, functional capacity is measured and expressed quantitatively; symptoms alone are virtually never sufficient for a determination of disability. Furthermore, a conclusion by a treating physician that his or her patient is unable to work does not determine the presence of disability.

Third, does the impairment meet or exceed the listed medical and legal eligibility criteria? The Social Security regulations list a number of impairments for each major body system.[38] Within each system, specific diseases are listed, followed by the findings that must be present to confirm the diagnosis and by the measures of disease severity that support a presumption of a disabling impairment. Under the concept of "medical equivalency," nonlisted disorders may be considered equal to listed ones. Fourth, can the individual perform his or her previous work? Finally, can the disability applicant do any other available work?[39]

The presumably objective evaluation of impairment is only one factor in any disability determination. Other factors that can substantially influence decisions include ability to work with others, transportation issues, gender, education, training, expertise, experience, employability and local or national availability of suitable employment.[36]

CAUSATION IN SCIENCE AND MEDICINE

During the past century, the roles of causation and uncertainty in the philosophy of scientific investigation have evolved considerably. Quantitative ("classical") mechanics and the laws of motion and acceleration (mathematically expressed by Newton and epistemologically explained by Locke) theorized a limited power of one object to produce directional change in another via collision. Thus, mechanical contacts between particulate objects provided the basis for a mechanical notion of causation known as "corpuscularianism."[40] Along with "positivism" (the belief that scientific knowledge unceasingly expands), corpuscularian concepts of causation increasingly influenced legal approaches to scientific evidence in the eighteenth, nineteenth, and early twentieth centuries.[41]

Hempel summarized the positivism-corpuscularian view of scientific theory as a relationship between a "covering law" (one of a set of deductive principles), and an "*explanandum*" (the phenomenon that the covering law was to explain).[42] The nature of that relationship (the "*explanans*" or ultimate explanation) was usually expressed in causal language. Thus, according to Hempel, science progresses as deductive reasoning applies ever-expanding covering laws to more and more phenomena, enrolling them into causal chains which, in turn, connect previously unexplained phenomena. Uncertainty results only when a covering law cannot be applied to a phenomenon. Hempel further argued that deductive reasoning outweighs inductive reasoning as the primary method of causal explanation, of prediction and of knowledge in general.

The development of calculus, matrix analysis, quantum mechanics and the theory of relativity in this century undermined Newtonian (classical) mechanics and corpuscularian approaches to scientific evidence. Statistical relationships and inductive reasoning, which rely on random sampling and probability calculation, were increasingly accepted as bases for causal propositions.[43] Medicine, like modern physics, recognized the validity, importance and indispensability of "probabilistic reasoning" in the language of scientific expla-

nation. The concept of causation had to be expanded beyond the straitjacket of deductive, either/or, "causal-chain" analysis.

Today, progress in science is not viewed as steady accumulation of phenomena under the "covering laws" of deductive reasoning. Instead, the emphasis is on inductive/probabilistic reasoning and production of evidence to support or deny the validity of a particular hypothesis. The potential medicolegal significance of this shift in emphasis is best seen by examining how modern science addresses uncertainty, which is no longer viewed simply as phenomena outside the "covering laws" of deductive reasoning. Hermeneutic analysis, or the study of methodologic principles of interpretation, has concluded that scientists consciously use hypothesis testing to confront uncertainty. To distinguish levels of uncertainty, scientists choose among competing theories to formulate testable hypotheses which can be accepted or rejected following statistical analysis of experimental or epidemiologic data. Science progresses as some theories and hypotheses provide better (but not necessarily ultimate) causal explanations than others.[44] Thus it is theory (not the deductive, logical universe of the corpuscularian model) that frames uncertainty, provides context, and forms the basis of modern scientific inquiry. Theories and the explanations they offer are not expected to eliminate all uncertainty. Nevertheless, the process of inductive framing, testing and rejection of hypotheses based on statistical evidence is now well accepted as a better paradigm of scientific thought than pure, deductive causal-chain analysis.

If causality is a matter of theory, and if theories are modified over time, then causality is not a simple either/or proposition. The probability that one event caused another can be increased or decreased, depending on how well new evidence fits with the guiding theory. Thus, every scientific cause is packed with contingencies and assumptions of the theory which guides the underlying research. This paradigm clearly displaces one which simply states that something either is or is not a cause of something else.[40]

Thus concepts of causation have been modified to allow for probability. By contrast, the expression or articulation of causation has not. The language of causation still centers on deductive, causal chains. Confusion arises when a scientific explanation is framed in deductive, causal-chain terms, but the evidence to support that explanation is summarized by a probability statement. (Many scientists admit that the language of causal concepts they use often expresses inductive/probabilistic reasoning as deductive reasoning.) Therefore, the metaphor of science as a constantly growing causal chain is no longer appropriate. Unfortunately, this idea has not gained a strong foothold in U.S. jurisprudence. Thus current scientific concepts of causation continue to be poorly communicated in current legal articulation of causation.

If causation is, at least in part, a probabilistic concept, then decision-makers must deal with degrees, types and/or levels of uncertainty. Jurists and legislators, unlike physicians and scientists, are uncomfortable with this task because they are less familiar with the nature of uncertainty in statistical and epidemiological evidence. At least three kinds of uncertainty have been analyzed.[40] The first concerns issues of *transscience*, the second concerns the significance of *confidence intervals*, and the third concerns problems associated with *individual attributions based on group characteristics*. Some elaboration of these specific issues will show how uncertainty in probabilistic causation creates problems for regulatory or judicial decision-makers.

Transscientific issues are issues cast in scientific terms which cannot be resolved by science.[45] For example, many assume that mutagenesis is a marker for carcinogenesis, that animal models of carcinogenesis always apply to humans, or that the high-dose region of a dose-response curve can be extrapolated to the low-dose end in the absence of data in the low-dose region.[46] In contrast to the uncertainty that is characteristic of much of science, in which "the answer" is accompanied by some level of unpreventable statistical noise or uncertainty, transscientific questions are uncertain because ethical, technological or informational constraints prevent scientists from performing appropriate experiments to test their hypotheses.[47] Transscience is typically distinguished from mechanistic science, which is characterized by consensus theories, well-established hypotheses, hundreds or thousands of repetitions of test protocols and noncontroversial interpretation of data.[48]

To prove a causal connection between two factors, researchers try to disprove a null hypothesis, which states that no connection exists. In general, most data are expected to cluster about a mean in a characteristic way. The *confidence interval* is arbitrarily defined as the range within which the mean of a study parameter lies 95% of the time. With fewer data points, the scatter or standard deviation from the mean increases, thereby widening the confidence interval. Even if data allow rejection of the null hypothesis, a wide confidence interval suggests the results are not completely reliable, creating significant uncertainty.

Large, well-controlled epidemiologic studies permit conclusions only about a *group*, not the *individual*. Decision-makers should explicitly recognize that application to individuals of summary statistics concerning a sampled population is always accompanied by substantial uncertainty.

The ontologic framework of scientific materialism, which displaced vitalism many centuries ago, continues to dominate Western biomedical concepts of disease, causation and pathogenesis.[49] Realistic views of this ontology hold that the integration of insights derived from epidemiology, basic science and clinical science remains the best way to generate and test causal hypotheses.[50] To support an opinion with reasonable medical or scientific certainty that exposure to an environmental agent(s) is a cause of a disease, illness or disorder, the overwhelming majority of scientists, physicians and epidemiologists demand that the following criteria be satisfied[51,52]:

1) The prevalence and incidence rate of the disorder should be significantly higher in those exposed to the hypothesized cause than in controls not so exposed (the cause may be present in the external environment or as a defect in host responses).

2) Exposure to the hypothesized cause should be more frequent among those with the disorder than in controls without the disorder when all other risk factors are held constant.

3) In the course of time, the disorder should follow exposure to the hypothesized causal agent.

4) A spectrum of host responses should follow exposure to the hypothesized agent along a logical biologic gradient from mild to severe.

5) A measurable host response following exposure to the hypothesized cause: a) should have a high probability of appearing in those lacking this response before exposure, or b) should increase in magnitude if present before exposure. This response pattern should occur infrequently in persons not so exposed.

6) Experimental reproduction of the disorder should occur more frequently in animals or humans appropriately exposed to the hypothetical cause than in those not so exposed; this exposure may be deliberate in volunteers, experimentally induced in the lab, or demonstrated in a controlled regulation of natural exposure.

7) Elimination or modification of the hypothesized cause or of the vector carrying it should decrease the incidence of the disorder.

8) Prevention or modification of the host's response on exposure to the hypothesized cause should decrease or eliminate the disorder.

9) All of the relationships and findings should make biologic and epidemiologic sense.

Importantly, the number of these criteria that must be satisfied in the mind of any expert before he or she will render an opinion supporting a causal connection between exposure to agent X and onset of effect (or injury) Y varies from just one to all nine. There is no reliable evidence indicating consistency in the use of these criteria among individual experts or among members of a particular scientific discipline or medical specialty. Furthermore, experts typically do not identify those principles of causation analysis which underlie the basis of their opinions. This failure to make explicit the methodology of causation analysis has created much confusion in workers' compensation, product liability, toxic tort, hazardous waste and adverse drug reaction litigation.

Even if all of the above criteria are met, the alleged causal link between environmental agent(s) and a person's health problem becomes merely a possibility. The case-specific causation analysis must now be undertaken. Assuming the causative agent(s) can be identified, the expert must: 1) establish actual and biologically significant exposure; and 2) link the exposure to a reproducible, reasonably well-defined disorder. "Exposure" does not typically mean "in the vicinity of" for purposes of scientific causation analysis. There must be some evidence of inhalation, absorption or ingestion by an individual of measurable quantities of specific substance(s). Assuming some credible evidence of exposure, the expert typically identifies a reproducible, reasonably well-defined, measurable health effect. Not all effects, however, are adverse or detrimental to an individual, and, of course, not all adverse effects constitute disease (in medicine or in law).

Several mistakes of inference should be avoided by those attempting to assign cause-and-effect relationships.[53] For example, although anecdotes and case reports can suggest testable hypotheses, they should not, by themselves, provide a basis for causal inference, especially in the absence of unbiased selection of subjects, examination of patients for other explanations of the adverse event, and measurement of the frequency of the same adverse event in appropriate control patients.

Bias in the selection of experimental subjects should also be avoided. Findings in clinic populations that are not randomly selected may not be representative of (or apply to) the general population. The phenomenon known as Berkson's paradox (selection bias) is frequently overlooked by those attempting causally to relate environmental exposures to rheumatologic conditions.[54]

Many people, and some medical and legal professionals, fall into the trap of attributing an adverse effect to a procedure, mishap or medication simply because the event occurred sometime after the performance of the procedure or the administration of the drug. This fallacy of logic is known as *post hoc, ergo propter hoc*, which loosely translated means "if condition B temporarily follows situation A, then A must have caused B." Just because one sees a lot of worms and toads on the sidewalk after a thunderstorm does not mean it has been raining worms and toads.[53]

Interpretations of population means or averages must be made with caution. Some data sets display a Gaussian (bell-shaped) distribution, while others manifest biphasic or other distributions. Calculations of averages for the latter population distributions can be misleading, for example, when estimating future costs based on "average" survival times.

Finally, the role of statistical associations and correlation coefficients in the proof of causality remains controversial.[55] In particular, *meta-analysis,* or the use of formal statistical techniques to provide a "quantitative synthesis" of a body of separate but similar experiments or studies, has provoked substantial disagreement in many disciplines.[56] Critics of meta-analysis warn that: 1) meta-analysis itself is not an experiment; 2) it is difficult to avoid mixing the results of well-designed studies with poorly designed ones; 3) the investigator never knows if she's included all the relevant studies; 4) overlooking unpublished "negative" studies may produce bias towards "positive" results; 5) investigators often erroneously assume that exposure conditions are equal among the studies; 6) meta-analysis often abandons quantitative scientific evaluation of the magnitude of some effects; 7) inconsistent use of statistical methods to report the results of meta-analyses decreases the ability both to extrapolate (decreases external validity) and to undertake comparative risk assessment. The role of meta-analysis as a tool for proof of causation in environmental tort, product liability and workers' compensation cases remains to be determined.

CAUSATION IN THE LAW

In or out of the workplace, the role of environmental agents in compensable human injury remains highly controversial. Identification of a particular agent as the cause of injury or damage is seldom straightforward and often impossible. This is especially true when attempts are made to prove injuries that remain latent for years, are associated with diverse risk factors and/or occur at background levels even without any apparent cause.

To probe the controversy surrounding toxic tort and hazardous substance litigation, one must understand the traditional legal approach to causation. First, alleged wrongful conduct must be a *cause-in-fact* of harm. Proof of "factual causation" usually involves proof of logical relationships between events linked in a deductive "causal chain." Cause-in-fact corresponds to the use of causation in everyday language. It is also called "but for" or "*sine qua non*" causation, suggesting that the consequences would have been different if the cause-in-fact had not occurred. Courts, however, must often deal with multiple-cause events, and experienced jurists recognize that harm is not necessarily the result of antecedent individual events. In addition, courts which confront excessively long causal chains must decide where a causal chain should end. Thus the concept of *proximate cause* evolved to allow a jurist to discriminate between many so-called causes-in-fact and to incorporate policy-making into identification of the cause or causes which the legal system holds ultimately responsible for harm.[57]

A third notion of causation—*probabilistic causation*—has also evolved over the last century.[58,59] Probabilistic causation relies on probabilistic reasoning rather than on simple, deductively derived causal chains. Problems have arisen, however, because, as explained below, probabilistic reasoning serves two analytically distinct purposes in legal proceedings.

Traditionally, a plaintiff has two tasks known as burdens of proof. First, he or she must meet the *burden of production* by providing factual evidence for each element of a particular cause-of-action (for example, negligence, battery and so on). Second, he or she has a *burden of persuasion*. That is, he or she must convince the jury that his or her version of the facts is worthy of their collective belief with a minimum level of certainty, as defined by a standard of persuasion. The four commonly used standards are: 1) "beyond a reasonable doubt" in criminal cases; 2) "by clear and convincing evidence" in some civil cases; and 3) "more likely than not" or 4) "by a preponderance of the evidence" in most civil cases, including toxic torts and occupational disease claims.

Qualitative concepts of probability (as embodied in the above standards) have long and explicitly influenced jury deliberations as to whether or not plaintiff has met his burden of *persuasion.* By contrast, in conventional personal injury litigation, probability and inductive reasoning have not explicitly played a role in fact-finding *per se.* That is, the facts themselves, defined as elements on which one party has the burden of *production,* are generally deemed true or false—with a probability of either 0 or 1.[60] For example, the light was either red or green, the brakes either did or did not work, or the pedestrian either did or did not fall.

Among the elements of a case which the plaintiff has the burden of proving is causation-in-fact. This element is common to toxic tort, hazardous waste, occupational disease and conventional traumatic injury claims. As noted above, causation-in-fact probability is not an issue in most conventional injury cases. The jury simply decides which version of the facts it believes in an all-or-none, yes-or-no fashion, with no room for intermediate probabilities. Causation evidence is not expressed probabilistically.

This is not so in late twentieth-century environmental claims where, given the frequent impossibility of proving individual causation, statistical causation evidence (expressed probabilistically) is required as a factual estimate of defendant's contribution to plaintiff's risk.[61] For example, the issue in a typical trauma case may be whether or not a car could have stopped at a red light.[60] Evidence might be heard on speed, braking ability and driver reaction time for that particular vehicle (car X). The jury then finds that car X either could or could not have stopped. However, in the absence of facts concerning the individual car, undisputed evidence may show that of 100 cars chosen at random, 55 would have been able to stop. As to whether or not plaintiff has met the burden of production, the jury could find either way, depending on how it responds to probabilistic (statistical) evidence. Jury response is, in turn, likely to be influenced by judicial instructions on inferences to be drawn from group-based information.

The jury may believe that 55% of cars could have stopped, but have no idea whether car X is among that group. Thus, the jury would say plaintiff had not met the burden of production. Alternatively, the jury may believe that 55% of cars could have stopped and may infer that car X (assuming it is not atypical) more likely than not would have stopped since most cars would have. This finding, however, incorporates a leap of faith from established fact about a population to a conclusion about a particular car.

The propriety of this kind of mental leaping is one of the most controversial aspects of toxic tort and occupational disease cases, where causation often cannot be properly formulated as a yes-or-no fact. Instead, parties rely on evidence of increased risk or enhanced probability of disease which may or may not be attributable to defendant's conduct. The inquiry becomes one of the existence and magnitude of a fact probability. Therefore, understanding the dual nature of probability—as both a factual statistical quantity (fact probability) and a measure of strength of belief (belief probability)—becomes important. Unfortunately, fact probability and belief probability have not been kept analytically distinct. Courts have "collapsed" the requirements for burden of production and burden of persuasion into one test that blurs plaintiff's twofold task of defining not only the facts or elements to be proven but also the amount of credence to be accorded a fact in support of a finding.[60] When a judge tells a jury that "plaintiff must show that causation is more likely than not," she or he risks confusion. Does she or he mean that the fact of causation which plaintiff must prove (burden of production) is not traditional true-or-false (100% versus 0%) causation but only the existence of a statistical probability of causation greater than 50%? Or does she or he refer to the burden of persuasion guided by a standard of belief that causation is "more likely than not" true; that is, does the jury believe a knowable fact with more than 50% confidence?

Concern over haphazard and unrecognized transfer of "preponderance of evidence" or "more likely than not" standards from the burden of persuasion to the burden of factual proof (burden of production) involves more than idle semantics. The adverse effects of failure to undertake a deliberate, two-step, probabilistic analysis include: 1) undue preference for particular probabilities of causation found in one epidemiologic study, especially when meta-analysis of multiple studies is not possible or available; 2) unrecognized lowering of the burden of production with concomitant stiffening of the burden (standard) of persuasion; 3) inappropriate fixation on simplistic quantitative rules such as the "more than 50% likelihood" rule; and 4) poorly reasoned opinions because courts fail to explain exactly how they apply the "more than 50%," "more likely than not" rule.[60]

Courts that apply the rule only to fact probabilities essentially seek a yes-or-no belief in a more-than-50% fact probability. By contrast, traditional courts that apply the rule only to belief probabilities seek a more-than-50% belief in a yes-or-no fact. In toxic tort/occupational disease claims where both fact probability and belief probability are issues, there are at least two other approaches. Courts could apply the "more likely than not" standard jointly, reducing alleged fact probability by a factor reflecting the jury's doubt about its truth. By contrast, the rule could be applied sequentially to require only a more-than-50% belief in a fact probability which itself may barely exceed the more-than-50% threshold. It is important to see that joint application stiffens the causation burden-of-production/burden-of-persuasion, while sequential application substantially lessens the causation production/persuasion requirements.[60] The point here is that, regardless of approach, a court that deals with causal indeterminacy characteristic of toxic tort/occupational disease claims should be explicit about what it is doing, especially if defendant's culpability of conduct or duty to prevent risk is factored into determination of the causation issue.

Causation in Workers' Compensation

Both work-related and non-work-related disorders may have multiple contributing causes. In occupational disorders, the determination of causes impacts on prevention as well as compensation. Regarding prevention, it may not matter whether lung cancer in asbestos workers is due to smoking or asbestos or both, because reasonable people may consider the reduction or removal of both as important public health priorities.[62] By contrast, compensating asbestos workers who smoke and develop lung cancer can be more controversial because many systems award full compensation even though only a part of the cause in an individual case is due to occupational factors. Jurisdictions vary in the minimum percentage contribution required of the occupational component. With any cutoff point, however, some workers are overcompensated while others are undercompensated. Sliding-scale awards in proportion to the percentage of work-related causality have been proposed.[63]

Some commentators have challenged the concept that financial awards to disabled patients should depend on proof of causation rather than proof of need.[64] They contend that requiring proof of causation generates a privileged class of disabled within the community, a situation that is rather more illogical when occupational causality is only part of the origin of disability in a particular individual.

WHEN ARE SCIENCE EXPERTS REALLY EXPERT?

In environmental rheumatology, proving causation generally requires proof of: 1) *exposure* (to an identified, potentially harmful substance) that is sufficient to cause injury or harm; 2) a demonstrable *relationship* between the substance and the harm; 3) a *diagnosis* of such harm in plaintiffs; 4) *expert opinion* that harm to plaintiff is consistent with exposure to the substance; and 5) that the *defendant was responsible* for the etiologic agent of the harm diagnosed in the plaintiff.

Of great importance are the standard and/or criteria used by a particular court to screen for the admissibility of scientific studies and expert opinions. At least three methods of screening have been adopted by federal appellate courts. These are: 1) the "pure" *Frye* approach; 2) the relevance approach; and 3) the discretionary approach.

In an attempt to shift the decision on admissibility entirely to the scientific community, many courts have relied on *Frye v. United States,*[65] which provided that: "The thing from which the deduction is made must be sufficiently established to obtain general acceptance in the particular field in which it belongs." To apply the *Frye* rule, courts must determine

1) what must be accepted; 2) who must accept the "thing" involved; and 3) how the general acceptance will be established.

In deciding what to accept, courts clearly disagree. Some demand that the expert's conclusion be generally accepted. Others require only that the theory, principle or reasoning behind the conclusion be generally accepted. Still others demand that the technique(s) or methodology used to reach the conclusion be generally accepted. Finally, an occasional court has even required that a particular application of a theory or methodology for a particular purpose be generally accepted.

In deciding who must accept the "thing" involved, courts can focus on: 1) the expert him/herself; 2) those who developed or espouse the theory or principle; 3) those who developed or espouse the technique or methodology; 4) the entire scientific community; or 5) members of the relevant branches of that community.

How general acceptance is to be established is usually a question of law for the trial court. Even courts that have rejected *Frye* insist that judicial screening of proposed experts remains a necessity.

Unlike *Frye,* the general relevance standard admits all opinion testimony from qualified experts, so long as it satisfies the relevance requirement of Federal Rule of Evidence (FRE) 401.[66] The "any tendency" test of FRE 401 requires the court to balance the probative value of the evidence against identified, countervailing dangers or prejudice. Once the proponent proves relevance, the burden shifts to the opponent to show otherwise. Some courts adopting the relevance test for expert testimony may, however, undertake a preliminary "reliability" determination using *Frye* standards. Nevertheless, shifting the burden to require prove of irrelevance may enhance the likelihood of admissibility of expert testimony.

In the discretionary approach, courts determine the probativity of evidence by balancing reliability, relevance and helpfulness against prejudice, confusion and waste of time. (General acceptance is but one element of reliability under this approach.) The "helpfulness" standard has been described as a "let it all in" or "hands-off" or "noninterventionist" approach. The idea is that judges have no special competence to resolve complex and refractory issues raised by attempts to link low-level exposure to toxic chemicals and human disease. On questions such as these, which stand at the frontier of scientific inquiry, if experts are willing to testify that such a link exists, some courts believe it is for the jury to decide whether to credit such testimony. Thus the federal circuits have been split on how to handle expert evidence generally, and on how to apply *Frye* specifically.

The ascent of inductive/probabilistic reasoning, the inability of courts clearly to articulate their approaches to causation issues, and the liberalization of courtroom rules of evidence have facilitated growth of unorthodox research activity described by some as "pathological science," "junk science" or the "science of things that aren't so." Characteristic features of junk science include: 1) dependence on experiments at the threshold of detectability or at the lowest margins of statistical significance; 2) use of selectively incomplete data and claims of great accuracy to convert random noise into an apparent meaningful pattern; 3) effects often independent of intensity (despite the fact that dose-response is the best sanity check in real science); and 4) a tendency to cling to trivial and/or false discoveries with inappropriate tenacity.[67]

Courts contribute (perhaps unwittingly) to the development of nontraditional science as they: 1) decide factual issues that mainstream scientists still consider unresolved; 2) award judgments on the strength of scientific claims few scientists would endorse; and 3) decide what is good and bad science and what causes what on the way to resolving who should pay whom. Many argue, however, that courts must increasingly intervene because individuals, professional societies, government agencies, insurance company labs and standard-setting organizations cannot be trusted. This skepticism, which arose over the last 30 years, led the law to shift attention from technologist to technology.[68] Before 1960, the focus was on behavior of the professional. Was he or she negligent? Did he or she use reasonable care? Were the activities appropriate for the place where conducted? Today, however, the emphasis has shifted to the underlying science and technology. Was the workplace, the drug or the medical device designed, manufactured or labeled in a "defective" fashion? Thus courts now resolve tough scientific questions that used to be resolved on nonscientific grounds.

As they tackle scientific issues, modern courts also support junk science if they tend to admit any expert testimony relevant to a case. The "let it all in" approach has several effects.[67] First, it increases the risk of expert witness malpractice.[69,70] Second, it decreases the value of replication, reinforcement, consensus, peer review and standards in science, as authority is transferred from professional communities to individual scientists. Third, it pressures (or at least enables) courts to take new, fringe claims of cause and effect seriously and to use presumptions, burdens of proof and other niceties of legal procedure to favor isolated, "innocent victims" over wealthy, culpable defendants. Fourth, it facilitates verdicts (transfers of wealth) based on evidence that has nothing to do with traditional cause-and-effect relationships. For example, as noted above, it appears that issues in toxic tort, product liability and occupational disease litigation may increasingly be reoriented around the question of risk.

We live in a society that values the right of an individual to be left to do or be whatever he or she is able to do or be, without interference by others. A person has the right to smoke, to eat certain foods and to expose himself knowingly to "private risks." By contrast, many would argue that individual freedom also mandates reduction of unknowing exposures to hazardous substances. To reach this goal, however, the observations in this chapter suggest the need for further refinement and reform of tort, workers' compensation and product liability law. Continuing efforts by the legal system

to address the role of environmental agents in compensable human injury should include: 1) experimentation with advisory panels of scientific or medical experts who can accommodate probabilistic evidence of causation in both regulatory and courtroom settings; and 2) more precise articulation by decision-makers of the basis for their approaches to causation and the measure of damages.

THE DAUBERT DECISION

The Federal Rules of Evidence (FRE) were adopted in 1975. Subsequently at least 37 states have adopted their own codified rules of evidence modeled closely on the FRE.[71] For scientific evidence, the most relevant of the rules are found in Article VII of the FRE in a section known as "Opinions and Expert Testimony."[72] Prior to 1993, some federal appellate courts had applied Rule 702 of the FRE (which authorizes scientific testimony whenever it will assist the trier of fact to understand the evidence or to determine a fact in issue) to medical and scientific experts.[73] In 1993, the Supreme Court of the United States ruled that judges must serve as evidentiary gatekeepers who determine whether proffered evidence is scientifically valid and relevant.[74,75] The Court suggested several factors for judges to consider in determining whether to admit a particular theory or technique: Is the theory or hypothesis testable? Has it been tested? Has the theory or technique been subjected to peer review and publication? For a particular scientific technique or methodology, what is the known or potential rate of error? What (if any) are the standards that control the technique's operation? To what extent is the theory or technique generally accepted in the scientific community?

The *Daubert* case involved an interpretation of the FRE; therefore the decision binds only the federal courts. Nevertheless, the decision has already influenced state courts grappling with novel scientific evidence.[71] Any rheumatologist seeking to testify about scientific or medical matters that are novel or not generally accepted should be prepared to address each of the concerns articulated by the Supreme Court.[76] In addition, rheumatologists functioning as experts should remember that[77]:

- In qualifying a physician to offer testimony, courts are typically more concerned with degree of familiarity with the pertinent subject matter than with title or specialty designation.

- Regarding causation analysis, courts like to hear from nonphysicians, especially in toxic tort and product liability cases.

- In general, experts cannot offer legal conclusions or express opinions about the credibility of other witnesses.

- In general, expert testimony that a conclusion is "possible" does not suffice to meet the standard for admissibility with respect to the party who bears the burdens of production and persuasion.[78] "A doctor's testimony that a certain thing is enough is possible is no evidence at all. His opinion as to what is possible is no more valid than the jury's own speculation as to what is or is not possible.[78]

SUMMARY

Rheumatologic "disorders" are litigated in toxic tort, disability, workers' compensation and products liability cases. In all four legal arenas, the plaintiff (or claimant) must prove that the defendant's act (or failure to act) caused the legally cognizable injury. The first part of this chapter underscored the wide spectrum of views and definitions of compensable injury that can influence dispute resolution in cases involving potentially environmentally associated rheumatologic disorders. The second part of the chapter emphasized the equally wide range of approaches to the proof of causation in such cases. In the absence of uniform application of consensus criteria for the proof of causation, the fact finder's definition of compensable injury ultimately determines the nature and strength of the evidence required as proof of the cause of that injury. For example, the judge or jury who views a breast implant, arthritis or other rheumatologic plaintiff as a victim of outrageous conduct or as a person experiencing unwarranted fear or excessive risk of future harm may not see the relevance of or accord significant weight to expert scientific or medical testimony concerning the presence (or absence) of biochemical or morphologic abnormalities. Similarly, the judge or jury who views an alleged rheumatologic disorder as psychic injury or as a disability may not demand that the plaintiff's evidence fulfill even one of the rigorous scientific or medical criteria traditionally required for "proof" that agent X causes disease Y or objectively verifiable outcome Z.

Where powerful forces constantly influence the transfer of wealth from one party to another, people will seek to expand or contract the concept of compensable injury. Thus, in caring for patients whose health problems may be causally related to environmental exposures, physicians should expect to encounter remarkably disparate views of injury and of the type of evidence needed to prove both the existence and cause of that injury. Health professionals participating in the legal process must make strenuous and consistent efforts to educate other participants about important differences between fact and belief, deductive and inductive reasoning, evidence-based opinion and speculation, and between science by consensus and science by expostulation or protest.

REFERENCES

[1]Huber P. Injury litigation and liability insurance dynamics. *Science.* 1987;238:31–35.

[2]Blumenberg AB. Medical monitoring funds: The periodic payment of future medical surveillance expenses in toxic exposure litigation. *Hastings Law J.* 1992;43:661–730.

[3]Keeton WP. *Prosser & Keeton on Torts.* St. Paul, MN: West Publishing Co., 1984;608–615.

[4]Cardwell MS. Reproduction patients. In: *American College of Legal Medicine: Legal Medicine: Legal Dynamics of Medical Encounters.* 3d edition. St. Louis: Mosby, 1995;432–455.

[5]See generally *American College of Legal Medicine: Legal Medicine: Legal Dynamics of Medical Encounters.* 3d edition. St. Louis: Mosby, 1995.

[6]Hood JB, Hardy BA. *Workers' Compensation and Employee Protection Laws.* St. Paul, MN: West Publishing Co., 1984;70.

[7]Bond TR. Causation concepts in workers' compensation law. In: Simon WH, Ehrlich GE, eds. *Medicolegal Consequences of Trauma.* New York: Marcel Dekker, Inc., 1993;1–29.

[8]See, e.g., *McWilliams v. Union Pac. Resources Co.,* 569 So.2d 702 (Ala. 1990).

[9]See, e.g., *Meadows v. Union Carbide Corp.,* 710 F.Supp. 1163 (N.D.Ill. 1989).

[10]See, e.g., *Eagle-Picher Industries, Inc. v. Liberty Mutual Insurance Co.,* 829 F.2d 227 (1st Cir. 1987).

[11]See, e.g., *Evenson v. Osmose Wood Preserving Company of America,* 899 F.2d 701 (7th Cir. 1990).

[12]See, e.g., *Hagerty v. L & L Marine Services, Inc.,* 788 F.2d 315 (5th Cir. 1986).

[13]Consortium refers to the conjugal fellowship of husband and wife and the right of each to the company, cooperation, affection and aid of the other. See, e.g., *Shedrick v. Lathrop,* 106 Vt. 311, 172 A. 630.

[14]See, e.g., *Gooding v. University Hospital Building, Inc.,* 445 So.2d 1015 (Fla. 1984).

[15]Graubard SR. Preface to the issue "Risk." *Daedalus.* 1990; 119(4):v–vi.

[16]Priest GL. The current insurance crisis and modern tort law. *Yale Law J.* 1987;96:1521–1590.

[17]See, e.g., *Miller v. Campbell County,* 854 P.2d 71 (Wyo. 1993); *Ball v. Joy Technologies, Inc.,* 958 F.2d 36 (4th Cir. 1991), *cert. denied,* 112 S.Ct. 876, 116 L.Ed.2d 780 (1992).

[18]See, e.g., *Sterling v. Velsicol Chemical Corporation,* 855 F.2d 1188 (6th Cir. 1988).

[19]See, e.g., *Payton v. Abbott Labs,* 386 Mass. 540, 437 N.E.2d 171 (1982).

[20]See, e.g., *Potter v. Firestone Tire & Rubber Co.,* 15 Cal.App.4th 490, 274 Cal.Rptr. 885 (1990), *reversed in part, affirmed in part,* 25 Cal.Rptr.2d 550, 863 P.2d 795 (1993).

[21]See, e.g., *Johnson v. West Virginia University Hospitals, Inc.,* 413 S.E.2d 889 (W.Va. 1991).

[22]See, e.g., *Lejeune v. Rayne Branch Hosp.,* 556 So.2d 559 (La. 1990).

[23]Hoffman AC. Medical malpractice. In: *American College of Legal Medicine: Legal Medicine: Legal Dynamics of Medical Encounters.* 3d ed.). St. Louis: Mosby, 1995;129–140.

[24]*Black's Law Dictionary.* 6th edition. 1990;461–462 offers a smorgasbord of definitions of disability found in the law. Disability is generally defined as the want of legal capability to perform an act. The term is also used to indicate an incapacity for the full enjoyment of ordinary legal rights; thus persons under age, insane persons and convicts are said to be under legal disability. Sometimes the term is used in a more limited sense, as when it signifies an

impediment to marriage, the restraints placed upon clergymen by reason of their spiritual avocations, or lack of legal qualifications to hold office.

As used in connection with workers' compensation acts, disability is a composite of (1) actual incapacity to perform the tasks usually encountered in one's employment and the wage loss resulting therefrom (*i.e.* impairment of hearing capacity), and (2) physical impairment of the body that may or may not be incapacitating. *Russell v. Bankers Life Co.,* 46 Cal.App.3d 405, 120 Cal.Rptr. 627, 633.

Statutory definition of a "disability," for social security benefits purposes, imposes three requirements: (1) that there be a medically determinable physical or mental impairment which can be expected to result in death or to be a long-continued and indefinite duration (at least 12 months); (2) that there be an inability to engage in any substantial gainful employment; (3) that the inability be by reason of the impairment. 42 U.S.C.A. §§ 416(I)(1), 423(d). *Pierce v. Gardner,* C.A.Ill., 388 F.2d 846, 847. Inability to work without some pain or discomfort does not necessarily satisfy the test of disability. *DeFontes v. Celebrezze,* 226 F.Supp. 327, 330 (D.C.R.I.). However, pain by itself or pain in conjunction with other injuries may be the basis for "disability" within meaning of the Social Security Act. *Farmer v. Weinberger,* 368 F.Supp. 1, 5 (D.C.Pa).

Absence of competent physical, intellectual, or moral powers; impairment of earning capacity; loss of physical function that reduces efficiency; inability to work. *Rorabaugh v. Great Eastern Casualty Co.,* 117 Wash. 7, 200 P.2d 587, 590.

Under the Uniform Probate Code, an incapacitated person is one who is impaired by reason of physical disability.

GENERAL CLASSIFICATION

Disability may be either *general* or *special;* the former when it incapacitates the person for the performance of all legal acts of a general class, or given to them their ordinary legal effect; the latter when it debars him from one specific act. *Disability* may also be either *personal* or *absolute;* the former where it attaches to the particular person, and arises out of his *status,* his previous act, or his natural or juridical incapacity; the latter when it originates with a particular person, but extends also to his descendants or successors. The term *civil* disability is used as equivalent to *legal* disability, both these expressions meaning disabilities or disqualifications created by positive law, as distinguished from *physical* disabilities. A *physical* disability is a disability or incapacity caused by physical defect or infirmity, or bodily imperfection, or mental weakness or alienation; as distinguished from *civil* disability, which relates to the civil *status* or condition of the person, and is imposed by the law.

Partial disability. Under workers' compensation law, incapacity in part from returning to work performed before an accident. Such exists if employee is unable to perform duties in which he was customarily engaged when injured or duties of same or similar character, nature or description, but is able to engage in gainful activity at some job for which he is fitted by education, training or experience. *Daney v. Argonaut Ins. Co.,* La.App., 421 So.2d 331, 338.

Permanent disability. Incapacity forever from returning to work formerly performed before accident, though this incapacity may be either total or partial.

Temporary disability. Temporary, as distinguished from permanent, disability is a condition that exists until the injured employee is as far restored as the permanent character of the injuries will permit.

Total disability. Total disability to follow insured's usual occupation arises where person is incapacitated from performing any substantial part of his ordinary duties, though still able to perform a few minor duties and be present at his place of business. "Total disability" within an accident policy does not mean absolute physical disability to transact any business pertaining to insured's occupation, but disability from performing substantial and material duties connected with it. The term may also apply to any impairment of mind or body rendering it impossible for insured to follow continuously a substantially gainful occupation without seriously impairing his health, the disability being permanent when of such nature as to render it reasonably certain to continue throughout the lifetime of the insured.

[25]Engelberg AL. Disability and workers' compensation. *Occupational Health.* 1994;21:275–289.

[26]42 U.S.C. §§ 12101 *et seq.* (1992).

[27]Langer CS. Title I of the Americans with Disabilities Act. In: Snyder JW, Klees JE, eds. *Occupational Medicine: State of the Art Reviews—Law and the Workplace.* Philadelphia: Hanley & Belfus, Inc., 1996;11(1):5–16.

[28]The ADA defines major life activities as "those basic activities that the average person in the general population can perform with little or no difficulty." Examples of major life activities include walking, speaking, breathing, hearing, learning, caring for oneself, performing manual tasks, working, sitting, standing, lifting, reaching, thinking, concentrating, reading and interacting with others.

[29]Transvestism, transsexualism, pedophilia, exhibitionism, compulsive gambling, kleptomania, pyromania, current illegal drug use and associated psychoactive substance use disorders are specifically excluded from the category of protected disability under the ADA.

[30]29 C.F.R. 1630.2(h).

[31]29 C.F.R. 1630.2(h). Impairment of the mind is medically defined by diagnostic labels that do not remain constant. The American Psychiatric Association officially adopts a system of classification of mental disorders. This system is subject to periodic revisions as the state of knowledge expands, and is published in a *Diagnostic and Statistical Manual of Mental Disorders.* The current version is known as DSM-IV (1994). The DSM-IV states that it is to be used for diagnosis and treatment by mental health professionals and not for legal purposes. In practice, attorneys, insurers, compensation professionals and forensic experts commonly refer to DSM-IV. A useful mnemonic device for recalling the major categories of mental disorders found in DSM-IV is MADCAPS F. DISEASES: M = medical (general) disorders; A = anxiety disorders; D = dementia, delirium and cognitive disorders; C = childhood disorders; A = adjustment disorders; P = personality disorders; S = sleep disorders; F = factitious disorders; D = dissociative disorders; I = impulse control disorders; S = somatoform disorders; E = eating disorders; A = affective (mood) disorders; Se = sexual and gender identity disorders; s = schizophrenia and other psychoses.

[32]Federal regulations do not provide an exhaustive list of specific impairments covered by the ADA; instead, they define the types of

conditions that constitute an impairment. The decision to characterize a condition as an impairment is made without regard to medications, prostheses or other mitigating measures, even if those interventions decrease or eliminate the adverse effect of that condition. By contrast, the ADA specifically states that homosexuality, bisexuality, age *per se,* pregnancy *per se,* normal deviations of height, weight or strength, handedness, eye color, hair color, personality traits and environmental, cultural or economic disadvantages that may predispose to illness or disease are *not* included in the statutory definition of impairment.

[33]Title II of the Social Security Act established the Social Security disability insurance program. Workers are entitled to coverage provided that they meet the disability insured status requirements of the Act, which are based on the worker's age and the quarters of coverage credited to him by the Social Security Administration. Title XVI established the Supplemental Security Income Program, which provides benefits to disabled individuals with minimal income and assets.

[34]Carey TS, Hadler NM. The role of the primary physician in disability determination for Social Security Insurance and workers' compensation. *Ann Int Med.* 1986;104:706–710.

[35]Rubinstein HL. Workers with disabilities. In: Last JM, Wallace RB, eds. *Public Health and Preventive Medicine.* 13th edition. Norwalk: Appleton & Lange, 1992;559–564.

[36]See 20 C.F.R. 404.1505 and 20 C.F.R. 416.905. Gibofsky A, Hirsh HL. Impaired and disabled patients. In: *American College of Legal Medicine: Legal Medicine: Legal Dynamics of Medical Encounters.* 3d edition. St. Louis: Mosby, 1995;531–533.

[37]20 C.F.R. 404.1520 and 20 C.F.R. 416.920. Claimants for disability benefits must file an application with their local Social Security office. When a claim is denied in whole or in part, the claimant may request that the application be reconsidered; if it is again denied or if the claimant disagrees with a determination that is only partially favorable, an appeal may be taken to the Office of Hearings and Appeals of the U.S. Dept. of Health and Human Services. Over 300,000 appeals are adjudicated annually by administrative law judges in regional offices throughout the country. See 20 C.F.R. 404.907–404.922, 404.929–404.961, 404.1512–404.1516, 416.1407–416.1422, 416.1429–416.1461 and 416.912–416.916.

[38]Social Security Administration. *Disability Evaluation under Social Security.* Social Security Administration Pub. No. 05–10089, Washington, DC: U.S. Dept. of Health and Human Services, 1986

[39]Resources that contain general information on Social Security disability claims include 20 C.F.R. §§ 404.130–404.133 and §§ 404.1501–404.1694. See also Social Security Administration. *Social Security Handbook.* 11th edition. Washington, DC: U.S. Dept. of Health and Human Services, 1993.

[40]Brennan TA. Causal chains and statistical links: The role of scientific uncertainty in hazardous substance litigation. *Cornell Law Rev.* 1988;73:469–533.

[41]Brennan TA, Carter RL. Legal and scientific probability of causation of cancer and other environmental diseases in individuals. *J Health Pol Pol'y Law.* 1985;10:33.

[42]Hempel C. Aspects of scientific explanation. In: *Aspects of Scientific Explanation and Other Essays in the Philosophy of Science,* 1965;331–410.

[43]Suppes F. *The Structure of Scientific Theories.* 1977;4.

[44]Kuhn T. *The Structure of Scientific Revolutions.* 1961;60.

[45]Weinberg AM. Science and trans-science. *Minerva.* 1972;10:209.

[46]See Wagner WE. The science charade in toxic risk regulation. *Columbia Law Rev.* 1995;95:1614–1723.

[47]McGarity TO. Substantive and procedural discretion in administrative resolution of science policy questions: Regulating carcinogens in EPA and OSHA. *Geo Law J.* 1979;67:729–769.

[48]Black B, *et al.* Science and the law in the wake of *Daubert:* A new search for scientific knowledge. *Texas Law Rev.* 1994;72:715–765.

[49]Whitehead AN. *Science and the Modern World.* London: Free Association Books, 1985;22.

[50]Renton A. Epidemiology and causation: A realist view. *J Epidemiol Community Health.* 1994;48:79–85.

[51]Black B, Lillienfeld D. Epidemiologic proof in toxic tort litigation. *Fordham Law Rev.* 1984;52:732–785.

[52]Hill AB. The environment and disease: Association or causation? *Proc R Soc Med.* 1965;58:295–300.

[53]Caldwell JR. Silicone and silliness: Probabilistic prevarication in the legal arena. *J Fla Med Assn.* 1994;81:596–598.

[54]Berkson J. Limitations of the application of fourfold table analysis to hospital data. *Biometrics.* 1946;2:47–53.

[55]Compare Feinstein AR. Meta-analysis: Statistical alchemy for the 21st century. *J Clin Epidemiol.* 1995;48:71–79 with Liberati A. "Meta-analysis: Statistical alchemy for the 21st century": Discussion. A plea for a more balanced view of meta-analysis and systematic overviews of the effect of health care interventions. *J Clin Epidemiol.* 1995;48:81–86.

[56]Mann C. Meta-analysis in the breech. *Science.* 1990;249:476–480.

[57]Borgo S. Causal paradigms in tort law. *J Legal Stud.* 1979;8:419–455.

[58]Calebresi G. Concerning cause and the law of torts: An essay for Harry Kalven, Jr. *U Chi Law Rev.* 1975;43:69. Calabresi argues that "a causal link exists between an act or activity and an injury when we conclude on the basis of the available evidence that the recurrence of that act or activity will increase the *chances* that the injury will also occur."

[59]Shavell S. An analysis of causation and the scope of liability in the law of torts. *J Legal Stud.* 1980;9:463–516.

[60]Gold S. Causation in toxic torts: Burdens of proof, standards of persuasion, and statistical evidence. *Yale Law J.* 1986;96:376–402.

[61]Rosenberg P. The causal connection in mass exposure cases: A "public law" vision of the tort system, *Harv Law Rev.* 1984;97: 851–929. Rosenberg has argued that all evidence, even if styled "particularistic," involves inference from observed probability patterns. Of course, most rational conclusions are reached by applying a logical process of inference. If one sees another slip and fall on ice, one infers that the ice caused the fall, because one "knows" that people tend to fall more on ice than on dry sidewalks. The high *belief probability* about the cause of this particular pedestrian's fall depends crucially on individual observation as well. The fact that we see the ice overwhelms any inference one might have made from a table listing the relative frequencies of causes of falls. The power of particularistic proof to generate belief probabilities regardless of known fact probabilities strongly suggests that particularistic and group-based evidence be treated differently.

[62]Muir DCF. Cause of occupational disease. *Occup Environ Med.* 1995;52:289–293.

[63]Muir DCF. Compensating occupational diseases: A medical and legal dilemma. *Can Med Assoc J.* 1993;148:1903–1905.

[64]Stapleton J. *Disease and the Compensation Debate.* Oxford: Clarendon Press, 1986.

[65]293 F. 1013, 1014 (D.C. Cir. 1923).

[66]Rule 401 states that "relevant evidence means evidence having any tendency to make the existence of any fact that is of consequence to the determination of the action more probable or less probable than it would be without the evidence."

[67]Huber P. Pathological science in court. *Daedalus.* 1990;119(4):97–110.

[68]Priest GL. The new legal structure of risk control. *Daedalus.* 1990;119(4):207–227.

[69]See e.g., *Mattco Forge, Inc. v. Arthur Young & Co.,* 5 Cal.App.4th 392, 6 Cal.Rptr.2d 781 (1992); *Murphy v. A.A. Mathews,* 841 S.W.2d 671 (Mo. 1992).

[70]Moenssens AA, Starrs JE, Henderson CE, Inbau FE. Expert evidence and testimony. In: *Scientific Evidence in Civil and Criminal Cases.* 4th edition. Westbury, NY: Foundation Press, Inc. 1995;94–100. At present, the law does little to regulate the quality of expert testimony. Solutions offered by the legal and scientific communities to curb expert abuses include: capping expert witness fees, pre-screening experts, using only court-appointed experts, self-regulation, adhering to a strict code of ethics, peer review, a science court and liability in tort for expert witness malpractice.

[71]Bohan TL, Heels EJ. The case against *Daubert:* The new scientific evidence "standard" and the standards of the several states. *J Forensic Sci.* 1995;40:1030–1044.

[72]The Federal Rules of Evidence with the greatest impact on medical and scientific experts are:

Rule 702. Testimony by Experts. If scientific, technical, or other specialized knowledge will assist the trier of fact to understand the evidence or to determine a fact in issue, a witness qualified as an expert by knowledge, skill, experience, training, or education, may testify thereto in the form of an opinion or otherwise.

Rule 703. Bases of Opinion Testimony by Experts. The facts or data in the particular case upon which an expert bases an opinion or inference may be those perceived by or made known to the expert at or before the hearing. If of a type reasonably relied upon by experts in the particular field in forming opinions or inferences upon the subject, the facts or data need not be admissible in evidence.

Rule 705. Disclosure of Facts or Data Underlying Expert Opinion. The expert may testify in terms of opinion or inference and give reasons therefore without prior disclosure of the underlying facts or data, unless the court requires otherwise. The expert may in any event be required to disclose the underlying facts or data on cross-examination.

Rule 401. Definition of Relevant Evidence. "Relevant evidence" means evidence having any tendency to make the existence of any fact that is of consequence to the determination of the action more probable or less probable than it would be without the evidence.

Rule 402. Relevant Evidence Generally Admissible; Irrelevant Evidence Inadmissible. All relevant evidence is admissible, except as otherwise proscribed by the Supreme Court pursuant to statutory authority. Evidence which is not relevant is not admissible.

Rule 403. Exclusion of Relevant Evidence on Grounds of Prejudice, Confusion, or Waste of Time. Although relevant, evidence may be excluded if its probative value is substantially outweighed by the danger of unfair prejudice, confusion of the issues, or misleading the jury, or by considerations of undue delay, waste of time, or needless presentation of cumulative evidence.

[73]See e.g., *United States v. Downing,* 753 F.2d 1224 (3d Cir. 1985).

[74]See *Daubert v. Merrell Dow Pharmaceuticals,* 113 S.Ct. 2786, 125 L.Ed.2d 469 (1993).

[75]Gold JA, Zaremski MJ, Lev ER, Shefrin DH. *Daubert v. Merrell Dow:* The Supreme Court tackles scientific evidence in the courtroom. *JAMA.* 1993;270:2964–2967.

[76]Gold JA. The occupational physician as expert witness. In: Snyder JW, Klees JE, eds. *Occupational Medicine: State of the Art Reviews—Law and the Workplace.* Philadelphia: Hanley & Belfus, Inc. 1996;11(1):145–151.

[77]See Piorkowski JD. Medical testimony and the expert witness. In: *American College of Legal Medicine: Legal Medicine: Legal Dynamics of Medical Encounters.* 3d edition St. Louis: Mosby, 1995;141–155.

[78]See, e.g., *Cohen v. Albert Einstein Medical Ctr.,* 592 A.2d 720, 724 (Pa.Super. 1991), *appeal denied,* 602 A.2d 855 (Pa. 1992).

[79]Snyder JW. Medicolegal controversies in proof of causation and injury in occupational disease and toxic tort cases. In: Simon WH, Ehrlich G, eds. *Consequences of Trauma: Medicolegal Controversies.* New York: Marcel Dekker, Inc., 1993;365–395.

21

Surveillance and Monitoring of Environmentally Associated Diseases: Some Lessons from the Eosinophilia Myalgia Syndrome

Theodore Pincus and Daniel J. Clauw

The eosinophilia myalgia syndrome (EMS) was described in 1989 as an acute illness characterized by intense myalgia and eosinophilia associated with the use of L-tryptophan-containing products.[1-9] Several reports described the status of patients with EMS two to four years after its initial description.[10-14] These reports provided considerable information about long-term outcomes of EMS. However, the information is limited by a number of issues which include missing baseline data, ambiguities of surveillance criteria for EMS, patient selection for inclusion in long-term studies, and interpretation of late symptoms.

Some of the problems encountered in studies of long-term outcome of EMS may have resulted from the clear priority for acute surveillance to control an outbreak of a potentially severe disease. Nonetheless, it is likely that attention to matters in development of the surveillance database might have facilitated studies of long-term outcome in EMS without compromising effective surveillance.

This chapter discusses some of the principal problems encountered in clinical research concerning long-term outcomes of EMS, and proposes new approaches to surveillance and monitoring of environmentally associated diseases. It is recognized that an ideal program to monitor long-term outcomes of any acute or chronic disease is inevitably compromised by limitations of resources. Nonetheless, insight from studies of EMS can be extrapolated to the analysis of other environmental exposures and may suggest new approaches to surveillance, including identification and request for consent of patients for long-term monitoring, collection of formal quantitative data regarding pain, fatigue and other symptoms through patient questionnaires, and more specific classification criteria.

PROBLEMS IN STUDIES OF LONG-TERM OUTCOME IN EMS

Three categories of problems have adversely affected studies of long-term patient outcomes in EMS: limitations of data in the initial baseline surveillance database established at the Centers for Disease Control and Prevention (CDC); ambiguities of the initial surveillance criteria for EMS; and complexity in interpretation of symptoms years after disease onset (see Table 21-1).

Problems Resulting from Limitations of the Initial CDC Surveillance Database

The optimal approach to analysis of long-term outcomes in EMS would have been to account for all patients who were reported in the initial CDC database in 1989 and 1990.[15] However, this was not possible, in part because the database was (understandably) oriented primarily to acute events. Some of the more prominent shortcomings of this database that limit long-term monitoring of outcomes are reviewed briefly.

All Patients Were Entered Anonymously

All patients were anonymous in the case reports in the initial CDC database of 1407 patients. At that time, concerns about patient confidentiality, particularly with respect to HIV infection (an unrelated problem), were prominent, and it appeared appropriate not to identify patients by name or any other marker. However, the anonymity of patients required that subsequent attempts to contact them involve the reporting physicians. In 1996, more than 50% of physicians could not remember the patient with EMS whom he or she had reported seven years earlier (Pincus *et al.,* unpublished data). It is conceivable, if not likely, that the physicians were unable to remember less severely affected patients, thereby biasing long-term studies toward inclusion of patients with more severe disease.

No Consent was Requested from Patients for Long-Term Monitoring Studies

The absence of any identifier meant that no consent was requested for long-term monitoring. In large studies of long-

Table 21-1 Problems in studies of long-term outcomes in EMS

Problems resulting from limitations of the initial CDC surveillance database:
1. All patients were anonymous.
2. No consent was requested for participation in long-term monitoring studies.
3. Extensive identifying data for physicians were missing.
4. No baseline information concerning pain, fatigue, functional status psychological distress and other symptoms was obtained.
5. Selection bias is seen in patients available for long-term studies of EMS.

Problems with surveillance criteria for EMS:
1. Application of surveillance criteria as diagnostic criteria.
2. No exclusions for atopic and inflammatory rheumatic diseases.
3. Evidence of a new acute disease not required.
4. Myalgia is common in the general population.
5. Eosinophilia is unusual, but not rare, in the general population.

Problems in interpretation of symptoms years after onset of EMS:
1. Persistence of symptoms in patients with EMS not resulting from inflammation or objective residual damage.
2. Extensive somatic and cognitive symptoms years after acute EMS may be indistinguishable from those noted in patients with fibromyalgia.

---

term outcomes of patients with rheumatic diseases, it has been found that most are willing, if not anxious, to consent to participate in long-term studies.[16,17] After all, patients have a personal interest in results of studies designed to advance knowledge and treatment of their disease, particularly when long-term outcomes are poorly characterized or unknown, as was the case in EMS.

Although it is possible for reporting physicians to contact their patients long after onset of a disease in order to request consent for participation in long-term outcome studies, this procedure is suboptimal because physician offices have little experience in (and time for) this type of activity, and it is often difficult to locate patients after long periods. A direct contact for consent at baseline by a research organization with experience in longitudinal studies results in considerably higher patient enrollment rates and maintenance of patient contact for long-term studies. Centers with experience in longitudinal studies recognize issues of confidentiality and privacy, and have effective procedures to locate patients who may have moved to another address or died.

Extensive Physician Identifying Data Were Missing

The information entered into the surveillance database itself was quite incomplete. For example, the first name, address or telephone number was not recorded for more than 50% of the physicians reporting cases. Extensive searches of

physician directories led to apparent recognition of about 85% of these physicians (Pincus *et al.* 1996, unpublished data). However, it was not possible to identify the reporting physician to inquire about long-term outcomes for more than 10% of cases.

No Formal Baseline Information Concerning "Subjective" Symptoms Was Available

The acquisition of medical information is generally focused on "objective" data in the biomedical model.[18] The biomedical paradigm has been spectacularly successful in acute diseases, including epidemiologic surveillance of acute infectious diseases, in which critical information has been provided through laboratory cultures and serologic tests. Little need is seen to collect formal quantitative data concerning "subjective" symptoms such as pain, fatigue, functional status, psychological distress or other symptoms in most acute diseases. In chronic diseases, however, neither the patient nor the health professional can recall accurately the patient's clinical status months or years earlier. If no data are recorded at baseline, it is not possible to assess improvement or progression of clinical status with regard to these variables.

Quantitative assessment of these symptoms can be accomplished through patient self-report questionnaires.[17,19–21] The absence of any formal baseline information to quantitate pain, fatigue, functional status and psychological distress has limited assessment of changes in status and outcome in EMS.

Critical Selection is Seen in Patients Available for Long-Term Studies of EMS

Three important sources of selection limit the representative nature of patients for studies of long-term outcomes in EMS:

1) Only patients who could be remembered by their physician and could be contacted for follow-up are available from the initial CDC surveillance database;

2) The database involved a passive surveillance system for initial case reporting by a physician;

3) nearly all studies of long-term outcome in EMS have involved patients selected for continuing to see a physician about EMS[10–14]

The available reports are preferable to no follow-up information, but selection bias of patients must be recognized. All patients included in reports of late outcomes, with the possible exception of one cohort of patients monitored in South Carolina,[10,14] were under continuing care of a rheumatologist or a physician with a particular interest in EMS two to four years after presentation.

It is possible to attempt to determine the representative nature of a patient cohort by analyzing differences between the cohort being followed and the entire population of persons with the illness. In the case of EMS, several population-based studies were performed that identified a representative sample of all patients with EMS in a certain region. If one of these cohorts had been compared to the CDC cohort, clearer understanding of the representative nature of the CDC database might be available.

Furthermore, the establishment of unexposed "control" or comparison groups at the onset of the EMS epidemic would have been valuable. Several such cohorts were identified in the original epidemiologic studies that demonstrated the association between EMS and L-tryptophan, including individuals who were exposed to L-tryptophan but did not develop EMS. However, no measures were taken to ensure that these persons could be contacted for follow-up evaluation. If these individuals were available for study now, a better capacity to delineate further risk factors for developing EMS might be available.

Further data concerning the natural history of individuals who were taking L-tryptophan but did not become ill would also have been valuable. Several studies have suggested that individuals consuming L-tryptophan in 1989 were not representative of the general population, as these individuals had more frequent insomnia, myalgia, depression or other symptoms that prompted them to take L-tryptophan. Thus, to characterize fully late symptoms in patients with EMS, it would be important to know what symptoms might be anticipated in people who took L-tryptophan but never developed EMS. If the symptoms of such a group could be compared to those of a representative group of patients with EMS, long-term problems could be more accurately assessed.

Problems with Surveillance Criteria for EMS

The initial surveillance criteria for EMS established by the CDC were eosinophilia greater than 1000×10^9/L, severe myalgia, and lack of explanation for eosinophilia on the basis of a malignant or infectious disease.[3,15] More than 2,000,000 people in the United States were taking L-tryptophan.[1,4,7,22,23] This large number of individuals at potential risk for development of EMS led to establishment of surveillance criteria in relative haste.

In retrospect, problems have been recognized in application of the original CDC surveillance criteria for EMS that may not have been apparent at the time of the acute outbreak. These include the following:

Application of Surveillance Criteria as Diagnostic Criteria

Although the criteria were established as "surveillance," rather than "diagnostic," they were applied in diagnosis. This phenomenon has also been seen in application of "classification" criteria to many rheumatic diseases, including rheumatoid arthritis or systemic lupus erythematosus, in which a simple pathogenomic physical or laboratory abnormality is not available.[24]

No Exclusions for Allergic and Inflammatory Rheumatic Diseases

No exclusions were designated in the surveillance criteria for patients with allergic and inflammatory rheumatic diseases that may be associated with eosinophilia, including atopic disorders, Churg-Strauss vasculitis, angioedema with eosinophilia[25] and other nonmalignant hypereosinophilia-associated syndromes.

Evidence of a New Acute Disease Not Required

Certain patients with eosinophilia and severe myalgia could have received a diagnostic label of EMS in the absence of evidence for an acute new disease with clinical features of EMS.

Myalgia is Common in the General Population

Population-based studies suggest that approximately 10% of the U.S. population suffer from chronic widespread pain and nearly 20% suffer from chronic regional pain.[26] About 2% of the U.S. population, including 3.4% of women aged 40 to 49 and 5.6% of women aged 50 to 59 meet formal criteria for fibromyalgia, that is, widespread muscle pain and 12 specific tender points on physical examination.[26] Many individuals with fibromyalgia or other chronic widespread or regional pain syndromes have severe enough myalgia to meet this component of the definition of EMS. This was unusual in the acute presentation of EMS, but the clinical picture of many patients with "late EMS" is indistinguishable from that of patients with fibromyalgia.

Eosinophilia is Unusual, but Not Rare, in the General Population

Textbooks of medicine imply that eosinophilia (greater than 1000×10^9/L eosinophils) indicates a significant allergic, immunologic or neoplastic disease. However, a study of 38,086 people in Vancouver who had random blood differential counts identified 42 people who had absolute eosinophil counts greater than 1000×10^9/L.[27] In general, there was no explanation for the eosinophilia in these individuals. Additional laboratory tests were ordered for only about half of the patients, and many patients had no apparent illness.[27]

These data suggest that eosinophilia greater than 1000×10^9/L may be found in about one in 1000 individuals in the general population, many of whom apparently have no symptoms or disease. While confirming the relative rarity of eosinophilia, the data nonetheless may be interpreted to suggest among 2,000,000 individuals, the number exposed to L-tryptophan, 20,000 (1%) would be anticipated to have eosinophilia by chance alone. Furthermore, about 1000 would have concurrent fibromyalgia and eosinophilia by coincidence.

These observations have led some observers to raise the question of whether a unique disease picture of EMS exists at all.[28–30] The authors feel that many, if not most, patients reported in the original CDC database of 1407 EMS cases did have an acute *de novo* disease, with eosinophilia and a characteristic clinical picture of acute debilitating myalgia in the absence of preexisting inflammatory rheumatic diseases. An imperfect set of surveillance criteria with limited specificity does not negate the existence of a new condition. Nonetheless, certain problems appear intrinsic to clinical criteria to describe syndromes that cannot be diagnosed according to a pathognomonic laboratory test, such as a culture, biopsy or blood test. Such problems emerge even in well-described entities such as rheumatoid arthritis.[24] The definition of any disease according to a set of criteria appears inevitably associated with misclassification of certain patients.

Problems in Interpretation of Symptoms Years after Onset of EMS

Persistence of Symptoms in Patients with EMS Not Resulting from Inflammation or Residual Damage

EMS was described as an acute disease characterized by clinical signs of acute inflammation, such as severe myalgia, pleuritis and neuritis, as well as an elevated eosinophil count.[31] After six to 12 months, most patients had no evidence of continuing inflammation.[12] Nonetheless, many patients reported persistent symptoms, including myalgia, severe fatigue, paresthesia, muscle weakness, arthralgia and muscle cramps.

In certain cases, persistent symptoms could be attributed to residual damage that resulted from acute inflammation affecting the skin, lungs, nervous tissue and/or other organs. However, most patients who reported extensive late symptoms had no detectable evidence of tissue injury. Therefore, many symptoms in chronic EMS appear to involve neither acute inflammation nor objective residual damage. Some patients with chronic EMS may have fibromyalgia or other types of affective spectrum disorders[32] that, in some cases, antedated the onset of EMS.

Extensive Somatic and Cognitive Symptoms Years after Acute EMS are Indistinguishable from Those Noted in Patients with Fibromyalgia, and May Be Seen Without an Acute Episode

The biomedical model suggests that somatic symptoms reflect somatic disease, and the severity of symptoms in an individual patient reflects the severity of disease. This is seen in acute somatic illnesses, particularly those managed within a hospital. However, in long-term outpatient patient care, the setting of most medical care at this time, experienced clinicians recognize that the presence of many somatic symptoms does not necessarily indicate severe somatic disease. Indeed, many somatic symptoms may suggest the absence of a severe somatic disease and the presence of somatization and other related disorders.[33]

In one outpatient study, 85% of symptoms could not be explained by laboratory tests, radiographs or other studies.[34] A large proportion of symptoms seen in primary care may reflect somatization rather than demonstrable somatic disease.[35,36]

These observations may be pertinent to reports of somatic symptoms in patients with EMS years after the acute inflammatory stage of the disease. Many of the symptoms reported by patients with EMS, such as headache, gastrointestinal distress, chest pain and dyspnea, commonly are seen in affective spectrum disorders and are indistinguishable from those seen in patients with fibromyalgia.[32] Thus, the report of many somatic symptoms by patients with EMS is not necessarily related to a severe somatic disease, and may result from the processes that cause symptoms in conditions such as fibromyalgia.

PROPOSED APPROACHES TOWARD IMPROVED SURVEILLANCE AND MONITORING

Several lessons learned from studies of EMS may be instructive toward new approaches to surveillance and monitoring of patients with environmentally associated syndromes. The suggestions (Table 21-2) are presented according to three requirements for effective studies of long-term outcomes: a comprehensive baseline database, a protocol to monitor patients, and defined long-term outcomes.

Baseline Database

Baseline Case Reports Should Include Patient Identification

It is recognized that an individual with a disease whose case is reported to a state health department or to the CDC should retain the privilege of remaining anonymous. However, most people who have a chronic rheumatic or other disease have an obvious interest in trying to learn as much as possible about the disease, including its natural history and long-term prognosis.

Patients understand that there may be advantages to allowing health organizations and professionals to contact them for information about their disease and/or to perform follow-up studies, and generally give consent to being included in a

Table 21-2   Requirements for a database to monitor patients with chronic rheumatic disease over long periods

---

Comprehensive baseline database:
1. Baseline case reports should include patient identification.
2. Baseline database should be complete, particularly with respect to physician and patient data, and should be reviewed within a short period to complete missing data.
3. Baseline data should include patient self-report questionnaire data concerning functional status, pain, fatigue, psychological distress and other symptoms.

Protocol to monitor patients periodically:
1. Consent should be obtained from patients at baseline for further contact for follow-up studies.
2. A method to monitor patients periodically by mail should be implemented.

Defined long-term outcomes assessment:
1. Define outcomes for long-term assessment.
2. Use patient self-report questionnaires to assess outcome.

---

database to monitor long-term outcomes.[17] A monitoring program may include a semi-annual newsletter to update patients, which may be cost-effective in reducing visits to health professionals.[37] Therefore, it would be reasonable to include patient identification in an initial surveillance database concerning a new disease.

The Baseline Database Should Be Complete and Should Be Reviewed Within a Short Period

It is understandable that missing data concerning patients and reporting physicians is common in a surveillance database of an acute disease, because the primary objective is to assemble data quickly to understand etiology, pathogenesis and clinical consequences of the disorder. However, an effort to complete missing data through a state health department or reporting physician, preferably within a few weeks after receiving a case report, could have averted the problem that fewer than 50% of physicians in the CDC EMS database had a complete address and telephone number recorded.

Of course, a similar effort could be directed to identifying the *patients* by name, address, and telephone number, with consent for long-term monitoring. Studies of long-term outcomes are much more likely to be effective if the primary contact is the patient rather than a physician or health professional. The patient has a strong incentive to complete questionnaires or other activities required to assemble the database, whereas physicians may not have time to complete questionnaires or to contact patients. It is recognized that longitudinal databases in which all data are supplied by patients are effective to monitor long-term outcomes of rheumatic and other diseases.[16,17]

Baseline Data Should Include Patient Self-Report Questionnaire Data

Patient self-report questionnaires to characterize and monitor clinical status allow the physician to quantitate pain, level of functional capacity, fatigue and psychological distress, which cannot be assessed by laboratory tests or imaging procedures.[17,19,38–42] Although these data may be viewed as subjective, in that they are the observations of the patient, they can represent valid and reliable quantitative scores that are highly reproducible.[21] The data can be used to compare patient status from one visit to the next and to compare patients in different clinical settings.[17]

The health assessment questionnaire (HAQ)[38] and its derivatives, the modified health assessment questionnaire,[19,41,43] the Clinical Health Assessment Questionnaire (CLINHAQ),[17] the Arthritis Impact Measurement Scales (AIMS),[39] the McMaster Toronto Arthritis Patient Preference Disability Questionnare (MACTAR)[44] and the Short Form 36 (SF-36)[45] are of documented value to monitor clinical status in patients with rheumatic diseases. Scores for functional status and helplessness on the HAQ and its derivative tests are effective to document long-term functional declines,[46] identify work disability[47] and predict premature mortality in patients with rheumatoid arthritis.[20,48] Availability at baseline of patient questionnaire data concerning functional status, pain, fatigue and psychological distress, as well as somatic and cognitive symptoms, presents major advantages for long-term studies of patients with rheumatic diseases.

Method to Monitor Patients Periodically

Consent Should Be Obtained from Patients for Further Contact

At the time a patient is reported to a public health agency, a request could be made for consent for designated investigators to contact the patient for future follow-up studies. The patient must be assured that all data will remain confidential, and procedures to maintain confidentiality and privacy by the agency compiling the initial database should be explained. It should also be made clear that the patient may refuse consent with no consequences for medical care and may refuse any subsequent request for follow-up information even if consent is given at the time of request.

Nonetheless, it is ethically appropriate to provide the patient with an opportunity to participate in a properly conducted long-term monitoring program. Accurate compilation of long-term outcome data may be of direct benefit to the patient, and the absence of such information can contribute to uncertainty, psychological distress and expenses of inappropriate medical testing in future care.

A Method to Monitor Patients Periodically by Mail Should Be Implemented

In monitoring patients with rheumatic diseases over a period of 15 years it has been recognized that optimal follow-up should include biannual patient contact.[17] Using this procedure, 1421 patients with rheumatoid arthritis have been monitored and follow-up data collected for 1387 (97.6%) five years later[16] and 92% 10 years later. Patients who do not complete written questionnaires are telephoned and asked to complete a structured oral questionnaire to review their status.

A major concern with this type of follow-up is the cost incurred. Although the costs of an individual patient completing a questionnaire are minimal, additional expenses are incurred in printing, postage, data entry and data analysis. For example, it is estimated that monitoring 1000 patients requires $50,000 to $100,000 annually. These costs are relatively small in relation to the costs of assembling the initial database. Therefore, we estimate that the costs to monitor 1400 EMS patients in the CDC database for 10 years would have involved about $70,000 to $140,000 annually. The incremental cost of long-term follow-up should be addressed while assembling the initial database.

Outcome Assessment

Define Outcomes for Long-Term Assessment

In theory, data needed to analyze long-term patient outcomes should be found in a standard medical history, physical examination, laboratory tests, radiographs and other imaging procedures available from a standard medical record. However, this is not usually the case, for two reasons:

1) The most important outcomes in rheumatic disease include the capacity to perform usual activities, work outside the home and participate in social and recreational activities, with freedom from pain, fatigue and psychological distress. The medical record rarely includes a formal assessment of these problems.

2) It is quite expensive and pragmatically difficult to conduct a full-scale history, physical examination, laboratory tests and radiographs on patients for research studies years after baseline.

Fortunately, the important outcomes, such as functional disability, pain, fatigue, work status and psychological distress, can be accurately assessed through a patient self-report questionnaire.

Use of Patient Self-Report Questionnaires to Assess Outcomes

As noted above, long-term outcomes of patients with many diseases can be characterized through mailed self-report questionnaires almost as well, and sometimes even more effectively, than through a complete standard medical follow-up examination. Self-report questionnaires may be viewed as a method to translate information from the medical history into quantitative and reproducible scientific data for comparison with data collected of a later time. The validity (measures what is thought to be measured) and reliability (reproducibility) of patient self-report questionnaires are as great as most serological laboratory tests or reading of radiographs.[21,42]

Although most studies of self-report questionnaires have been conducted in patients with rheumatoid arthritis, such questionnaires are also useful in systemic lupus erythematosus (SLE), osteoarthritis (OA), systemic sclerosis and fibromyalgia.[43] The highest scores for functional limitations were found in patients with RA, and the highest scores for pain and psychological distress in patients with fibromyalgia.[41] A ratio of the pain score (pain visual analog scale score [PVAS]) to the functional limitation score (difficulties in activities of daily living [DADL]) is a useful adjunct to distinguish patients with a noninflammatory condition such as fibromyalgia from patients with an inflammatory rheumatic disease.[41]

Clear limits are seen regarding the utility of patient self-report questionnaires in analyses of chronic diseases. Patient self-report of diagnosis is frequently incorrect.[49,50] Most physical findings, such as joint swelling, skin tightening or purpura, require assessment by a health professional. Fortunately, recognition of physical findings, as well as abnormal laboratory tests or imaging data, is generally most important as baseline diagnostic data, rather than outcome data. Outcomes such as functional or work disability may be assessed without physical examination, laboratory tests or diagnostic imaging tests. Therefore, monitoring patient outcomes through mail and telephone follow-up studies can be as effective as evaluating patients by comprehensive physical examinations, laboratory and radiographic studies, and at considerably lower expense than a visit to a research center.

SUMMARY

It is suggested that surveillance of environmentally associated diseases should include identification of patients, with consent for long-term monitoring, formal assessment of patient functional status, pain, psychological distress and other symptoms at baseline, and a plan to monitor patients periodically by mail or telephone to assess preselected long-term outcomes.

REFERENCES

[1]Hertzman PA, Blevins WL, Mayer J, Greenfield B, Ting M, Gleich GJ. Association of the eosinophilia-myalgia syndrome with the ingestion of tryptophan. *N Engl J Med.* 1990;322:869–973.

[2]Kaufman L, Gruber BL, Gregersen PK. Clinical follow-up and immunogenetic studies of 32 patients with eosinophilia-myalgia syndrome. *Lancet.* 1991;337:1071–1074.

[3]Centers for Disease Control. Eosinophilia-myalgia syndrome—New Mexico. *MMWR.* 1989;38:765–767.

[4]Varga J, Peltonen J, Uitto J, Jimenez S. Development of diffuse fasciitis with eosinophilia during L-tryptophan treatment: Demonstration of elevated Type I collagen gene expression in affected tissues: A clinicopathologic study of four patients. *Ann Intern Med.* 1990;112:344–351.

[5]Silver RM, Heyes MP, Maize JC, Quearry B, Vionnet-Fuasset M, Sternberg EM. Scleroderma, fasciitis, and eosinophilia associated with the ingestion of tryptophan. *N Engl J Med.* 1990;322:874–881.

[6]Kaufman LD, Seidman RJ, Phillips ME, Gruber BL. Cutaneous manifestations of the L-tryptophan-associated eosinophilia-myalgia syndrome: A spectrum of sclerodermatous skin disease. *J Am Acad Dermatol.* 1990;23:1063–1069.

[7]Glickstein SL, Gertner E, Smith SA, *et al.* Eosinophilia myalgia syndrome associated with L-tryptophan use. *J Rheumatol.* 1990; 17:1534–1543.

[8]Freundlich B, Werth VP, Rook AH, *et al.* L-Tryptophan ingestion associated with eosinophilic fasciitis but not progressive systemic sclerosis. *Ann Intern Med.* 1990;112:758–762.

[9]Clauw DJ, Nashel DJ, Umhau A, Katz P. Tryptophan-associated eosinophilic connective-tissue disease: A new clinical entity? *JAMA.* 1990;263:1502–1506.

[10]Kamb ML, Murphy JJ, Jones JL, *et al.* Eosinophilia-myalgia syndrome in L-tryptophan-exposed patients. *JAMA.* 1992;267:77–82.

[11]Gaudino E, O'Loughlin T, Kaufman LD, Masur DM, Krupp LB. A longitudinal study of cognitive functioning in the eosinophilia-myalgia syndrome. *Neurology* 1993;34:248.

[12]Hertzman PA, Clauw DJ, Kaufman LD, *et al.* The eosinophilia-myalgia syndrome: Status of 205 patients and results of treatment 2 years after onset. *Ann Intern Med.* 1995;122:851–855.

[13]Campbell DS, Morris PD, Silver RM. Eosinophilia-myalgia syndrome: A long-term follow-up study. *South Med J.* 1995;88: 953–958.

[14]Sullivan EA, Kamb ML, Jones JL, *et al.* The natural history of eosinophilia-myalgia syndrome in a tryptophan-exposed cohort in South Carolina. *Arch Intern Med.* 1996;156:973–979.

[15]Swygert LA, Maes EF, Sewell LE, Miller L, Falk H, Kilbourne EM. Eosinophilia-myalgia syndrome: Results of national surveillance. *JAMA.* 1990;264:1698–1703.

[16]Callahan LF, Cordray DS, Wells G, Pincus T. Formal education and five-year mortality in rheumatoid arthritis: Mediation by helplessness scale scores. *Arthritis Care Res.* 1996;9:463–472.

[17]Wolfe F, Pincus T. Data collection in the clinic. *Rheum Dis Clin North Am.* 1995;21:321–358.

[18]Engel GL. The need for a new medical model: A challenge for biomedicine. *Science.* 1977;196:129–136.

[19]Pincus T, Callahan LF, Brooks RH, Fuchs HA, Olsen NJ, Kaye JJ. Self-report questionnaire scores in rheumatoid arthritis compared with traditional physical, radiographic, and laboratory measures. *Ann Intern Med.* 1989;110:259–266.

[20]Pincus T, Brooks RH, Callahan LF. Prediction of long-term mortality in patients with rheumatoid arthritis according to simple questionnaire and joint count measures. *Ann Intern Med.* 1994;120: 26–34.

[21]Pincus T. Documenting quality management in rheumatic disease: Are patient questionnaires the best (and only) method? *Arthritis Care Res.* 1996;9:339–348.

[22]Slutsker L, Hoesly FC, Miller L, Williams LP, Watson JC, Fleming DW. Eosinophilia-myalgia syndrome associated with exposure to tryptophan from a single manufacturer. *JAMA.* 1990;264:213–217.

[23]Eidson M, Philen RM, Sewell CM, Voorhees R, Kilbourne EM. L-tryptophan and eosinophilia-myalgia syndrome in New Mexico. *Lancet.* 1990;335:645–648.

[24]Pincus T, Callahan LF. How many types of patients meet classification criteria for RA? (editorial). *J Rheumatol.* 1994;21:1385–1389.

[25]Hertzman PA, Kaufman LD, Love LA, *et al.* The eosinophilia-myalgia syndrome—guidelines for patient care. *J Rheumatol.* 1995;22:161–163.

[26]Wolfe F, Ross K, Anderson J, Russell IJ, Hebert L. The prevalence and characteristics of fibromyalgia in the general population. *Arthritis Rheum.* 1995;38:19–28.

[27]Brigden ML, Horak MG. Incidence and clinical significance of unsuspected eosinophilia discovered by automated wbc differential counting. *Laboratory Med.* 1993;24:173–176.

[28]Spitzer WO, Haggerty JL, Berkson L, *et al.* Continuing occurrence of eosinophilia myalgia syndrome in Canada. *Br J Rheumatol.* 1995;34:246–251.

[29]Horwitz RI, Daniels SR. Bias or biology: Evaluating the epidemiologic studies of L-tryptophan and the EMS. *J Rheumatol.* 1996;23S:60–72.

[30]Shapiro S. Epidemiologic studies of the association of L-tryptophan with the EMS: A critique. *J Rheumatol.* 1996;23S:44–59.

[31]Kaufman LD. The eosinophilia-myalgia syndrome: Current concepts and future directions. *Clin Exp Rheumatol.* 1992;10:87–91.

[32]Hudson J, Pope H. Fibromyalgia and psychopathology: Is fibromyalgia a form of "affective spectrum disorder?" *J Rheumatol.* 1989;16:S15–22.

[33]Hudson JI, Pope HG Jr., Carter WP, Daniels SR. Fibromyalgia, psychiatric disorders, and assessment of the longterm outcome of EMS. *J Rheumatol.* 1996;23S:37–43.

[34]Kroenke K, Mangelsdorff AD. Common symptoms in ambulatory care: Incidence, evaluation, therapy, and outcome. *Am J Med.* 1989; 86:262–266.

[35]Kaplan C, Lipkin M Jr, Gordon GH. Somatization in primary care: Patients with unexplained and vexing medical complaints. *J Gen Intern Med.* 1983;3:177–190.

[36]Katon W, Lin E, Korff MV, Russo J, Lipscomb P, Bush T. Somatization: A spectrum of severity. *Am J Psychiatry.* 1991;148:34–40.

[37]Lorig KR. Arthritis patient education: What we know, what clinicians can do. In: Wolfe F, Pincus T, eds. *Rheumatoid Arthritis: Pathogenesis, Assessment, Outcome, and Treatment.* New York: Marcel Dekker, Inc., 1994;449–462.

[38]Fries JF, Spitz P, Kraines RG, Holman HR. Measurement of patient outcome in arthritis. *Arthritis Rheum.* 1980;23:137–145.

[39]Meenan RF, Gertman PM, Mason JH. Measuring health status in arthritis: The Arthritis Impact Measurement Scales. *Arthritis Rheum.* 1980;23:146–152.

[40]Meenan RF, Pincus T. The status of patient status measures. *J Rheumatol.* 1987;14:411–414.

[41]Callahan LF, Pincus T. The P-VAS/D-ADL ratio: A clue from a self-report questionnaire to distinguish rheumatoid arthritis from noninflammatory diffuse musculoskeletal pain. *Arthritis Rheum.* 1990;33:1317–1322.

[42]Wolfe F, Pincus T. Standard self-report questionnaires in routine clinical and research practice—an opportunity for patients and rheumatologists. *J Rheumatol.* 1991;18:643–646.

[43]Callahan LF, Smith WJ, Pincus T. Self-report questionnaires in five rheumatic diseases: Comparisons of health status constructs and associations with formal education level. *Arthritis Care Res.* 1989;2:122–131.

[44]Tugwell P, Bombardier C, Buchanan WW, Goldsmith CH, Grace E, Hanna B. The MACTAR Patient Preference Disability Questionnaire—an individualized functional priority approach for assessing improvement in physical disability in clinical trials in rheumatoid arthritis. *J Rheumatol.* 1987;14:446–451.

[45]McHorney CA, Ware JE Jr, Raczek AE. The MOS 36-Item Short-Form Health Survey (SF-36): II. Psychometric and clinical tests of validity in measuring physical and mental health constructs. *Med Care.* 1993;31:247–263.

[46]Pincus T, Callahan LF. Rheumatology function tests: Grip strength, walking time, button test and questionnaires document and predict longterm morbidity and mortality in rheumatoid arthritis. *J Rheumatol.* 1992;19:1051–1057.

[47]Callahan LF, Bloch DA, Pincus T. Identification of work disability in rheumatoid arthritis: Physical, radiographic and laboratory variables do not add explanatory power to demographic and functional variables. *J Clin Epidemiol.* 1992;45:127–138.

[48]Pincus T, Wolfe F, Callahan LF. Updating a reassessment of traditional paradigms concerning rheumatoid arthritis. In: Wolfe F, Pincus T, eds. *Rheumatoid Arthritis: Pathogenesis, Assessment, Outcome, and Treatment.* New York: Marcel Dekker, Inc., 1994; 1–74.

[49]Star VL, Scott JC, Sherwin R, Lane N, Nevitt MC, Hochberg MC. Validity of self-reported rheumatoid arthritis in elderly women. *J Rheumatol.* 1996;23:1862–1865.

[50]Kvien TK, Glennas A, Knudsrod OG, Smedstad LM. The validity of self-reported diagnosis of rheumatoid arthritis: Results from a population survey followed by clinical examinations. *J Rheumatol.* 1996;23:1866–1871.

Subject Index

Page numbers followed by *t* and *f* indicate tables and figures, respectively.

A

Acebutolol, lupus-like disease induced by, 84*t*, 85
Acute phase reactants, 13
Acute phase response, 13
Adverse events. *See also* Safety surveillance
  mandatory reporting, 213
  report, essential elements in, 215
  voluntary reporting, MedWatch Program for, 212*t*, 213
Agranulocytosis, drug-induced, immunogenetic associations with, 36*t*
Alcohol
  gout and, 129–132
  myopathy or myositis caused by, 14
Aldomet. *See* Methyldopa
Alfalfa seeds/sprouts, disease associated with, 27, 94–95
Allergens, and fibromyalgia, 162
Allergies, and fibromyalgia, 162
Allopurinol
  autoimmunity produced by, 21*t*
  with cytotoxic therapy, 134
Alpha-interferon, lupus-like disease induced by, 84*t*
Americans with Disabilities Act
  disability and, 222
  impairments covered by, 222, 231
  major life activities in
    definition, 230
    and disability, 222
  mental impairment defined in, 222, 230–231
  physical impairment defined in, 222
Amine compounds, implicated in SSc-like conditions, 77, 78*f*

Aminoglutethimide, lupus-like disease induced by, 84*t*
Aminorex fumarate, pulmonary hypertension associated with, 105–106
Amiodarone, autoimmunity produced by, 21*t*
ANA. *See* Antinuclear antibodies
Analytical study, 4
Androgenicity, in smokers, and rheumatoid arthritis, 121
Anemia, in rheumatic disease, 14
Anergy, 21
Anilides, in toxic oil syndrome, 46–51
Aniline, chemical structure, 78*f*
Anorexigen, pulmonary hypertension associated with, 105–106
Antiarrhythmics, lupus-inducing, 84*t*
Antibiotics
  and exacerbation of SLE or initiation of SLE flares, 94
  lupus-inducing, 84*t*
Antichromatin antibodies, in drug-induced lupus, 87–88
Anticonvulsants
  and exacerbation of SLE or initiation of SLE flares, 94
  lupus-inducing, 84*t*, 85
Anti-dDNA antibodies, in drug-induced lupus, 87–88
Anti-DNA antibody, in systemic lupus erythematosus, 12, 15
Antigen-presenting cell(s), and immune tolerance, 21
Antihistone antibodies, in drug-induced lupus, 85
Antihypertensives, lupus-inducing, 84*t*
Anti-inflammatory agents, lupus-inducing, 84*t*
Anti-La (SSB), in autoimmune disorders, 12

Antinuclear antibodies
  conditions associated with, 11–12, 12*t*
  in dermatomyositis, 16
  in drug-induced lupus, 85, 86*t*, 87
  screening test for, 12
  in systemic lupus erythematosus, 11–12, 15
  in systemic sclerosis, 15
Antipsychotics
  lupus-inducing, 84*t*
  lupus-like disease induced by, 84*t*
Anti-Ro (SSA), in autoimmune disorders, 12
Antithyroidal drugs, lupus-inducing, 84*t*
Antituberculous drugs, and uric acid underexcretion, 133
Apoptosis
  defects, induction
    in etiopathogenesis of environmentally associated rheumatic disease, 37, 38*t*
    and impaired immune tolerance, 21
  defects, in etiopathogenesis of xenobiotic-induced autoimmunity, 24
Apresoline. *See* Hydralazine
Atenolol, lupus-like disease induced by, 84*t*
Atopy, eosinophilia with, 14
Augmentation mammoplasty. *See* Silicone breast implants
Autoantibodies
  in drug-induced lupus, 87, 88*f*
  in rheumatic disease, 12, 13*t*, 16
Autoantigens, novel, formation, in etiopathogenesis of xenobiotic-induced autoimmunity, 22–23
Autoimmune disorder(s)
  diagnosis, 14
  diagnostic criteria for, 14
  immunogenetic associations with, 36*t*